Interventional Management of Chronic Visceral Pain Syndromes

Interventional Management of Chronic Visceral Pain Syndromes

Edited by

DANIEL J. PAK, MD
Assistant Professor of Clinical Anesthesiology
New York-Presbyterian Hospital
Weill Cornell Medicine
New York, NY, United States

R. JASON YONG, MD
Assistant Professor of Anesthesia
Brigham and Women's Hospital
Harvard Medical School
Boston, MA, United States

KRISHNA B. SHAH, MD
Assistant Professor of Anesthesiology
Baylor St. Luke's Medical Center
Baylor College of Medicine
Houston, TX, United States

ELSEVIER

Publisher: Dolores Meloni
Acquisitions Editor: Michael Houston
Editorial Project Manager: Billie Jean Fernandez
Production Project Manager: Sreejith Viswanathan
Cover Designer: Alan Studhome

3251 Riverport Lane
St. Louis, Missouri 63043

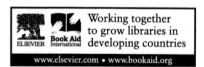

List of Contributors

Newaj Abdullah, MD
Resident Physician
Department of Anesthesiology
Baylor College of Medicine
Houston, TX, United States

Mark Abumoussa, MD
Resident Physician
Department of Anesthesia & Perioperative Medicine
Medical University of South Carolina
Charleston, SC, United States

Heena S. Ahmed, MD
Resident Physician
Department of Anesthesiology
Baylor College of Medicine
Houston, TX, United States

Rana AL-Jumah, MD
Resident Physician
Department of Anesthesiology
Baylor College of Medicine
Houston, TX, United States

Mansoor M. Aman, MD
Division of Pain Medicine
Department of Anesthesiology
Advocate Aurora Health
Oshkosh, WI, United States

Jessica Beatty, MD
Resident Physician
Department of Anesthesiology
University of Colorado School of Medicine
Aurora, CO, United States

Alina Boltunova, MD
Resident Physician
Department of Anesthesiology
NewYork-Presbyterian Hospital
New York, NY, United States

Joel Ehrenfeld, MD
Resident Physician
Department of Anesthesiology
NewYork-Presbyterian Hospital
New York, NY, United States

Christine S. Haddad, MD, PhD
Fellow Physician
Department of Anesthesia, Critical Care &
    Pain Medicine
Massachusetts General Hospital
Harvard Medical School
Boston, MA, United States

David Hao, MD
Resident Physician
Department of Anesthesia, Critical Care &
    Pain Medicine
Massachusetts General Hospital
Harvard Medical School
Boston, MA, United States

Cathy He, MD
Interventional Pain Physician and Anesthesiologist
Private Practice
Baltimore, MD, United States

Josianna Henson, MD
Fellow
Pain Medicine
Department of Anesthesiology
University of Colorado School of Medicine
Aurora, CO, United States

M. Gabriel Hillegass, MD
Associate Professor of Anesthesiology
MUSC Health University Medical Center
Medical University of South Carolina
Charleston, SC, United States

Ronnie M. Ibrahim, MD
Resident Physician
Department of Anesthesia, Critical Care &
    Pain Medicine
Massachusetts General Hospital
Harvard Medical School
Boston, MA, United States

Benjamin L. Katz, MD, MBA
Resident Physician
Department of Anesthesia, Critical Care &
    Pain Medicine
Massachusetts General Hospital
Harvard Medical School
Boston, MA, United States

Ammar Mahmoud, MD
Division of Pain Medicine
Department of Anesthesiology
Northern Light Eastern Maine Medical Center
Bangor, ME, United States

Anokhi D. Mehta, MD
Fellow
Department of Anesthesiology
Brigham and Women's Hospital
Harvard Medical School
Boston, MA, United States

Neel D. Mehta, MD
Associate Professor of Clinical Anesthesiology
NewYork-Presbyterian Hospital
Weill Cornell Medicine
New York, NY, United States

Vwaire Orhurhu, MD
Fellow
Department of Anesthesia, Critical Care &
    Pain Medicine
Massachusetts General Hospital
Harvard Medical School
Boston, MA, United States

Daniel J. Pak, MD
Assistant Professor of Clinical Anesthesiology
New York-Presbyterian Hospital
Weill Cornell Medicine
New York, NY, United States

Samantha Royalty, MD
Resident Physician
Department of Anesthesiology
Baylor College of Medicine
Houston, TX, United States

A. Sassan Sabouri, MD
Assistant Professor of Anaesthesia
Massachusetts General Hospital
Harvard Medical School
Boston, MA, United States
Visiting Professor
Anesthesiology
Shahid Beheshti Medical University
Tehran, Iran

Javier Sanchez, MD
Resident Physician
Department of Anesthesiology
NewYork-Presbyterian Hospital
Weill Cornell Medicine
New York, NY, United States

Meron Selassie, MD
Assistant Professor of Anesthesiology
MUSC Health University Medical Center
Medical University of South Carolina
Charleston, SC, United States

Krishna B. Shah, MD
Assistant Professor of Anesthesiology
Baylor St. Luke's Medical Center
Baylor College of Medicine
Houston, TX, United States

Matthew A. Spiegel, MD
Resident Physician
Department of Anesthesiology
NewYork-Presbyterian Hospital
New York, NY, United States

Kim A. Tran, MD
Resident Physician
Department of Anesthesiology
Baylor College of Medicine
Houston, TX, United States

Trudy Van Houten, PhD
Assistant Professor
Anatomy and Neurobiology
Boston University School of Medicine
Boston, MA, United States

Clinical Instructor in Radiology
Brigham and Women's Hospital
Boston, MA, United States

Narayana Varhabhatla, MD
Assistant Professor of Anesthesiology
UCHealth University of Colorado Hospital
University of Colorado School of Medicine
Aurora, CO, United States

R. Jason Yong, MD
Assistant Professor of Anesthesia
Brigham and Women's Hospital
Harvard Medical School
Boston, MA, United States

Salim Zerriny, MD
Resident Physician
Department of Anesthesiology
Critical Care, and Pain Medicine
Brigham and Women's Hospital
Harvard Medical School
Boston, MA, United States

Contents

CHAPTER 1

Epidemiology of Chronic Visceral Pain Syndromes

HEENA S. AHMED, MD • KRISHNA B. SHAH, MD • DANIEL J. PAK, MD

INTRODUCTION

Chronic visceral pain is estimated to affect over 20% of the global population, and it is one of the most common reasons why patients seek medical attention.[1] More than 12 million physician visits each year in the United States are for abdominal pain, with functional gastrointestinal disorders, such as irritable bowel syndrome, representing the vast majority of these complaints.[2,3] Globally, chronic female pelvic pain has been reported to affect up to 25% of reproductive-age women.[4] In the outpatient setting, up to 47% of chest pain is categorized as noncardiac in nature.[5]

Additionally, chronic pain is widely prevalent in patients with visceral malignancies, with 52% of patients experiencing pain irrespective of disease stage and the percentage increasing to 71% in patients with advanced disease.[6] Given the unpredictable and worsening nature of pain with disease progression, it is perhaps one of the most feared symptoms in patients battling cancer. Furthermore, with improved diagnostic tools and advancements in cancer treatment, there is a growing population of survivors who face the unexpected burden of treatment-related chronic pain syndromes, such as chemoradiotherapy-induced neuropathies and postsurgical pain.

Given its vague clinical presentation and potential concomitant factors, the diagnosis and management of visceral pain has a substantial economic impact. About 35%–41% of emergency visits for nonspecific abdominal pain are admitted to the hospital for further diagnostic evaluation.[7,8] Chronic pancreatitis is estimated to cost the healthcare system approximately 150 million dollars in the United States annually.[9] Chronic pelvic pain is the single most common indication for referral to women's health services, accounting for 20% of all outpatient appointments and resulting in $881.5 million spending per year in the United States alone.[4] The economic impact for gastrointestinal disease is also high with an estimated $15–$20 billion a year in healthcare costs.[10] Aside from the direct healthcare costs from chronic visceral pain, there is also a substantial economic impact from indirect costs associated with decreased productivity, lost workdays, and increased risk of long-term disability.[1]

CLINICAL FEATURES AND NEUROTRANSMISSION

Visceral pain is characterized by diffuse and poorly localized pain due to low-density innervation of visceral structures relative to the sensory innervation of other tissues and divergence of the sensory inputs as they ascend in the peripheral and central nervous systems.[1] Clinically, the mechanisms causing visceral pain vary widely and include distension of hollow organs, ischemia, traction on mesentery, muscular contractions of hollow organs, chemical irritants, and malignancies causing nerve compression among others.[2,11] Visceral pain can involve the thoracic, abdominal, or pelvic organs and can also produce nonspecific motor, autonomic, and affective responses.[1]

Most viscera receive dual afferent innervation through sympathetic and parasympathetic nerves that ultimately project to the central nervous system. During a noxious event, the spinothalamic tract and dorsal column are the two major ascending fiber tracts in the spinal cord that convey sensory input from the viscera to the brain.[12] Subsequent projections to the ventromedial thalamus are closely linked to the emotional and autonomic responses triggered by pain, while projections to the ventral posterolateral thalamus contribute to information related to pain perception, including location and

Interventional Management of Chronic Visceral Pain Syndromes. https://doi.org/10.1016/B978-0-323-75775-1.00017-9

intensity. Visceral pain also preferentially has increased activity in the anterior cingulate cortex, which may explain the strong emotional response to visceral pain.[13] Furthermore, in response to persistent injury or inflammation, visceral afferents can lead to peripheral and central sensitization from increased neuron excitability. This leads to enhanced sensitivity as seen with hyperalgesia and an expanded area of referred pain as seen in some visceral pain syndromes such as irritable bowel syndrome, dyspepsia, and interstitial cystitis.[11]

PSYCHOSOCIAL IMPACT

The psychosocial impact of chronic visceral pain should be included as part of a comprehensive evaluation of the patient. As visceral afferent pathways have projections to the anterior cingulate cortex, there is a large emotional component of visceral pain that should be addressed in addition to the pain. Therefore, patients typically present with multiple vague and overlapping symptoms of visceral pain syndromes and concurrent mood disorders.

Visceral pain has a detrimental effect on quality of life.[14] The emotional effects of pain varies from patient to patient and can lead to depression, anxiety, sleep disturbances, fatigue, decrease in physical and cognitive functioning, sexual dysfunction, and changes in mood and personality. It can also have a detrimental effect on relationships with family members and colleagues at work.[1,15]

TREATMENTS

Due to the complexity and poor understanding of the mechanisms underlying many visceral pain syndromes, there are few treatment guidelines for providers to follow. Conservative management typically involves the use of nonopioid medications such as nonsteroidal antiinflammatory drugs, serotonergic agents, anticonvulsants, and acetaminophen among others.[1] Although opioid therapy is commonly utilized for malignancy pain syndromes, its use for chronic nonmalignant visceral pain syndromes remains controversial and can be provided at the discretion of the provider. As previously mentioned, the psychosocial impact of chronic visceral pain syndromes cannot be understated and thus, behavioral therapy modalities should be utilized when appropriate. When conservative measures have been ineffective, treatment options aimed at the spinal afferent pathway including pain blocks or surgical interventions can be considered. A multidisciplinary approach is typically required for the treatment of these patients.

This book aims to provide a comprehensive approach for treating chronic visceral pain syndromes including a review of pharmacologic agents, psychotherapy, physical therapy, injections, and advanced interventions.

REFERENCES

1. Sikandar S, Dickenson AH. Visceral pain: the ins and outs, the ups and downs. *Curr Opin Support Palliat Care.* 2012;6(1): 17–26. https://doi.org/10.1097/SPC.0b013e32834f6ec9.
2. Kocoglu H, Pirbudak L, Pence S, Balat O. Cancer pain, pathophysiology, characteristics and syndromes. *Eur J Gynaecol Oncol.* 2002;23(6):527–532.
3. Kamin RA, Nowicki TA, Courtney DS, Powers RD. Pearls and pitfalls in the emergency department evaluation of abdominal pain. *Emerg Med Clin North Am.* 2003; 21(1):61–72. https://doi.org/10.1016/S0733-8627(02) 00080-9.
4. Ayorinde AA, Bhattacharya S, Druce KL, Jones GT, Macfarlane GJ. Chronic pelvic pain in women of reproductive and post-reproductive age: a population-based study. *Eur J Pain.* 2017;21(3):445–455. https://doi.org/10.1002/ ejp.938.
5. Bosner S, Becker A, Hani MA, et al. Chest wall syndrome in primary care patients with chest pain: presentation, associated features and diagnosis. *Fam Pract.* 2010;27(4): 363–369. https://doi.org/10.1093/fampra/cmq024.
6. van den Beuken-van Everdingen MHJ, de Rijke JM, Kessels AG, Schouten HC, van Kleef M, Patijn J. Prevalence of pain in patients with cancer: a systematic review of the past 40 years. *Ann Oncol.* 2007;18(9):1437–1449. https:// doi.org/10.1093/annonc/mdm056.
7. Austin PD, Henderson SE. Biopsychosocial assessment criteria for functional chronic visceral pain: a pilot review of concept and practice. *Pain Med.* 2011;12(4):552–564. https://doi.org/10.1111/j.1526-4637.2010.01025.x.
8. Merskey H, Bogduk N, International Association for the Study of Pain, eds. *Classification of Chronic Pain: Descriptions of Chronic Pain Syndromes and Definitions of Pain Terms.* 2nd ed. IASP Press; 1994.
9. Lew D, Afghani E, Pandol S. Chronic pancreatitis: current status and challenges for prevention and treatment. *Dig Dis Sci.* 2017;62(7):1702–1712. https://doi.org/10.1007/ s10620-017-4602-2.
10. Kellerman R, Kintanar T. Gastroesophageal reflux disease. *Prim Care Clin Off Pract.* 2017;44(4):561–573. https:// doi.org/10.1016/j.pop.2017.07.001.
11. Mayer EA, Gebhart GF. Basic and clinical aspects of visceral hyperalgesia. *Gastroenterology.* 1994;107(1):271–293. https://doi.org/10.1016/0016-5085(94)90086-8.
12. Willis Jr WD. Dorsal root potentials and dorsal root reflexes: a double-edged sword. *Exp Brain Res.* 1999;124(4): 395–421. https://doi.org/10.1007/s002210050637.
13. Benzon HT, Raj PP, eds. *Raj's Practical Management of Pain.* 4th ed. Mosby-Elsevier; 2008.

14. Hsia RY, Hale Z, Tabas JA. A national study of the prevalence of life-threatening diagnoses in patients with chest pain. *JAMA Intern Med.* 2016;176(7):1029. https://doi.org/10.1001/jamainternmed.2016.2498.

15. Phillips CJ. The cost and burden of chronic pain. *Rev Pain.* 2009; 3(1):2—5. https://doi.org/10.1177/204946370900300102.

CHAPTER 2

Neuroanatomy and Mechanisms of Visceral Pain

BENJAMIN L. KATZ, MD, MBA • TRUDY VAN HOUTEN, PHD •
A. SASSAN SABOURI, MD

INTRODUCTION TO THE AUTONOMIC NERVOUS SYSTEM

The autonomic nervous system regulates integral body functions such as heart rate, blood pressure, respiratory rate, temperature, digestion, and pupillary response. The specific targets of autonomic efferent (motor) fibers are smooth muscle, cardiac muscle, and glands (Fig. 2.1). The autonomic nervous system includes three basic divisions: the sympathetic, parasympathetic, and enteric divisions. Although extrinsic sympathetic and parasympathetic input can moderate the actions of smooth muscles and glands in the gastrointestinal (GI) system, the intrinsic neurons of the enteric nervous system, which are distributed throughout the wall of the GI tract, can sustain digestive function in the absence of extrinsic input. In this chapter, we will review the autonomic nerves and plexuses responsible for normal function in the thorax and abdomen, as well as the physiological mechanisms of visceral pain.

SYMPATHETIC NERVOUS SYSTEM

General sympathetic nervous system functions include vasoconstriction, increased heart rate, inhibition of glandular secretion and smooth muscle contraction in organs, and contraction of smooth muscle sphincters.

Except for sympathetic nerve fibers that synapse directly on chromaffin cells in the adrenal medulla, all autonomic visceral efferent pathways consist of at least two neurons.

The nerve cell bodies of sympathetic presynaptic neurons are found in the lateral gray horn of spinal cord segments T1 through L2 (Fig. 2.2). The sympathetic chain, also known as the sympathetic trunk, consists of a series of interconnected ganglia that run from the base of the skull to the coccyx lateral to the vertebral column (Fig. 2.3). The sympathetic chain allows the axons of sympathetic presynaptic neurons to synapse at ganglia above or below their spinal cord segmental origin.

The myelinated axons of all sympathetic presynaptic neurons leave the spinal cord in the ventral roots of the thoracic, lumbar spinal nerves and enter the sympathetic trunk through white rami communicantes. Sympathetic visceral motor impulses may take several pathways at this point.

1. The axons of presynaptic sympathetic neurons carrying impulses to peripheral blood vessels, skin glands, and smooth muscles synapse at the sympathetic chain ganglia. The axons of the corresponding postsynaptic neurons then join spinal nerves through gray rami communicantes to reach their targets.
2. The axons of presynaptic sympathetic neurons carrying impulses to structures in the head and neck ascend within the sympathetic chain from upper thoracic spinal cord levels and synapse on cervical sympathetic ganglia. The axons of the corresponding postsynaptic neurons typically follow branches of the carotid arteries to their targets.
3. The axons of presynaptic sympathetic neurons carrying impulses to thoracic viscera such as the heart, lungs, and esophagus enter the ventral rami of spinal nerves and typically synapse at adjacent sympathetic chain ganglia. The axons of the corresponding postsynaptic neurons typically travel by direct branches to the cardiac, pulmonary, and esophageal autonomic plexuses.
4. The axons of most sympathetic presynaptic neurons to abdominal and pelvic viscera pass through the sympathetic trunk without synapsing, form distinct thoracic splanchnic or lumbar splanchnic nerves, and synapse at ganglia within one of the many autonomic nerve plexuses clustered around the major branches of the abdominal aorta. The axons

Interventional Management of Chronic Visceral Pain Syndromes. https://doi.org/10.1016/B978-0-323-75775-1.00020-9

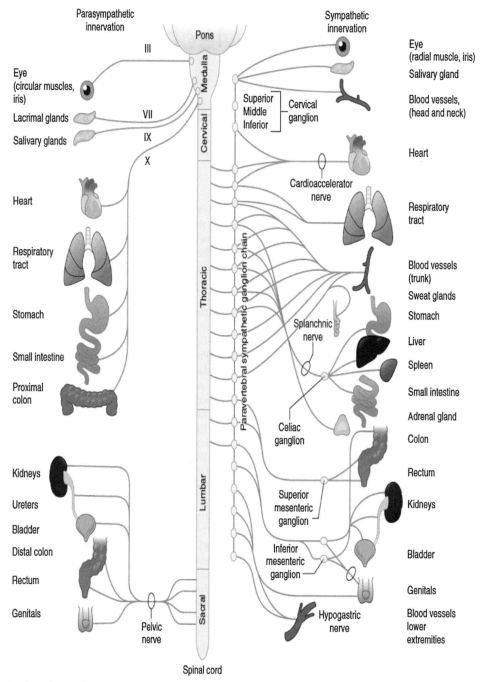

FIG. 2.1 Sympathetic and Parasympathetic Innervation of Various Organs. The autonomic nervous system has a diverse and extensive innervation to the thoracic, abdominal, and pelvic viscera. Please note that multiple pelvic nerves innervate the pelvic viscera. (Adapted from Glick, DB. The Autonomic Nervous System. Miller's Anesthesia. 7th ed. Philadelphia: Elselvier, 2010.)

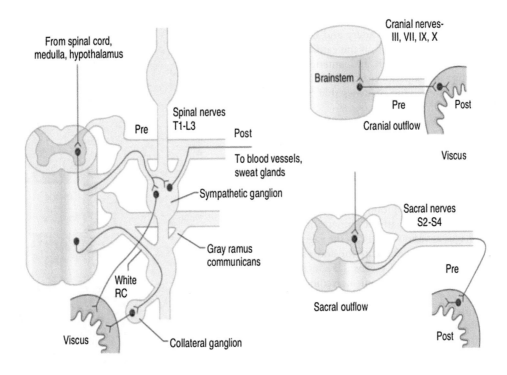

FIG. 2.2 **Autonomic Neuronal Organization: Sympathetic and Parasympathetic Pre- and Post-Ganglionic Nerves.** The sympathetic trunk consists of a series of interconnected ganglia whereas parasympathetic neurons are found in the brainstem visceral motor nuclei and in spinal cord segments S2 through S4. Please note that only sympathetic nerves to the thoracic viscera synapse in the sympathetic trunk. Sympathetic nerves to the abdominal and pelvic viscera synapse in the preaortic ganglia. (Adapted from Glick, DB. The Autonomic Nervous System. Miller's Anesthesia. 7th ed. Philadelphia: Elselvier, 2010.)

of the corresponding postsynaptic neurons typically follow the appropriate visceral branches of the aorta to reach their targets.

5. The axons of some lower lumbar presynaptic neurons carrying impulses to the distal portions of the urogenital organs and the perineal erectile tissue may descend in the sympathetic chain to synapse at the sacral sympathetic chain ganglia. The axons of the corresponding postsynaptic neurons, the "sacral splanchnic nerves," travel anteriorly by direct, and possibly vascular, branches to reach their targets.

PARASYMPATHETIC NERVOUS SYSTEM

The nerve cell bodies of presynaptic parasympathetic neurons are found in the brainstem visceral motor nuclei and in spinal cord segments S2 through S4. In general, parasympathetic nerves decrease heart rate, increase glandular secretion, and increase smooth muscle contraction.

The vagus nerve is one of the longest nerves in the body and contains parasympathetic fibers. It originates from the brain stem as the 10th cranial nerve. The right and left vagus nerves leave the cranial cavity through the jugular foramina and run inferiorly within the carotid sheath with the carotid arteries and internal jugular veins. Its visceral branches innervate glands as well as muscles of the cardiac, respiratory, and GI systems.

AUTONOMIC INNERVATION OF THORACIC ORGANS

The cardiac, pulmonary, and esophageal plexuses are mixed sympathetic and parasympathetic plexuses. The sympathetic contributions to these plexuses are typically from postsynaptic neurons with nerve cell bodies in the T1–T4 sympathetic trunk. The parasympathetic contributions are branches of the vagus nerve that synapse at ganglia within the plexuses or in the walls of thoracic organs.

The superficial portion of the cardiac plexus lies anterior to the right pulmonary artery and inferior to the aortic arch. The deep portion of the cardiac plexus lies posterior to the aortic arch and anterior to the tracheal bifurcation just superior to the carina. The plexuses then give rise to varying branches that reach the sinoatrial node to regulate heart rate.

The right and left pulmonary plexuses lie along the anterior and posterior surfaces of the mainstem bronchi and lung hila. Overall, the pulmonary plexus innervates the bronchial tree and visceral pleura, although the posterior pulmonary plexus innervates more than 70% of the lungs.[1]

An esophageal plexus is a group of nerve fibers with parasympathetic and sympathetic innervation that enter the esophagus at various levels. As the vagus nerve moves through the thorax, the anterior and posterior trunks become the esophageal plexus. Like most parasympathetic nerves, the preganglionic nerve fibers enter the wall of the organ and eventually synapse with postganglionic neurons. The vagus nerve components of the esophageal plexus contain nerve fibers that are both excitatory and inhibitory depending on the neurotransmitters released and their origin in the dorsal motor nucleus.[2]

AUTONOMIC INNERVATION OF ABDOMINAL AND PELVIC ORGANS

Sympathetic Innervation of Abdominal and Pelvic Organs

The greater (superior thoracic) splanchnic nerve typically consists of presynaptic fibers originating from the T5 to T9 spinal cord segments. However, nerve fibers can arise from levels as high as T1 and as low as T11 (Fig. 2.3). The greater splanchnic nerve is usually located anterolateral to the T12 vertebral body. The greater splanchnic nerve leaves the thorax, perforates the crura of the diaphragm, and enters the retroperitoneum where the presynaptic axons synapse on postsynaptic neurons in the celiac plexus. Postsynaptic sympathetic fibers from the celiac plexus typically follow arterial branches of the celiac trunk to the stomach, proximal duodenum, pancreas, spleen, and hepatobiliary organs. Some presynaptic sympathetic fibers in the greater splanchnic nerve synapse directly on chromaffin cells in the adrenal medulla.

The lesser splanchnic nerve typically consists of presynaptic fibers originating from the T9 to T11 spinal cord segments. Presynaptic fibers in the lesser splanchnic nerve typically synapse on postsynaptic neurons located in the celiac or superior mesenteric plexuses. Postsynaptic axons typically follow branches

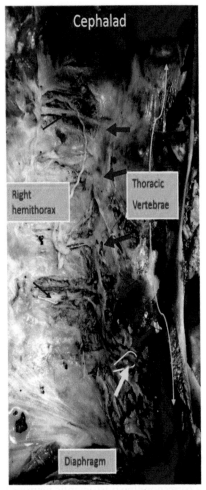

FIG. 2.3 Cadaver Dissection of the Thoracic Sympathetic Chain and Greater Splanchnic Nerve. The lungs and pleura have been removed to expose the thoracic sympathetic chain (*black arrows*). The greater (superior thoracic) splanchnic nerve has a clip around it (*yellow arrow*). The T5 intercostal nerve is located with a tie around it and they are marked with a *small black arrow*.

of the superior mesenteric artery to the distal duodenum, remaining small bowel, ascending colon, and transverse colon proximal to the splenic flexure.

The least splanchnic nerve typically consists of presynaptic fibers from T11 to T12 spinal cord segments. Presynaptic fibers in the least splanchnic nerve typically synapse on postsynaptic neurons located in the aortorenal ganglion. Postsynaptic axons follow the renal arteries to the kidneys.

The lumbar splanchnic nerves generally arise from L1 to L2 spinal cord segments. Presynaptic axons synapse on postsynaptic neurons in the inferior mesenteric plexus. Postsynaptic axons follow branches of the inferior mesenteric artery to the splenic flexure, descending colon, sigmoid colon, and proximal rectum. Postsynaptic axons also descend into the pelvis via direct branches, the hypogastric trunks, to reach the superior hypogastric plexus, inferior hypogastric plexus, and specific visceral plexuses on the lateral walls of the rectum and pelvic organs. Branches of the cervical (uterovaginal) or prostatic plexuses descend along the urethra to reach perineal erectile tissue.

Visceral afferent fibers from the GI tract typically return to the spinal cord along sympathetic visceral motor pathways.

Parasympathetic Innervation of Abdominal and Pelvic Organs

The left and right vagus nerves enter the abdomen on the esophagus, passing through the esophageal hiatus as the anterior and posterior branches of the esophageal plexus, respectively. The anterior branch innervates the intraabdominal esophagus and stomach. The posterior branch innervates the liver, biliary tree, gallbladder, and lesser omentum, and joins the celiac plexus. Vagal branches from the celiac plexus supply the small intestine and large intestine proximal to the splenic flexure. Postsynaptic parasympathetic neurons are situated in the wall of the gut in the myenteric (Auerbach) and submucosal (Meissner) plexuses (Fig. 2.2).

Abdominal and Pelvic Autonomic Nerve Plexuses

A series of intercommunicating nerve plexuses and ganglia surround the major branches of the abdominal aorta (Fig. 2.4). The axons of presynaptic sympathetic neurons reach the aortic plexuses via the thoracic and lumbar splanchnic nerves and synapse at sympathetic ganglia within the plexuses. The axons of sympathetic postsynaptic neurons follow blood vessels to the abdominal organs.

The axons of presynaptic parasympathetic fibers from the vagus nerve and pelvic splanchnic nerves run through the plexuses without synapsing and reach the abdominal organs either through direct branches or branches on blood vessels.

Celiac Plexus

The celiac plexus is a large network of sympathetic and parasympathetic nerve fibers surrounding the celiac axis at the T12−L1 vertebral levels (Fig. 2.5). The greater and lesser splanchnic nerves supply the sympathetic contribution to the celiac. The parasympathetic contribution consists of a small contribution from the anterior vagal trunk and a larger contribution from the posterior vagal trunk. The celiac ganglia can vary considerably in size. Nerve fibers leaving the celiac plexus typically follow branches of the celiac axis to the stomach, liver and biliary system, pancreas, and proximal duodenum. Laterally, the celiac plexus is associated with the aorticorenal and gonadal autonomic plexuses. Inferiorly, the celiac plexus is associated with the superior mesenteric plexus.

Superior and Inferior Mesenteric Plexus

The superior mesenteric plexus is a mixed sympathetic and parasympathetic plexus surrounding the superior mesenteric artery. The sympathetic contribution to the superior mesenteric plexus is primarily from the lesser thoracic splanchnic nerve (T10−T11). The parasympathetic contribution is primarily from the posterior branch of the vagus nerve. The inferior mesenteric plexus and associated ganglia surround the inferior mesenteric artery. The sympathetic contribution to the plexus is primarily from the lumbar splanchnic nerves. The parasympathetic contribution is from the pelvic splanchnic nerves (S2−S4).

Intermesentric Plexus

The intermesenteric plexus is situated between the superior and inferior mesenteric artery on the abdominal aorta. Sympathetic nerve fibers from the thoracic and lumbar splanchnic nerves and parasympathetic fibers from the vagus nerve contribute to this plexus.

Superior Hypogastric Plexus

The superior hypogastric plexus lies at the L5−S1 vertebral level and consists primarily of postganglionic sympathetic axons from lumbar splanchnic nerves descending from the inferior mesenteric plexus and preganglionic pelvic splanchnic nerves ascending from sacral spinal cord levels through the left and right hypogastric nerves (Fig. 2.6). From the superior hypogastric plexuses, the left and right hypogastric nerves descend into the pelvis to the inferior hypogastric plexus.

Inferior Hypogastric Plexus

The inferior hypogastric plexus, also known as the pelvic plexus, is a paired plexus that can be found on the lateral surfaces of the rectum. This plexus supplies the pelvic organs, giving rise to the prostatic plexus in men and uterovaginal plexus in women. The contributors include the superior hypogastric plexus, the sacral splanchnic nerves, and the pelvic splanchnic nerves.

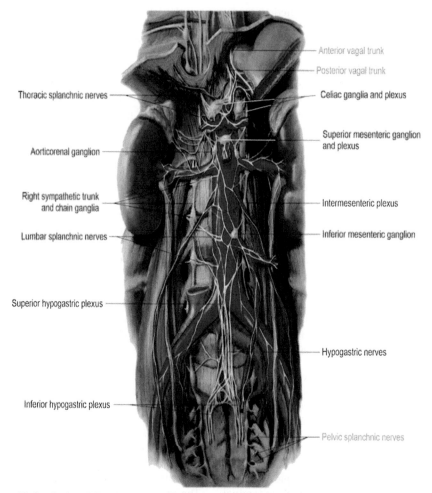

Anterior vagal trunk

Posterior vagal trunk

Celiac ganglia and plexus

Thoracic splanchnic nerves

Superior mesenteric ganglion and plexus

Aorticorenal ganglion

Right sympathetic trunk and chain ganglia

Intermesenteric plexus

Lumbar splanchnic nerves

Inferior mesenteric ganglion

Superior hypogastric plexus

Hypogastric nerves

Inferior hypogastric plexus

Pelvic splanchnic nerves

FIG. 2.4 **Abdominal and Pelvic Autonomic Nerve Plexuses.**   Abdominal and pelvic autonomic nerve plexuses are distributed extensively in the retroperitoneal space. *Red labels* indicate sympathetic contribution, *blue labels* indicate parasympathetic contributions, and *black labels* indicate mixed sympathetic and parasympathetic components. (Modified from Netter Atlas of Human Anatomy. Elsevier.)

The pelvic plexus consists of sympathetic nerve fibers that descended in the hypogastric nerves with additional contributions from the sacral sympathetic trunk ("sacral splanchnic nerves"), and parasympathetic fibers from the pelvic splanchnic nerves or hypogastric plexuses. Injury to the hypogastric nerves can cause pelvic organ dysfunction.

VISCERAL SENSORY INNERVATION
Sensation from abdominal and pelvic organs and the adjacent visceral pleura is conveyed by visceral afferent fibers. Sensation from the parietal peritoneum and body wall is conveyed by somatic afferent fibers. The

nerve cell bodies of both visceral afferent and somatic afferent fibers are located within the dorsal root ganglion. Central processes of visceral and somatic afferent nerve cell bodies enter the spinal cord and synapse on interneurons that transmit pain and sensation via various tracts that lead to the brainstem and cerebral cortex. The nerve fibers involved in pain are almost exclusively A-delta and C fibers.

The visceral afferent pathway from the abdominal and pelvic viscera and adjacent visceral pleura consists of a single neuron. The peripheral processes of the visceral afferent nerve fibers from most of the GI tract travel with sympathetic visceral efferent fibers. The peripheral processes of visceral afferent fibers pass through

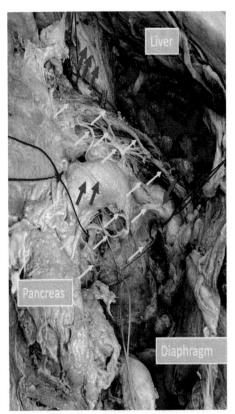

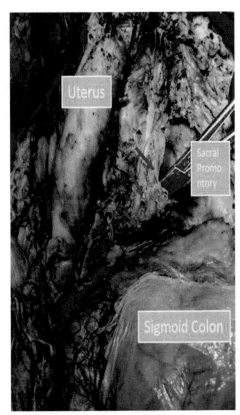

FIG. 2.5 **Anatomy of the Celiac Plexus.**   After opening the lesser sac (omental bursa) and mobilization of the liver, pancreas, and spleen, the celiac plexus is exposed as a diffuse nerve plexus around the celiac trunk. *One red arrow* and *black suture* (right) around it localizes the left gastric artery. *Two red arrows* with *black suture* (left) around it isolated the splenic artery. Both arteries approach the celiac trunk (with a *blue tie* around it). *Small yellow arrows* show the distribution of the celiac plexus. *Three red arrows* show the common hepatic artery (*black suture* at top of image).

FIG. 2.6 **The Superior Hypogastric Plexus.**   The superior hypogastric plexus (*red arrows* and over the surgical instrument) lies anterior to the sacral promontory within the retroperitoneal space. Uterus and sigmoid colon were mobilized to expose the plexus.

the autonomic plexuses surrounding the aorta, follow splanchnic nerves to the sympathetic trunk, leave the sympathetic trunk through white rami communicantes and enter the dorsal roots of spinal nerves and dorsal root ganglion. Like somatic afferent neurons, the nerve cell bodies of visceral afferent neurons lie within the dorsal root ganglion. The central processes of these nerve cell bodies continue through the dorsal root, reach the spinal cord, and synapse on interneurons within the cord. No synapse occurs in the dorsal root ganglion. Visceral afferent fibers from the distal colon and pelvis typically return to the spinal cord with parasympathetic efferent fibers that originate from the sacral nerve roots Table 2.1 below summarizes the innervation of the various visceral organs.

Liver and Biliary System

The sensation from the liver and biliary systems is conveyed by both somatic and visceral sensory nerve fibers. Sensory impulses return to the CNS by following sympathetic visceral pathways through the celiac plexus and thoracic splanchnic nerves, and by following parasympathetic pathways through the vagus nerve.

Stomach

Sensory impulses from the stomach follow sympathetic pathways through the celiac plexus and through T7–T9 spinal nerve roots and by following parasympathetic pathways through the vagus nerve.

Pancreas

Sensory impulses from the pancreas follow sympathetic pathways through the celiac plexus and T6–T10 spinal nerve roots and by following parasympathetic pathways through the vagus nerve.

TABLE 2.1
Summary of Visceral Sensation From the Gastrointestinal Tract.[18]

Organ	Visceral Afferents Traveling with Sympathetic Efferent Fibers	Visceral Afferents Traveling With Parasympathetic Efferent Fibers
Liver and biliary tract	T5–T10 via celiac plexus	Vagus nerve
Stomach	T7–T9 via celiac plexus	Vagus nerve
Pancreas	T6–T10 via celiac plexus	Vagus nerve
Small bowel	T9–L1 via celiac plexus	Vagus nerve
Cecum, ascending and transverse colon	T9–L1 via celiac plexus	Vagus nerve
Descending colon	T9–T12 via celiac plexus	S2–S4 via pelvic nerves
Sigmoid, rectum	T11–L1 via inferior hypogastric plexus	S2–S4 via pelvic nerves

Small Intestine, Cecum, and Ascending and Transverse Colon

Sensory impulses from the small bowel, cecum, and ascending and transverse colon follow sympathetic pathways through the celiac plexus and through T9–L1 spinal nerve roots and by following parasympathetic pathways through the vagus nerve.

Descending Colon, Sigmoid, and Rectum

The descending colon receives sympathetic innervation from the T9 to T12 nerve roots via the celiac plexus. The sigmoid colon and rectum receive sympathetic innervation via the inferior hypogastric plexus from the T11 to L1 nerve roots. At this point forward in the GI tract, sacral nerves S2-S4 provide parasympathetic innervation.

PHYSIOLOGY OF VISCERAL PAIN

Abdominal pain is one of the most common reasons a person may seek consultation with a physician. Depending on symptoms and presentation, the differential diagnosis can be vast. Although some portion of abdominal pain resolves with diagnosis and treatment, a substantial portion of cases can become chronic. Chronic abdominal pain is difficult to manage because our understanding of the pathogenesis of the pain and visceral sensation is incomplete.

Functional Organization of the Autonomic Nervous System

The central nervous system ultimately receives and processes pain signals from the abdominal viscera. Nerves that innervate the viscera project to the CNS via sympathetic and parasympathetic nerve fibers. However, the course a pain signal takes from origin to CNS is not necessarily direct. As outlined previously in this chapter, the course of a pain signal can involve nerves intrinsic and extrinsic to the abdominal organs before finally reaching the spinal cord and the rest of the CNS.

Cholinergic, Adrenergic Preganglionic, and Postganglionic Synapsis

The autonomic nervous system is complex, with various synapses throughout the body. In general, the presynaptic neurons of both sympathetic and parasympathetic nerves contain nicotinic acetylcholine (cholinergic) receptors. The sympathetic and parasympathetic efferent nerves differ when it comes to postganglionic receptors. The sympathetic postganglionic nerves release catecholamines, which act upon adrenergic receptors. The adrenergic receptors contain multiple subtypes that are found in the various end organs. Parasympathetic nerves release acetylcholine, which activates nicotinic acetylcholine receptors. Of course, there are exceptions that warrant discussion. The first exception is sweat glands, which are innervated by both sympathetic and parasympathetic nerves. Both divisions release acetylcholine and contain cholinergic receptors. The other exception is the adrenal medulla, which contains nicotinic acetylcholine receptors, the activation of which ultimately causes catecholamine release.

Neurotransmitters: Acetylcholine, Catecholamines

Acetylcholine (AcCh): is the neurotransmitter released at all autonomic preganglionic nerve endings as well as parasympathetic postganglionic endings at the neuromuscular junction. The AcCh receptors at the autonomic ganglia are of the nicotinic class, and they are the same class that is found at the neuromuscular junction. Muscarinic class receptors are found at all cholinergic efferent cells. Stimulation of muscarinic receptors in the heart is inhibitory and in the GI tract is excitatory to increase gut motility.

Catecholamines [Norepinephrine (NE) and Epinephrine (EP)]: NE is the neurotransmitter predominantly found at the sympathetic postganglionic nerve ending. NE and EP are also released from the adrenal medulla into the bloodstream to reinforce their neurotransmission properties. There are two classes of adrenergic receptors, Alpha (α) and Beta (β). Stimulation of α receptors generally results in an excitatory response such as vasoconstriction or smooth muscle contraction, including sphincters of the GI tract and urinary bladder. In the pancreas, α stimulation inhibits insulin and exocrine secretion. Stimulation of β2 adrenergic receptors leads to hepatic glycogenolysis and has inhibitory effects on GI tract motility.

PAIN MECHANISMS

Pain arising from the visceral organs is extraordinarily complex and can be produced by various stimuli including traction, distention, compression, hypoxia or ischemia, chemical stimuli, etc. However, not every stimulus is perceived as painful and nociceptors can become sensitized to ongoing stimuli.[19] This occurs because various nociceptors are modulated by a variety of inflammatory and antiinflammatory mediators that ultimately lead to the generation of action potentials if the signal is strong enough to overcome an intrinsic threshold.[20] In addition, various hormones can affect abdominal pain and sensation.[21] The characteristics of visceral pain are often complex. The origin of an abdominal visceral pain can be initiated from either the visceral or parietal peritoneum or both. The parietal peritoneum is usually innervated by somatic nerves that contain cell bodies in the dorsal root ganglia. This allows for localization of the pain to a specific area. The visceral peritoneum and visceral organs themselves have a significant amount of autonomic innervation, which leads to more vague or referred pain.

Nociception and Visceral Nociceptors

Visceral nociception is caused by a variety of stimuli and causes several downstream effects depending on the intensity of the stimulus. The abdominal viscera nociceptors include chemo, thermo, and mechanoreceptors. Visceral afferent nerves utilize neuropeptides such as calcitonin gene-related peptide (CGRP), somatostatin,

vasoactive intestinal peptide, and substance P.[3] Organ distention, ischemia, and inflammation can all cause varying responses depending on the intensity of the stimuli. The afferent fibers come in two varieties, sympathetic and parasympathetic afferents. Based on studies, it seems the parasympathetic afferent nerves may modulate pain signaling rather than directly conveying pain signals.[4] The sympathetic afferents seem to be responsible for carrying pain signals back to the spinal cord.[5] However, vagal afferent nerves may also respond to some of the same neurotransmitters that affect the sympathetic afferents, like serotonin, adenosine triphosphate, prostaglandins, and capsaicin.[6] The activation of vagal afferents by visceral stimulation associated with the substances mentioned causes symptoms like nausea and vomiting, as some of these nerves project to the brainstem. This may help to explain the connection between pain and some of these autonomic responses.[7–9]

Theories of Visceral Pain

Visceral pain, while ubiquitous, is poorly understood. This lack of understanding is due to the complexity of the interactions between the visceral organs, the autonomic nervous system, and the central nervous system. For example, not all visceral organs respond to stimuli, some organs are more sensitive than others, and not all stimuli will cause pain. In addition, emotions and stress can affect visceral pain via the hypothalamic–pituitary–adrenal axis.[10,21] Therefore, multiple factors play a role in the development of visceral pain. Visceral pain signals can be transmitted to multiple locations within the central nervous system and can converge with somatic afferents, which can lead to referred pain and modulation of signals within the CNS. Dysregulation can also occur and lead to hyperalgesia.[22] Physical responses to visceral pain like spasms can also arise. More recent studies suggest that the microbiome of the gut can modulate pain[11] and that probiotics can lead to improved pain in IBS patients.[12–14] On the other hand, pathogenic bacteria may contain or secrete substances that cause inflammation and pain.[15,16,23]

Referred Pain

Pain from visceral organs is often described as a deep pain that is poorly localized and often felt in an area that differs from its true origin. This phenomenon is described as referred pain. Referred pain occurs because autonomic afferent fibers pass through the multiple plexuses before synapsing at a level that may be completely different from its origin. A classic example is an appendicitis. The pain of appendicitis starts as a dull, centrally located periumbilical pain. The physiology behind this pain is such that the visceral afferent autonomic nerves "sense" the pain and send signals through enteric prevertebral ganglia that eventually enter the spinal cord at various levels. This results in poorly localized pain. However, once the inflammation associated with appendicitis spreads to include the parietal pleura, the pain is sensed as right lower quadrant pain. This occurs because the somatic afferents more directly enter the spinal cord and register as pain via the spinothalamic tract.

Viscerosomatic convergence describes the communications between visceral neurons and somatic neurons. Afferent visceral neurons may have less spinal cord terminations than their somatic counterparts, and thus synapse with somatic neurons before signals entering the CNS.[18] This may also help explain the concurrence of visceral and somatic pain. Viscerovisceral convergence occurs when the pain from one visceral organ is referred to another. Afferent nerve fibers from the various visceral organs converge as they approach the CNS.

Noxious Stimuli to Trigger Visceral Pain

Population-based studies have revealed that noxious stimuli in young patients can lead to abdominal pain later in life.[17] The theory behind chronic pain is that the stimulus leads to visceral hyperalgesia. Interestingly, noxious stimuli to the sites of referred pain can also cause hyperalgesia at the level of the spinal cord, which can lead to visceral hyperalgesia. This phenomenon is referred to as somatovisceral convergence.

REFERENCES

1. Weijs TJ, Ruurda JP, Luyer MD, Cuesta MA, van Hillegersberg R, Bleys RL. New insights into the surgical anatomy of the esophagus. *J Thorac Dis.* 2017;9(Suppl 8):S675.
2. Goyal RK, Chaudhury A. Physiology of normal esophageal motility. *J Clin Gastroenterol.* 2008;42(5):610.
3. Coelho AM, Fioramonti J, Buéno L. Systemic lipopolysaccharide influences rectal sensitivity in rats: role of mast cells, cytokines, and vagus nerve. *Am J Physiol Gastrointest Liver Physiol.* 2000;279(4):G781–G790.
4. Dubin AE, Patapoutian A. Nociceptors: the sensors of the pain pathway. *J Clin Invest.* 2010;120(11):3760–3772.
5. Ness TJ, Fillingim RB, Randich A, Backensto EM, Faught E. Low intensity vagal nerve stimulation lowers human thermal pain thresholds. *Pain.* 2000;86:81–85.
6. Mazzone SB, Undem BJ. Vagal afferent innervation of the airways in health and disease. *Physiol Rev.* 2016;96(3):975–1024.
7. Andrews PL, Sanger GJ. Abdominal vagal afferent neurones: an important target for the treatment of gastrointestinal dysfunction. *Curr Opin Pharmacol.* 2002;2(6):650–656.
8. Rudd JA, Nalivaiko E, Matsuki N, Wan C, Andrews PL. The involvement of TRPV1 in emesis and anti-emesis. *Temperature.* 2015;2(2):258–276.
9. Bulmer DC, Roza C. Visceral pain. In: *The Oxford Handbook of the Neurobiology of Pain.* 2018.
10. Heinricher MM. Pain modulation and the transition from acute to chronic pain. In: *Translational Research in Pain and Itch.* Dordrecht: Springer; 2016:105–115.
11. Camilleri M, Boeckxstaens G. Dietary and pharmacological treatment of abdominal pain in IBS. *Gut.* 2017;66(5):966–974.
12. Hadizadeh F, Bonfiglio F, Belheouane M, et al. Faecal microbiota composition associates with abdominal pain in the general population. *Gut.* 2018;67(4):778–779.
13. Pokusaeva K, Johnson C, Luk B, et al. GABA-producing Bifidobacterium dentium modulates visceral sensitivity in the intestine. *Neuro Gastroenterol Motil.* 2017;29(1):e12904.
14. Harper A, Naghibi M, Garcha D. The role of bacteria, probiotics and diet in irritable bowel syndrome. *Foods.* 2018;7(2):13.
15. Chiu IM, Heesters BA, Ghasemlou N, et al. Bacteria activate sensory neurons that modulate pain and inflammation. *Nature.* 2013;501(7465):52.
16. Sengupta JN. Visceral pain: the neurophysiological mechanism. In: *Sensory Nerves.* Berlin, Heidelberg: Springer; 2009:31–74.
17. Gebhart GF. Visceral pain—peripheral sensitisation. *Gut.* 2000;47(suppl 4):iv54–iv55.
18. Gold MS, Gebhart GF. Nociceptor sensitization in pain pathogenesis. *Nat Med.* 2010;16(3):1248–1257.
19. Janig W. Neurobiology of visceral afferent neurons: neuroanatomy, functions, organ regulations and sensations. *Biol Psychol.* 1996;42(1–2):29–51.
20. Sagami Y, Shimada Y, Tayama J, Nomura T, SatakeM, Endo Y. Effect of a corticotropin releasing hormone receptor antagonist on colonic sensory and motor function in patients with irritable bowel syndrome. *Gut.* 2004;53:958–964.
21. Gebhart GF, Bielefeldt K. Physiology of visceral pain. *Comprehensive Physiol.* 2011;6(4):1609–1633.
22. Sikandar S, Dickenson AH. Visceral pain—the ins and outs, the ups and downs. *Curr Opin Support Palliat Care.* 2012;6(1):17.
23. Wood JN, ed. *The Oxford Handbook of the Neurobiology of Pain.* Oxford University Press; 2018.

FURTHER READING

1. Wood JD, Alpers DH, Andrews PLR. Fundamentals of neurogastroenterology. *Gut.* 1999;45(suppl 2):II6–II16.
2. Elias M. Cervical sympathetic and stellate ganglion blocks. *Pain Physician.* 2000;3(3):294–304.
3. Chung IH, Oh CS, Koh KS, Kim HJ, Paik HC, Lee DY. Anatomic variations of the T2 nerve root (including the

nerve of Kuntz) and their implications for sympathectomy. *J Thorac Cardiovasc Surg.* 2002;123(3):498–501.

4. Zaidi ZF, Ashraf A. The nerve of Kunz: incidence, location and variations. *J Appl Sci Res.* 2010;6:659–664.

5. Oh CS, Chung IH, Ji HJ, et al. Clinical implications of topographic anatomy on the ganglion impar. *Anesthesiology.* 2004;101:249–250.

6. Toshniwal GR, Dureja GP, Prashanth SM. Transsacrococcygeal approach to ganglion impar block for management of chronic perineal pain: a prospective observational study. *Pain Physician.* 2007;10:661–666.

CHAPTER 3

Female Pelvic Pain

MANSOOR M. AMAN, MD • AMMAR MAHMOUD, MD

INTRODUCTION

Chronic pelvic pain (CPP) in women is defined as noncyclical pain lasting greater than 6 months and can affect all ages. It is associated with impairment in sexual function and emotional and behavioral health. Patients present with symptoms suggestive of pelvic floor, urinary, bowel, sexual, or gynecological dysfunction. These include dysmenorrhea, dyspareunia, dysuria, and pain along the groin, vagina, or perineum. Among the many sources of CPP commonly seen in clinical practice are endometriosis, pelvic inflammatory disease, nonmalignant adnexal masses, vulvodynia, pudendal neuralgia, neuropathic postsurgical, and myofascial pain along the pelvic brim. Pain that fails to improve with established treatment algorithms for well-defined disease processes may be deemed refractory.

The World Health Organization estimates the global prevalence of CPP to be 5.7%–26.6%.[1] This number is likely an underrepresentation given many countries do not have data to report. Determining an underlying etiology to develop an effective treatment plan often requires a multidisciplinary team approach including primary care physicians, gynecology, urology, gastroenterology, behavioral health, and pain management specialists.

CPP is often associated with endometriosis; however, many patients do not have an obvious source for pain.[2] A study across 10 countries demonstrated an average diagnostic delay of 6.7 years for endometriosis in women with predominantly CPP symptoms, and this was longer in women with elevated BMI.[3] Physical limitations with activity and subfertility are accompanied by significant psychosocial impairment.[4,5] The economic burden stems primarily from the loss of productivity and decreased quality of life.[6,7] Pelvic inflammatory disease (PID) results from genital tract infections that cause inflammation[8] and is most frequently seen in women ages 15–25. The incidence is difficult to quantify, as it is not a reportable disease. Various demographic, clinical, and behavioral risk factors such as smoking have been identified as predictors of CPP after PID.[9] A sequela of PID are adhesions that may be associated with pain and may result in mechanical obstruction of the gastrointestinal tract or torsion of reproductive organs. Nonmalignant adnexal masses such as leiomyomas, tubo-ovarian cyst have a high lifetime incidence ranging between 5% and 71% based on age, ethnicity, BMI, and comorbidities such as diabetes and hypertension.[10,11] Vulvodynia has prevalence 8%[12] and often goes underdiagnosed as demonstrated by an incidence of 4.2%.[13]

This chapter will focus on refractory pelvic pain that has failed to improve with conventional medical management of the primary diagnosis being treated.

ETIOLOGY AND PATHOGENESIS

Unlike acute pain that is caused by inflammation, trauma, or infection resulting in afferent nociceptive input, the underlying etiology of CPP is complex with varying neuropathic, somatic, visceral, and musculoskeletal contributions (Fig. 3.1). The pathogenesis is genetic, endocrine, behavioral, and central nervous system mediated.

Genetic mechanisms are inferred by the increased incidence of other chronic pain syndromes in patients with CPP.[14,15] The endocrine system has also been implicated in the pathogenesis of CPP as dysregulation of sex hormones is associated with certain disease states such as endometriosis and can modulate nociception and pain perception.[16,17] The behavioral mechanism suggests an underlying trigger such as a negative emotional experience.[18-20] Central sensitization may

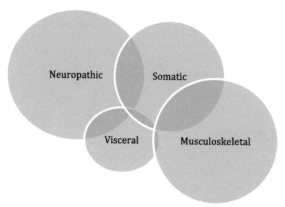

FIG. 3.1 Contributions of several overlapping pain mechanisms account for the variable clinical presentation of CPP.

develop and lead to an amplified pain response and reduced nociceptive thresholds of the dorsal horn neurons. This can lead to sensory disturbances and organ malfunction. Visceral stimuli that are normally subthreshold can be perceived and processed as noxious stimuli, an example of visceral hyperalgesia.

Many of the structures in the pelvis receive their innervation from the superior hypogastric plexus, which is located in the retroperitoneum and situated bilaterally along the anterior surface of the L5 vertebral body. It comprises sympathetic and parasympathetic visceral afferent and efferent projections.[21] The caudal ends of the sympathetic chains then converge to form the ganglion impar, which provides sympathetic innervation to pelvic viscera as well as carry both sympathetic and nociceptive fibers from the perineum, distal rectum, perianal region, and distal urethra among others. Parasympathetic innervation of the pelvis originates from the S2 to S4 roots via the pelvic splanchnic nerves. Somatic innervation, including afferent sensory fibers, also arises from the S2–S4 nerve roots.

CLINICAL PRESENTATION

There may be a myriad of signs and symptoms upon presentation. Patients report abdominopelvic pain that is deep, nagging, aching, cramping, sharp, burning, or lancinating. The pain may radiate along the back, groin, or thighs in a nondermatomal pattern. Patients often describe dysmenorrhea, menometrorrhagia, dysuria, pain along the pelvic brim, or vulva upon palpation. Dyspareunia is particularly taxing on both the patient and their sexual partner.

DIAGNOSIS

A comprehensive history and physical examination remain the mainstay for initial diagnosis. Common causes that may result in persistent pelvic pain should be evaluated and ruled out. A focused psychosocial history looking for recent stressors such as loss of a family member or prior negative experiences should be obtained to evaluate for coexisting depression and anxiety. An organ-based review should be detailed with attention to urologic, gastrointestinal, gynecological, and musculoskeletal involvement. Finally, red flag signs indicating systemic disease, including postmenopausal bleeding, postcoital bleeding, pelvic mass, involuntary weight loss, and hematuria, should be excluded.

Should there be symptoms suggestive of a well-known disease, treatment of the causing disease is initiated according to specific guidelines and best practices. In the majority of patients without an identifiable disease process, subspecialty consultation should be considered if organ-specific symptoms predominate. Without organ-specific sources of pain, a consult to a pain management specialist is encouraged.

Commonly obtained imaging includes transabdominal and transvaginal ultrasound[22,23] and pelvic computed tomography (CT) scans that may be beneficial in evaluating any underlying pelvic masses. Diagnostic laparoscopy is considered the gold standard for diagnosis in patients with clinical concern for endometriosis, adenomyosis, and leiomyosis. Laboratory testing including LH, FHS, estradiol, urine analysis, vaginal swab, and stool culture may be considered if clinically appropriate.

DIFFERENTIAL DIAGNOSIS

The differential diagnosis should first seek to rule out infection and malignancy. The remaining causes of CPP may be divided by organ system. Urological pain syndromes include interstitial cystitis and urethral pain. Gynecologic causes include dysmenorrhea, endometriosis, PID, adnexal masses, and injuries related to childbirth. Gastrointestinal sources include hemorrhoids, anal fissures, and irritable bowel syndrome. Musculoskeletal and neuromuscular etiologies include pudendal neuralgia, pelvic floor muscular dysfunction, and vulvodynia.

PHYSICAL EXAM FINDINGS

Physical examination should be targeted at identifying the muscles, nerves, and organs likely responsible for the patient's pain to elucidate the source. There are few pathognomonic findings on examination of chronic pelvic pain patients. The abdomen should be inspected for any gross deformity or masses. Prior surgical incisions should be evaluated to ensure appropriate healing and for overlaying skin dysesthesia or allodynia. Gentle palpation with a single digit along the rectus sheath and obliques for point tenderness should be performed to assess the degree of musculoskeletal involvement. A Carnett's test is conducted with a patient lying supine while the examiner places a finger over the abdominal musculature. The patient is asked to elevate the legs or head to contract the rectus abdominis. A positive test resulting in increase in pain suggests a muscular, or nerve entrapment etiology opposed to true visceral pain. Deeper palpation can be useful in evaluating adnexal tenderness or masses.

Examination of external genitalia and speculum exam should be performed with care due to hyperalgesia or allodynia. Palpation along the pelvic brim musculature may elicit the pain due to trigger points along the obturator internus and externus muscles. Palpation along the ischial spine may reproduce a sharp neuropathic pain due to irritation of the pudendal nerve. A spine examination of the lumbar facet joints, sacroiliac joints, hip joints, and lower back and buttock musculature is helpful in ruling out predominant musculoskeletal sources of pain.

TREATMENT

A multimodal approach to treatment is often necessary and should incorporate physical and behavioral therapy, pharmacological treatment, interventional, and surgical management as necessary to ensure treatment success (Fig. 3.2).

Pharmacologic

Pharmacological treatment for CPP necessitates an individualized and interdisciplinary approach. A straightforward algorithmic approach is often unsuccessful due to the variable underlying etiologies and coexisting medical and psychosocial comorbidities. Treatment recommendations are often extrapolated from the treatment of other chronic pain conditions to help guide management.[2] Limited data surrounding the initial pharmacological treatment is available for women with CPP.

The first step in the pharmacological treatment of CPP focuses on identifying the underlying pain mechanism (somatic, neuropathic, visceral, sympathetic). These categories often overlap and demand a multimodal strategy to provide a synergistic analgesic effect thereby improving the likelihood of successful treatment. Initial pharmacological therapy is usually limited to nonsteroidal antiinflammatory drugs and muscle relaxants as they are generally well tolerated with limited side effects. Acetaminophen is often added if a

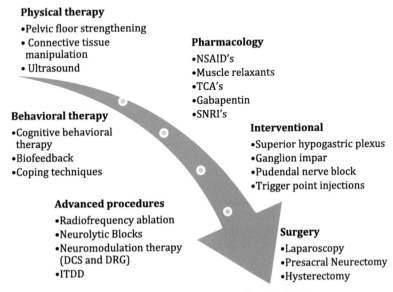

FIG. 3.2 Multimodal treatment options for CPP.

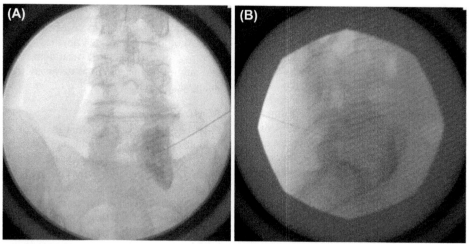

FIG. 3.3 **(A)** Anteroposterior view of unilateral superior hypogastric plexus block following contrast administration. **(B)** Lateral view with contrast at the anterior surface of the L5/S1 vertebral body.

predominantly somatic presentation is suspected, despite minimal evidence of efficacy.

Patients with predominantly neuropathic and sympathetic features are more likely to respond to tricyclic antidepressants, anticonvulsants (i.e., gabapentinoids), and selective norepinephrine reuptake inhibitors. Combination therapy with different neuropathic agents has been shown to be more effective in CPP. Specifically, gabapentin alone or in combination with amitriptyline resulted in greater pain relief than amitriptyline alone.[24]

For patients with cyclic exacerbation of their CPP, hormonal therapy with combined estrogen-progestin contraceptive, progestin-only contraceptives, or gonadotropin-releasing hormone analogs may be considered. Hormonal therapy should be managed by obstetrics and gynecology. Chronic opioid therapy is not recommended for the treatment of CPP.[2]

Injections

Interventional management should be considered to increase patient functionality and when conservative therapy has failed to provide adequate pain relief. Targeted injections can aid in the diagnostic evaluation and offer therapeutic benefits for patients with complex pain presentations. A careful review of the post-procedural pain diary may offer clinical insight by estimating the underlying pain process (visceral, neuropathic, or sympathetically mediated) and its degree of contribution to the presenting pain syndrome.

Superior hypogastric plexus block

The superior hypogastric plexus (SHP) contains both sympathetic and parasympathetic fibers located bilaterally along the anterior surface of the L5 vertebral body. Primary visceral afferents from the descending colon, rectum, bladder, ureters, uterus, and adnexal structures travel proximally alongside these sympathetic nerves and ganglia allowing them to be accessible for the diagnostic block. The SHP block is most commonly done with fluoroscopic guidance; however, CT can also be used. It is typically targeted from a posterior paramedian approach at the level of the lower one-third of the fifth lumbar vertebral body and upper one-third of the first sacral vertebral body with the needle tip advanced to the anterior vertebral body (Fig. 3.3). The SHP block has been demonstrated to be effective in the management of nononcological chronic pain due to endometriosis.[25,26] If the diagnostic block is successful, therapeutic neurolysis with alcohol and phenol have both been completed with improvement for patients with nonmalignant pelvic pain.[27]

Ganglion impar block

The termination of the sympathetic chains forms a single fused ganglion known as the Ganglion Impar (GI) or Ganglion of Walther. Primary visceral afferents from the perineum, distal rectum, distal urethra, vulva, perianal area, and distal one-third of the vagina travel alongside visceral sympathetic fibers converging at the GI.

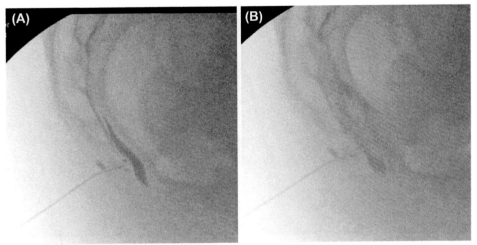

FIG. 3.4 **(A)** Lateral fluoroscopic view of ganglion impar block immediately following contrast administration. **(B)** Postmedication view.

Multiple approaches to target the ganglion impar have been described, but the most popular technique is the transcoccygeal approach due to its shortest trajectory. Although the patient is in the prone position, a spinal needle is placed through the sacrococcygeal ligament with the needle tip slightly posterior to the rectum (Fig. 3.4). Extra care should be taken to not advance needle tip into the rectum. Contrast is injected to confirm appropriate placement. Local anesthetic with or without steroids may be injected.

A retrospective study evaluated 83 patients for chronic refractory pelvic and perineal pain and offered a series of three ganglion impar blocks using 0.75% ropivacaine. Sixty-two patients completed the study with a statistically significant reduction in pain albeit transient.[28]

Currently, there are no studies describing the efficacy of radiofrequency ablation for chronic refractory pelvic pain. However, in a study of coccydynia patients who underwent conventional radiofrequency ablation at 80°C for 90 s, 90.2% reported pain relief at 6-month follow-up.[29] This procedure can be considered in patients with chronic pelvic pain who have a positive diagnostic GI block. Neurolysis and cryoablation may also be performed for longer-term relief.

Pudendal nerve block

The pudendal nerve originates from the ventral rami of the second through fourth sacral nerves and traverses the pelvis terminating into the inferior rectal nerve, perineal nerve, and dorsal nerve of the clitoris. The pudendal nerve is a major somatic nerve of the sacral

plexus with sensory, motor, and postganglionic sympathetic fibers. Injections can be performed using anatomical landmarks, fluoroscopic guidance, CT, or ultrasound. Unilateral or bilateral injections are performed depending on the laterality of the patient's pain.

When using the landmark technique in female patients, the transvaginal approach requires the patient to be placed in the lithotomy position. The ischial spine is palpated and the needle is guided toward the tip of the ischial spine. The needle is advanced through the vaginal mucosa until it reaches the sacrospinous ligament. With fluoroscopy or CT guidance, the patient is placed in the prone position and the needle is advanced to the tip of the ischial spine (Fig. 3.5). The needle is slightly withdrawn after contact with the ischial spine is made and medication is administered after negative aspiration rules out the intravascular injection.

In patients with a previous positive diagnostic block but short-term relief, pulsed radiofrequency ablation (PRF) may be performed, which is thought to be successful by neural modulation without affecting the motor or sensory nerve fibers.[30] PRF avoids the use of high temperatures compared to conventional continuous radiofrequency procedures. One study treated women with CPP from refractory pudendal neuralgia with transvaginal PRF at 42°C for 90 s for four courses of treatment. All of the women had significant decreases in their pain scores after at least one round of PRF.[31]

Trigger point injections

Local trigger points, indicative of tight pelvic floor muscles, can be elicited with a twitch response on

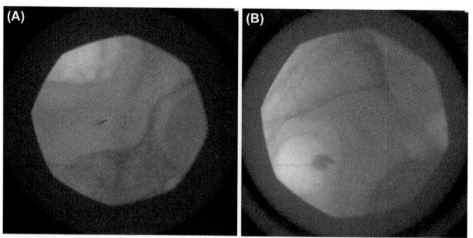

FIG. 3.5 **(A)** Anteroposterior fluoroscopic view of a unilateral pudendal nerve block before contrast administration. Final needle position is shown at the tip of the ischial spine. **(B)** Lateral view with contrast pooling at the level of the ischial spine.

transvaginal or transrectal exam. Patients with refractory trigger points despite pelvic floor therapy and medication management may be candidates for pelvic floor trigger point injections (TPI's). Injections targeting the obturator internus, iliopsoas, levator ani muscles, and suprapubic muscles, among others, have been reported.[32] Although the mechanism of action is not well established, it is believed that TPI's disrupt the reflex arcs and mechanics of abnormally contracted muscles and release endorphins. The injectate typically consists of local anesthetic with corticosteroid. For patients who do not receive long-lasting relief with traditional TPI's, botulinum injections may also be offered. Transvaginal injection with and without electromyographic guidance into the area of spasm with up to 200 units of botulinum toxin has been reported.[32]

Advanced Procedures
Dorsal root ganglion stimulation
The dorsal root ganglion (DRG) is an accessible neural structure in the spinal column that is intricately involved in the development and processing of chronic neuropathic pain.[33] The DRG houses the soma of sensory neurons and communicates with nerve roots. It is considered the intersection of somatic sensory and sympathetic afferents. Targeting this neural structure has been beneficial in the treatment of focal pains while limiting collateral unwanted stimulation in nearby areas. As such, DRG stimulation has shown promise when compared to traditional dorsal column stimulation (DCS) in difficult to capture areas such as the abdomen, groin, pelvis, knee, and foot.

Given the minimal cerebrospinal fluid along the neural foramen where the DRG is located, there is less dissipation of applied current. The programming parameters with this subparesthesia, paresthesia-independent therapy varies starkly from DCS with a median frequency of 20 Hz, pulse width 300 μs, and amplitude of 0.650 mA at 6 months postimplant.[34]

The Neuromodulation Appropriateness Consensus Committee on the best practices for Dorsal Root Ganglion stimulation recommends that DRG stimulation only be considered in the treatment of pelvic pain using strict selection criteria.[35] They describe that a clear mechanism of injury be ascertained, postsurgical or trauma related, and pain is categorized as being visceral or somatic. A history of sexual abuse or significant psychological comorbidity remains a relative contraindication to therapy until the patient receives adequate counseling and a behavioral health professional agrees that an implant is indicated. In this patient population, the decision to proceeding with DRG neuromodulation should truly be multidisciplinary involving gynecology, urology, psychology, and primary care. The use of DRG stimulation in the management of CPP is supported by level III evidence suggesting that the recommendations are based upon clinical experience-based opinions, descriptive studies, clinical observations, or reports of expert committees.

Various lead placement locations and combination arrays have been proposed when targeting DRG for CPP.[36,37] The L1 and S2 lead array has reported the most success ensuring coverage of lower abdomen, groin, and pelvis.[38,39] The L1 DRG is a confluence for three lumbar plexus nerves commonly implicated namely the ilioinguinal (L1-2), iliohypogastric (L1-2), and genitofemoral nerves (L1-2). Targeting the S2 DRG interrupts primary afferent input from the sacral plexus including the pudendal nerve (S2–S4) and sacral splanchnic sympathetic plexus. The DRG Focus paper also highlights other possible lead arrays that have been used to treat refractory CPP.[40]

Dorsal column stimulation

Conventional spinal cord stimulation delivers tonic stimulation via a fixed input of energy to the dorsal column of the spinal cord. Individual pulses at a constant amplitude, pulse width (duration), and frequency (interpulse gap) produce paresthesia over the area of pain at clinically relevant settings. DCS using low frequency (paresthesia based), high frequency (subparesthesia), and burst waveforms (subparesthesia) remains a well-recognized therapy with level-one evidence for use in complex regional pain syndrome, postlaminectomy, and other neuropathic pain conditions.[41–44] Data exclusively for pelvic pain is primarily case reports, case series, and small prospective studies.

A case series report described success as defined by at least 50% relief in pain and reduction in opioids when using low frequency, paresthesia-based DCS (lead tip at T11–T12 disc space) in the treatment of visceral pelvic pain stemming from multiple surgical explorations for endometriosis.[45] Stimulation of the conus medullaris for pudendal neuralgia[46] and high-frequency subparesthesia 10 kHz for neuropathic pelvic pain[47] also show promise for future studies. A lower lumbar epidural access would be recommended to achieve the lead tip at T11/T12 interspace or L1 for stimulation of the conus medullaris. The explant rate among pelvic pain patients remains high at 33%. The most common reason cited being the loss of therapeutic effect in 39% of explanted patients.[48]

Intrathecal drug delivery systems

Targeted drug delivery (TDD) into the intrathecal space confers the principal advantage of bypassing the blood–brain barrier resulting in superior analgesia while mitigating side effects.[49] Patients with focal nociceptive or neuropathic pain syndromes can be managed effectively when compared to patients with global pain complaints. Currently, there are no studies describing the efficacy of intrathecal drug therapy for chronic pelvic pain, but these patients can be considered for TDD should their pain be refractory to conservative medical management. FDA-approved medications for TDD include morphine, ziconotide, and baclofen. Consensus guidelines also provide guidance on the use of off label intrathecal medications such as hydromorphone, fentanyl, sufentanil, bupivacaine, and clonidine.[50]

The Polyanalgesic Consensus Conference recommends taking into consideration the patient's psychosocial status, pain characteristic, disease state, and prior treatment failures before trialing for intrathecal delivery systems. The trialing methodology may vary from institution to institution; however, a common approach is a single shot intrathecal trial in an outpatient setting. After a successful trial, permanent surgical implantation is performed and consists of an intrathecal catheter tunneled to a subcutaneous pump. There is no evidence-based data on the optimal intrathecal catheter tip location for chronic pelvic pain. Anecdotally, the catheter tip is commonly placed along the lower thoracic to upper lumbar vertebral levels (T10–L2). TDD is not without risk and physicians managing these systems must be well versed with both medical and surgical complications that may ensue.[51] Evidence focused on exclusively pelvic pain is lacking and clinical judgment must be exercised for patient selection.

Surgical Interventions

Surgical evaluation should be considered for women who continue to experience persistent pain and disability that is refractory to pharmacological and nonpharmacological therapy. Surgical management options include diagnostic laparoscopy, lysis of adhesions, presacral neurectomy, and hysterectomy. Surgical treatment should be sought out with caution in cases without identifiable and surgically correctable pathology. In the absence of any obvious pathology, surgical hysterectomy should be considered as a last resort for refractory and persistent pain as up to 40% of patients will have persistent pain and 5% will have new-onset or worsening pain.[52] Laparoscopic presacral neurectomy involves surgical excision of the SHP and traditionally targets midline dysmenorrhea. Presacral neurectomy has been demonstrated to provide long-term pain relief in patients with and without endometriosis.[53,54] Additionally, combined presacral neurectomy and laparoscopic treatment of endometriosis resulted in improved pain control when compared to laparoscopic endometriosis treatment alone for women with dysmenorrhea.[55]

Pelvic Floor Physical Therapy

Physical therapy should be considered in the multidisciplinary approach in the management of CPP. Myofascial dysfunction of the pelvic floor commonly occurs in patients with CPP and may overtime result in central sensitization phenomena that can worsen the pain.

Targeting the most likely ongoing etiology of pain is best accomplished through consultation with an experienced physical therapist with expertise in pelvic floor strengthening techniques, connective tissue manipulation, biofeedback, and ultrasound.

REFERENCES

1. Ahangari A. Prevalence of chronic pelvic pain among women: an updated review. *Pain Physician.* 2014;17(2): E141–E147.
2. Chronic pelvic pain: ACOG practice bulletin, number 218. *Obstet Gynecol.* 2020;135(3):e98–e109.
3. Nnoaham KE, Hummelshoj L, Webster P, et al. Impact of endometriosis on quality of life and work productivity: a multicenter study across ten countries. *Fertil Steril.* 2011; 96(2):366–373. e8.
4. Fourquet J, Gao X, Zavala D, et al. Patients' report on how endometriosis affects health, work, and daily life. *Fertil Steril.* 2010;93(7):2424–2428.
5. Ozkan S, Murk W, Arici A. Endometriosis and infertility. *Ann N Y Acad Sci.* 2008;1127(1):92–100.
6. Simoens S, Dunselman G, Dirksen C, et al. The burden of endometriosis: costs and quality of life of women with endometriosis and treated in referral centres. *Hum Reprod.* 2012;27(5):1292–1299.
7. Gao X, Yeh YC, Outley J, Simon J, Botteman M, Spalding J. Health-related quality of life burden of women with endometriosis: a literature review. *Curr Med Res Opin.* 2006; 22(9):1787–1797.
8. Jennings LK, Krywko DM. *Pelvic Inflammatory Disease (PID).* Treasure Island (FL): StatPearls Publishing; 2020.
9. Haggerty CL, Peipert JF, Weitzen S, et al. Predictors of chronic pelvic pain in an urban population of women with symptoms and signs of pelvic inflammatory disease. *Sex Transm Dis.* 2005;32(5):293–299.
10. Sparic R, Mirkovic L, Malvasi A, Tinelli A. Epidemiology of uterine myomas: a review. *Int J Fertil Steril.* 2016;9(4): 424–435.
11. Okolo S. Incidence, aetiology and epidemiology of uterine fibroids. *Best Pract Res Clin Obstet Gynaecol.* 2008;22(4): 571–588.
12. Reed BD, Harlow SD, Sen A, et al. Prevalence and demographic characteristics of vulvodynia in a population-based sample. *Am J Obstet Gynecol.* 2012;206(2):170.e1–170.e9.
13. Reed BD, Legocki LJ, Plegue MA, Sen A, Haefner HK, Harlow SD. Factors associated with vulvodynia incidence. *Obstet Gynecol.* 2014;123(2 Pt 1):225–231.
14. Kolesnikov Y, Gabovits B, Levin A, et al. Chronic pain after lower abdominal surgery: do catechol-O-methyl transferase/opioid receptor mu-1 polymorphisms contribute? *Mol Pain.* 2013;9:19.
15. Hawkins SM, Creighton CJ, Han DY, et al. Functional microRNA involved in endometriosis. *Mol Endocrinol.* 2011;25(5):821–832.
16. Heim C, Ehlert U, Hanker JP, Hellhammer DH. Psychological and endocrine correlates of chronic pelvic pain associated with adhesions. *J Psychosom Obstet Gynaecol.* 1999;20(1):11–20.
17. Wingenfeld K, Hellhammer DH, Schmidt I, Wagner D, Meinlschmidt G, Heim C. HPA axis reactivity in chronic pelvic pain: association with depression. *J Psychosom Obstet Gynaecol.* 2009;30(4):282–286.
18. Anda RF, Felitti VJ, Bremner JD, et al. The enduring effects of abuse and related adverse experiences in childhood. A convergence of evidence from neurobiology and epidemiology. *Eur Arch Psychiatr Clin Neurosci.* 2006; 256(3):174–186.
19. Raphael KG. Childhood abuse and pain in adulthood: more than a modest relationship? *Clin J Pain.* 2005; 21(5):371–373.
20. Savidge CJ, Slade P. Psychological aspects of chronic pelvic pain. *J Psychosom Res.* 1997;42(5):433–444.
21. Origoni M, Leone Roberti Maggiore U, Salvatore S, Candiani M. Neurobiological mechanisms of pelvic pain. *BioMed Res Int.* 2014;2014:903848.
22. Shwayder JM. Pelvic pain, adnexal masses, and ultrasound. *Semin Reprod Med.* 2008;26(3):252–265.
23. Joshi M, Ganesan K, Munshi HN, Ganesan S, Lawande A. Ultrasound of adnexal masses. *Semin Ultrasound CT MR.* 2008;29(2):72–97.
24. Sator-Katzenschlager SM, Scharbert G, Kress HG, et al. Chronic pelvic pain treated with gabapentin and amitriptyline: a randomized controlled pilot study. *Wien Klin Wochenschr.* 2005;117(21–22):761–768.
25. Wechsler RJ, Maurer PM, Halpern EJ, Frank ED. Superior hypogastric plexus block for chronic pelvic pain in the presence of endometriosis: CT techniques and results. *Radiology.* 1995;196(1):103–106.
26. Kanazi GE, Perkins FM, Thakur R, Dotson E. New technique for superior hypogastric plexus block. *Reg Anesth Pain Med.* 1999;24(5):473–476.
27. Richard III HM, Marvel RP. CT-guided diagnostic superior hypogastric plexus block and alcohol ablation treatment for nonmalignant chronic pelvic pain. *J Vasc Intervent Radiol.* 2013;24(4):S167–S168.
28. Le Clerc QC, Riant T, Levesque A, et al. Repeated ganglion impar block in a cohort of 83 patients with chronic pelvic and perineal pain. *Pain Physician.* 2017;20(6): E823–E828.
29. Adas C, Ozdemir U, Toman H, Luleci N, Luleci E, Adas H. Transsacrococcygeal approach to ganglion impar: radiofrequency application for the treatment of chronic intractable coccydynia. *J Pain Res.* 2016;9:1173–1177.
30. Rhame EE, Levey KA, Gharibo CG. Successful treatment of refractory pudendal neuralgia with pulsed radiofrequency. *Pain Physician.* 2009;12(3):633–638.
31. Frank CE, Flaxman T, Goddard Y, Chen I, Zhu C, Singh SS. The use of pulsed radiofrequency for the treatment of pudendal neuralgia: a case series. *J Obstet Gynaecol Can.* 2019; 41(11):1558–1563.
32. Fouad LS, Pettit PD, Threadcraft M, Wells A, Micallef A, Chen AH. Trigger point injections for pelvic floor myofascial spasm refractive to primary therapy. *J Endometriosis Pelvic Pain Disorders.* 2017;9(2):125–130.

33. International Neuromodulation Society 12th World Congress Neuromodulation: Medicine Evolving Through Technology June 6−11, 2015 Montreal, Canada. *Neuromodul Technol Neural Interface*. 2015;18(6):e107−e399.

34. Deer TR, Levy RM, Kramer J, et al. Dorsal root ganglion stimulation yielded higher treatment success rate for complex regional pain syndrome and causalgia at 3 and 12 months: a randomized comparative trial. *Pain*. 2017; 158(4):669−681.

35. Deer TR, Pope JE, Lamer TJ, et al. The Neuromodulation Appropriateness Consensus Committee on best practices for dorsal root ganglion stimulation. *Neuromodulation*. 2019;22(1):1−35.

36. Rowland DC, Wright D, Moir L, FitzGerald JJ, Green AL. Successful treatment of pelvic girdle pain with dorsal root ganglion stimulation. *Br J Neurosurg*. 2016;30(6): 685−686.

37. Liem L, Russo M, Huygen FJPM, et al. A multicenter, prospective trial to assess the safety and performance of the spinal modulation dorsal root ganglion neurostimulator system in the treatment of chronic pain. *Neuromodul Technol Neural Interface*. 2013;16(5):471−482.

38. Hunter CW, Yang A. Dorsal root ganglion stimulation for chronic pelvic pain: a case series and technical report on a novel lead configuration. *Neuromodulation*. 2019;22(1): 87−95.

39. Patel KV. Dorsal root ganglion stimulation for chronic pelvic pain [39T]. *Obstet Gynecol*. 2019;133:223S.

40. Hunter CW, Sayed D, Lubenow T, et al. DRG FOCUS: a multicenter study evaluating dorsal root ganglion stimulation and predictors for trial success. *Neuromodulation*. 2019;22(1):61−79.

41. Deer T, Slavin KV, Amirdelfan K, et al. Success Using Neuromodulation with BURST (SUNBURST) study: results from a prospective, randomized controlled trial using a novel burst waveform. *Neuromodulation*. 2018;21(1):56−66.

42. Kapural L, Yu C, Doust MW, et al. Comparison of 10-kHz high-frequency and traditional low-frequency spinal cord stimulation for the treatment of chronic back and leg pain: 24-month results from a multicenter, randomized, controlled pivotal trial. *Neurosurgery*. 2016;79(5):667−677.

43. Kapural L, Yu C, Doust MW, et al. Novel 10-kHz high-frequency therapy (HF10 therapy) is superior to traditional low-frequency spinal cord stimulation for the treatment of chronic back and leg pain: the SENZA-RCT randomized controlled trial. *Anesthesiology*. 2015;123(4): 851−860.

44. Kumar K, Taylor RS, Jacques L, et al. Spinal cord stimulation versus conventional medical management for neuropathic pain: a multicentre randomised controlled trial in patients with failed back surgery syndrome. *Pain*. 2007;132(1−2):179−188.

45. Kapural L, Narouze SN, Janicki TI, Mekhail N. Spinal cord stimulation is an effective treatment for the chronic intractable visceral pelvic pain. *Pain Med*. 2006;7(5): 440−443.

46. Buffenoir K, Rioult B, Hamel O, Labat JJ, Riant T, Robert R. Spinal cord stimulation of the conus medullaris for refractory pudendal neuralgia: a prospective study of 27 consecutive cases. *Neurourol Urodyn*. 2015;34(2):177−182.

47. Simopoulos T, Yong RJ, Gill JS. Treatment of chronic refractory neuropathic pelvic pain with high-frequency 10-kilohertz spinal cord stimulation. *Pain Pract*. 2018; 18(6):805−809.

48. Hayek SM, Veizi E, Hanes M. Treatment-limiting complications of percutaneous spinal cord stimulator implants: a review of eight years of experience from an academic center database. *Neuromodulation Technol Neural Interface*. 2015;18(7):603−609.

49. Deer TR, Pope JE, Hanes MC, McDowell GC. Intrathecal therapy for chronic pain: a review of morphine and ziconotide as firstline options. *Pain Med*. 2019;20(4): 784−798.

50. Deer TR, Pope JE, Hayek SM, et al. The Polyanalgesic Consensus Conference (PACC): recommendations on intrathecal drug infusion systems best practices and guidelines. *Neuromodulation*. 2017;20(2):96−132.

51. Deer TR, Pope JE, Hayek SM, et al. The Polyanalgesic Consensus Conference (PACC): recommendations for intrathecal drug delivery: guidance for improving safety and mitigating risks. *Neuromodulation*. 2017;20(2): 155−176.

52. Lamvu G. Role of hysterectomy in the treatment of chronic pelvic pain. *Obstet Gynecol*. 2011;117(5):1175−1178.

53. Jedrzejczak P, Sokalska A, Spaczynski RZ, Duleba AJ, Pawelczyk L. Effects of presacral neurectomy on pelvic pain in women with and without endometriosis. *Ginekol Pol*. 2009;80(3):172−178.

54. Liu KJ, Cui LQ, Huang Q, et al. Effectiveness and safety of laparoscopic presacral neurectomy in treating endometriosis-associated pain. *Zhongguo Yi Xue Ke Xue Yuan Xue Bao*. 2011;33(5):485−488.

55. Zullo F, Palomba S, Zupi E, et al. Effectiveness of presacral neurectomy in women with severe dysmenorrhea caused by endometriosis who were treated with laparoscopic conservative surgery: a 1-year prospective randomized double-blind controlled trial. *Am J Obstet Gynecol*. 2003; 189(1):5−10.

CHAPTER 4

Malignant Pelvic Pain

KIM A. TRAN, MD • SAMANTHA ROYALTY, MD • KRISHNA B. SHAH, MD • DANIEL J. PAK, MD

INTRODUCTION

It is estimated that approximately 60% of patients with malignancies encounter chronic pain, with 56%–82% of cases reporting inadequate pain control.[1] Colorectal cancer is the most common pelvic malignancy in both men and women. In 2018, over 1 million new cases were diagnosed in men and women.[2] When separated out by gender-specific malignancies, ovarian cancer had the highest incidence with 21,750 new cases.[3] Cervical cancer had the second highest incidence with about 13,800 new cases.[4] In men, however, prostate cancer was the most common pelvic malignancy with 164,690 new cases in 2018.[5] These malignancies along with many other causes of pelvic cancers can lead to malignant pelvic pain syndrome. With the progression of disease, malignant pelvic pain syndromes can be debilitating, limit functional status, and severely decrease quality of life. Chronic pain from increasing disease burden can present in multiple ways, including the mass effect from the primary tumor, invasion of nearby neurovascular structures, and metastatic disease to regional and distal sites. Furthermore, as improvements are made in diagnostic testing and treatments, there is a growing population of cancer survivors who face the unexpected burden of posttreatment chronic pain syndromes, such as radiation and chemotherapy-induced neuropathies.[1] The World Health Organization (WHO) describes a cancer pain ladder aimed at guiding nonopioid and opioid pharmacological treatments in a stepwise fashion.[6] When conservative therapy fails to provide adequate relief, interventional treatment options should be considered.

ETIOLOGY AND PATHOGENESIS

Pelvic malignancies can induce pain from intestinal obstruction, compression of neurovascular structures, and tumor infiltration to nearby viscera.[7] Extension to blood and lymphatic vessels leads to metastatic lesions, including involvement of the lungs, bone, and brain in patients with advanced-stage disease.

Female pelvic malignancies can involve the entire reproductive system including the vulva, vagina, uterus, fallopian tubes, and ovaries. These structures receive both sympathetic and parasympathetic innervation (Table 4.1). The superior hypogastric plexus, which is located in the retroperitoneum and situated bilaterally along the anterior surface of the L5 vertebral body, is part of the pelvic autonomic nervous system and receives its innervation from the T10–L2 nerve roots.[7] In women, the ovarian plexus branches from the superior hypogastric plexus and transmits nociceptive information from the uterus and cervix.[1] The caudal ends of the sympathetic chains then converge to form the ganglion impar, which provides sympathetic innervation to pelvic viscera as well as carry both sympathetic and nociceptive fibers from the perineum, distal rectum, perianal region, and distal urethra. Parasympathetic innervation of the pelvis originates from the S2–S4 roots via the pelvic splanchnic nerves. In women, this supplies the vagina, cervix, and lower portion of the uterus. Somatic innervation, including afferent sensory fibers, also arises from S2–S4 to innervate the vagina, perineum, and vulva.[7]

Malignancies specific to men affect structures such as the prostate, scrotum, testes, vas deferens, spermatic cord, tunica vaginalis, and penis. The pelvic organs in men are also innervated by sympathetic and parasympathetic fibers. The renal plexus contains sympathetic fibers that innervate the testes, vas deferens, and epididymis. The superior hypogastric plexus contains nerves that supply the prostate and bladder. The inferior hypogastric plexus, which is located presacrally and on the lateral aspects of the rectum ventral to the S2–S4 vertebrae, supplies the rectum as well as the prostate

Interventional Management of Chronic Visceral Pain Syndromes. https://doi.org/10.1016/B978-0-323-75775-1.00009-X

TABLE 4.1
Spinal Cord Level at Which the Autonomic Innervation Arises.

AUTONOMIC INNERVATION OF THE PELVIC ORGANS

Pelvic organ	Sympathetic innervation	Parasympathetic	Nerve plexus
Cervix	T10, T11, T12, L1	S2, S3, S4	Superior hypogastric plexus
Ovary	T10, T11, T12	S2, S3, S4	Superior and inferior hypogastric plexus
Uterus, fallopian tubes	T11, T12, L1	S2, S3, S4	Superior and inferior hypogastric plexus/Ovarian plexus
Testes	T10, T11, T12	S2, S3, S4	Renal/aortic plexus
Vas deferens, epididymis	T10, T11, T12, L1	S2, S3, S4	Renal/aortic plexus
Spermatic cord, tunica vaginalis	L1, L2	S2, S3, S4	Genitofemoral nerve
Prostate	L1, L2	S2, S3, S4	Superior and inferior hypogastric plexus
Bladder	T10, T11, T12, L1	S2, S3, S4	Superior and inferior hypogastric plexus
Rectum	T10, T11, T12, L1	S2, S3, S4	Inferior hypogastric plexus/ganglion impar

Sympathetic and Parasympathetic Innervation Originates at Different Spinal Cord Levels. These Fibers Travel Through Multiple Plexuses Listed in the Last Column.[1,42]

and bladder. The spermatic cord and tunica vaginalis are innervated by the genital branch of the genitofemoral nerve (L1−L2).[1]

Depression and pain are also highly related and overlapping in their symptoms and pathophysiology.[8] For instance, depression has been linked to higher levels of stress hormones and cytokines, which in turn increases inflammation and pain.[9] Chronic pain also causes changes in areas of the brain involved with mood regulation, such as the anterior cingulate cortex and prefrontal cortex, and can also worsen symptoms of depression, especially when it interferes with functional status, sleep, and sexual function.[10] Both pain and mood utilize serotonin, norepinephrine, and epinephrine, so treatments targeting these neurotransmitters have the potential to treat both.[11]

CLINICAL FEATURES

As previously discussed, pelvic malignancies can cause somatic, visceral, and neuropathic pain and present with a wide range of symptomatology. Therefore, a comprehensive history, including a detailed pain diary, is essential. Visceral pain tends to be diffused and poorly localized, while neuropathic pain may present with features of burning, numbness, allodynia, and hyperalgesia.[12]

The location of the pain varies from patient to patient and can include the low back, abdomen, pelvis, and lower extremities. Groin and penile pain can be referred from the kidneys, ureters, or testicles, as these are innervated by the T10−L1 nerve roots. Scrotal pain in men can be referred from the prostate, urethra, bladder, or seminal vesicle due to S2−S4 innervation. In women, uterine involvement often causes midline lower abdominal pain, while cervical involvement can cause lower back pain. Ovarian pain is less predictable and typically occurs late in the clinical course.[1]

In addition, being diagnosed with a malignancy and having to cope with chronic pain often cause mood disorders such as depression and anxiety. In a study of Veterans Affairs patients, symptoms of depression were found in approximately 25% of cancer patients. This commonly manifests as lack of energy and difficulty sleeping. Depressive symptoms are more common in cancer patients ranging from 41 to 88 years old. Lack of emotional support defined as having someone to talk to was also linked to depressive symptoms. Patients who report that pain interferes with their daily life are also more likely to have depression, emphasizing the importance of early pain management.[13] This is particularly important for patients who suffer chronic pelvic pain, given the impact that their pain syndrome may have on their sexual health and sexual identity.[14]

DIAGNOSIS

Pelvic pain can be caused by a variety of cancer and disease processes. The diagnostic process starts with a comprehensive history and physical exam. A thorough pain evaluation is critical. A detailed pain description should include the onset of pain, location, quality, intensity, duration, temporal characteristics, alleviating, and aggravating factors. A pain diary can assist with patient recall and recognizing pain patterns. Self-reported pain assessment tools are utilized on the initial encounter and reassessed on subsequent visits. The three most commonly used measures include numerical rating scale, visual analog scale, and adjective rating scale. It is also important to be aware that patients can have discrepancies in their behavior compared to the self-reported pain score due to coping mechanisms.[1] There are active and passive coping mechanisms. Active coping mechanisms include problem solving, collecting information and refocusing on the problem, and regulation of emotion. Passive coping mechanisms are avoidance and escape. Active coping has been shown to decrease the intensity of pain and overall improve the quality of life while passive coping can increase the perception of pain and decrease the quality of life.[15] Any psychological factors should be considered in an assessment when obtaining a self-reported pain score.[1]

Laboratory tests and diagnostic imaging are also typically obtained. Common laboratory tests include complete blood count, comprehensive metabolic panel, coagulopathy panel, magnesium, and phosphate. Ultrasound is often used as the initial imaging modality to identify gynecologic malignancies such as ovarian, uterine, and vaginal cancer. Computed tomography (CT) and magnetic resonance imaging (MRI) are commonly ordered to confirm the diagnosis and further assess location, mass characteristics, and stage. Other studies may be utilized to further assess for metastatic disease, including positron emission tomography scan and endoscopic procedures such as esophagogastroduodenoscopy, colonoscopy, and cystoscopy. Tumor markers assist with diagnosis and surveillance including prostate-specific antigen, cancer antigen 125 (CA-125), calcitonin, alpha fetoprotein, human chorionic gonadotropin, and carcinoembryonic antigen. A definitive diagnosis can be made with fine needle biopsy, core needle biopsy, excisional or incisional biopsy, and endoscopic biopsy.

PHYSICAL EXAM FINDINGS

Physical exam findings are often limited, and the patient's history and symptoms should guide the exam. A general exam provides useful information about a patient's level of distress, mood, nutritional status, and the ability to ambulate.[12] An abdominal exam may be significant for localized or diffuse tenderness. If rigidity and guarding are present, then this may be a sign of inflammation of the peritoneum. These signs can be caused by mass effect or intestinal obstruction secondary to a tumor. For patients with abdominal, pelvic, or urinary complaints, a rectal exam should be performed.[1] Rectal exam may be notable for an abnormal prostate, palpable masses, and fecal impaction that could be caused by infiltration of the malignancy into the rectum or mass effect causing compression of the rectum.[7] In women, an initial pelvic exam should include bimanual palpation of the uterus, vagina, cervix, and ovaries to evaluate for masses. Primary care or gynecologists typically provide detailed pelvic and rectal exam findings before the patient presenting to the interventional pain clinic.[1]

A comprehensive neurological exam should include deep tendon reflexes, sensory, and motor tests to further evaluate for peripheral and central nervous system involvement.[7] Red flag symptoms, including bowel/bladder dysfunction and persistent neurological deficits, should be urgently evaluated and treated. Dermatomal mapping of pain and numbness can also be useful when determining treatment plans.

Severe pain interfering with a patient's ability to bear weight may be indicative of a pathologic fracture. Fractures of the pelvis can be found on exam with point tenderness as well as pain with pelvic compression, thigh thrust, hip rotation, and single-leg hop. Pubic symphysis pain can occur in the anteromedial groin and presents as tenderness to palpation of the pubic symphysis or tubercle as well as pain during hip flexion with leg extension.[16] Sacroiliac joint involvement is assessed with provocative tests including distraction, thigh thrust, compression, FABER, and Gaenslen's test; the distraction test has the high positive predictive value of all the provocative tests.[12]

TREATMENT

Malignant disease is usually accompanied by refractory and recurrent pain. Behavioral and pharmacological treatments are often first-line therapy; however, interventional options should be considered early to avoid side effects associated with systemic therapies and to provide targeted pain relief. This includes sympathetic blocks/neurolysis, neuromodulation, and intrathecal drug delivery systems.

PHARMACOLOGIC AGENTS

The WHO provides a stepwise approach for alleviating cancer pain through nonopioid and opioid medications.[6] Step 1 uses nonopioids combined with adjuvant analgesics. If unable to provide adequate relief, Step 2 recommends starting a low potency opioid in addition to nonopioids and adjuvant analgesics. And Step 3 calls for higher potency opioids for severe cancer pain that is persistent and increasing.

Nonopioids medications are effective and have a relatively safe side-effect profile. The most common agents include acetaminophen, nonsteroidal anti-inflammatory drugs (NSAIDs), corticosteroids, antidepressants, and gabapentanoids.

NSAIDs are available in many formulations. Common NSAIDs used to treat pain include ibuprofen, meloxicam, naproxen, ketorolac, and celecoxib. The mechanism of action relies on the inhibition of cyclooxygenase 1 and 2, which decreases the amount of circulating inflammatory mediators that can activate the peripheral nociceptors.[17] The adverse effects of NSAIDs include toxicities involving the gastrointestinal, cardiovascular, hepatic, and renal systems.

Acetaminophen has been used for over 100 years. The mechanism is unclear, but its use is believed to inhibit the production of lipooxygenase and cylcooxygenase leading to a decreased amount of inflammatory mediators.[18] It is effective for treating mild pain with a maximum dose of 4 g for ages less than 60 with no liver disease. Higher daily doses can result in hepatoxicity and are more concerning in patients with a history of liver disease, alcohol use, and hepatitis.[17]

Corticosteroids provide analgesia primarily through the reduction of proinflammatory cytokines and eicosanoids. It also reduces tissue swelling, decreasing painful mass effects from tumor invasion. Oral dexamethasone is the preferred corticosteroid due to its high potency, long duration of action, and minimal mineralocorticoid effects. The recommended starting dose is 8 mg daily, but patients should be assessed regularly so that the lowest effective dose is prescribed.[19] Prolong use with high doses can lead to unwanted side effects including glucose intolerance, fluid retention, sleep disturbances, delirium, osteopenia, gastric ulcers, and worsening of psychiatric conditions.[17] These side effects can further worsen a patient's quality of life when combined with their already existing chronic pain.

Gabapentanoids, tricyclic antidepressants, and serotonin and norepinephrine reuptake inhibitors are commonly used to treat neuropathic pain. Few trials, however, have investigated the effectiveness of these medications specifically for the treatment of neuropathic malignancy syndromes. A comparative study between gabapentin, pregabalin, and amitriptyline showed that they are individually effective for the treatment of malignant neuropathic pain. Pregabalin was shown to be more effective at decreasing burning and dysesthesias. Over 4 weeks, dosing was increased to 1800 mg/day for gabapentin, 600 mg/day for pregabalin, and 100 mg/day for amitriptyline. Side effects should be monitored during up-titration including somnolence, dizziness, altered mental status, and edema.[20]

Opioids are still considered the mainstay treatment for moderate-to-severe cancer pain. Pure μ-agonists are preferred and most commonly used (morphine, fentanyl, hydromorphone, methadone, oxycodone, hydrocodone). It is important to recognize that individuals have varying responses to different μ-agonists, which has led practitioners to adopt opioid rotation to identify the most effective agent that minimizes side effects.[21] Therefore, while the WHO analgesic ladder generally recommends the use of weak opioids such as tramadol and codeine for moderate pain, more potent opioids such as oxycodone or morphine at lower doses should be considered as an alternative. When starting any opioids, patients should be monitored frequently to assess for side effects and efficacy of treatment. A reasonable starting dose for patients with moderate to severe pain is 30 mg of oral morphine milligram equivalents per day. Adverse effects of opioids are well known, including nausea, sedation, constipation, respiratory depression, and neurotoxicity.[22] If patients experience intolerable side effects or inadequate relief, opioid rotation should be considered. In these cases, the equianalgesic dose of the new opioid should be reduced by 20%−30% to account for incomplete cross-tolerance. Attention to a patient's neuropsychological function and tolerance to side effects is essential to provide individualized therapy.[21]

SYMPATHETIC BLOCKS

Superior hypogastric block, neurolysis: As previously mentioned, the superior hypogastric plexus is situated bilaterally at the level of the fifth lumbar vertebral body by the bifurcation of the common iliac vessels and receives innervation from the lumbar sympathetic chains and parasympathetic nerve fibers originating from the S2−4 nerve roots.[23] Descending projections of the superior hypogastric plexus reach the inferior hypogastric plexus, which is located anteriorly to the sacrum and the S2−S4 foramina. The superior hypogastric plexus, inferior hypogastric plexus, and the pelvic plexus then collectively provide innervation to the pelvic viscera, including the uterus, ovary, testes, ureter, prostate, bladder, rectum, and perineum. Therefore, the superior hypogastric plexus is a popular target for treating chronic pelvic pain syndromes.[24]

The superior hypogastric plexus is typically performed in the prone position. Under CT or fluoroscopic guidance, two needles are inserted with a paramedian approach and advanced anterolaterally until the tips sit at the anterior margin of the L5–S1 interspace. After aspiration of the needle to confirm negative intravascular injection, the injectate is given. Although providers may choose to initially perform a diagnostic block with local anesthetic, proceeding directly to a neurolytic block may be a viable alternative for patients with advanced disease. Neurolytic injections are typically done with 50%–100% ethanol or 4%–10% phenol, which causes necrotic damage to neural structures. Unlike phenol, ethanol has no local anesthetic effect and thus, it is recommended to inject local anesthetic 5 minutes before administering ethanol. A cohort study of 227 patients suffering from chronic pelvic pain associated with cancer demonstrated that superior hypogastric plexus neurolysis provided effective pain relief and a significant reduction in opioid usage in the majority of their patients.[25]

Ganglion impar block, neurolysis: The ganglion impar, or ganglion of Walther, is a retroperitoneal structure that is anterior to the coccyx. It contains nociceptive and sympathetic fibers of the perineum, rectum, anus, distal urethra, the lower third of the vagina, vulva, and scrotum. Ganglion impar neurolysis was first described in 1990 for the treatment of pain.

There are four main techniques used to access to this structure, including the anococcygeal, coccygeus-transverse, intercoccygeal, and transcoccygeal approaches.[26]

The transcoccygeal approach under fluoroscopy is the most popular because it allows the shortest needle trajectory while avoiding surrounding structures. Patients are placed in the prone position, and the needle is advanced through the sacrococcygeal ligament until the needle tip is anterior to the coccyx and posterior to the rectum. Contrast is used to verify correct needle placement. Diagnostic block with local anesthetic, neurolysis, cryoablation, and radiofrequency ablation of the plexus may then be performed. In a cohort of patients with perineal and pelvic cancer pain, 79% were found to have a reduction in morphine consumption 3 months following the ganglion impar block.[27]

NEUROMODULATION

The first two reported spinal cord stimulators (SCS) were placed by Norman Shealy in 1967 for a patient

with bronchogenic carcinoma and another for pelvic pain related to cancer. Interestingly, as the field of neuromodulation has advanced over the years, SCS devices have been used increasingly for the treatment of nonmalignant neuropathic pain and less for malignancy pain syndromes.[28]

The mechanism of SCS is not fully understood, though Melzack and Wall's "Gate Control" theory, has been used to describe pain perception and explain the therapeutic mechanism for SCS devices.[29] A delta and C fibers, which carry nociceptive signals, synapse within the dorsal horn of the spinal cord. Stimulation of A beta fibers, which carry nonpainful touch signals, at the same pain-generating regions then effectively "close the gate" for pain perception by inhibiting ascending nociceptive signals. This also reduces sympathetic activity and potentiate GABA receptors leading to an overall reduction in pain.[30]

SCS therapies can be considered for malignant pelvic pain syndromes if patients have failed conservative treatment and have a neuropathic component to their pain. Although no studies have specifically investigated the efficacy of SCS for pelvic malignancies, a recent Cochrane systemic review found in four case series totaling 92 patient with cancer pain syndromes, 80% endorsed a significant reduction in their pain, and another 50% had a reduction in opioid use.[31]

Perioperative paresthesia mapping is typically required to determine correct lead placement for traditional dorsal column stimulation during the trial phase. The pelvis is innervated by sensory neurons from the S1–S4 nerve roots, parasympathetic neurons from S1–S4, and sympathetic nerve fibers from T10–L1 levels.[32] Therefore, the treatment of chronic pelvic pain is aimed at these critical sites.

Dorsal root ganglion (DRG) stimulation can also be considered for these patients, which allows for focused stimulation of specific nerve roots. The number and the respective levels at which the leads are placed are dependent on the dermatomal distribution of the patient's pain. Furthermore, this particular technology has the added benefit of utilizing less overall energy and also less risk of unwanted paresthesia with positional changes compared to dorsal column stimulators. We would recommend DRG stimulation at the upper lumbar (L1, L2) and sacral (S2) nerve roots for patients suffering from refractory pelvic pain (Fig. 4.1).

Although dorsal column and DRG stimulation have been used for malignant cancer pain, a significant limiting factor in these patients is the need for long-term surveillance with MRI scans. Neuromodulation systems have limitations with regards to MRI use,

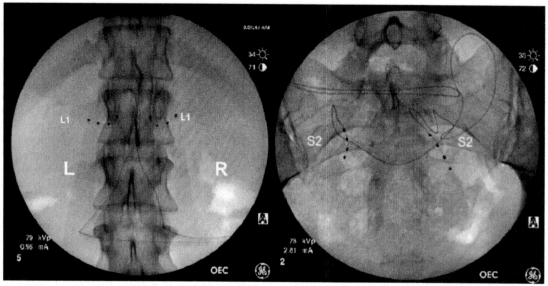

FIG. 4.1 Left: bilateral L1 DRG lead placement; right: bilateral S2 DRG lead placement.[43]

though with emerging technologies, most devices are at least MRI conditional. Specific compatibility restrictions should be reviewed with the manufacturer and patient before proceeding with any implant procedure.

INTRATHECAL DRUG DELIVERY SYSTEM

Intrathecal morphine was first reported for the treatment of cancer-related pain in 1978.[33] Intrathecal drug delivery system (IDDS) deliver medications directly into the intrathecal space through an indwelling catheter that is connected to a reservoir system implanted in a subcutaneous pocket typically in the abdomen (Fig. 4.2). The pump is then programmed to deliver a set dosage of medication at a continuous rate with the option of also providing scheduled and patient-controlled boluses. The catheter tip is placed according to the corresponding dermatomal distribution of the patient's pain; T9–T12 is typically targeted to obtain analgesia for pelvic pain. In a randomized controlled trial comparing IDDS with medical management in patients with refractory cancer pain, Smith et al. demonstrated a superior reduction in visual analog scale pain scores, reduced drug toxicity, and improved survival with IDDS.[34]

IDDS should be considered in patients with chronic pain that is refractory to traditional systemic opioids or those who are unable to tolerate its side effects (Fig. 4.3). Life expectancy greater than 3 months, ability to follow-up, intact immune system if on chemotherapeutic agents, and psychosocial status should also be considered.

Before proceeding with the implant, a trial of intrathecal opioids either by single-shot spinal injection or infusion via intrathecal catheter is often done to assess the potential benefit of the therapy and any side effects. Epidural catheter trials may also be pursued. It is important to note, however, that recent recommendations

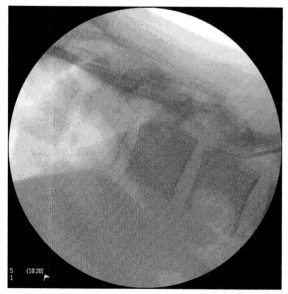

FIG. 4.2 **Catheter placement for intrathecal pump.** Advancement of intrathecal catheter shown on lateral fluoroscopic imaging.

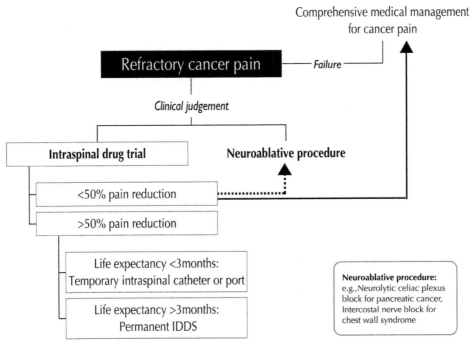

FIG. 4.3 Decision-making algorithm for IDDS.[44]

from the Polyanalgesic Consensus Conference, indicate that a trial may not be required for cancer patients with advanced disease and limited survival time.[35]

FDA approved intrathecal medications include ziconotide, morphine, and baclofen. Additive and off-label medications include fentanyl, bupivacaine, clonidine, and hydromorphone among others. Drug combinations, typically a combination of an opioid with either bupivacaine or clonidine, are also utilized for mixed nociceptive and neuropathic pain disorders. Titration of intrathecal medication depends on the disease process. Patients with advanced disease may require aggressive titration of their intrathecal medication. Patient Therapy Manager can also be considered in this patient population for breakthrough pain. Adverse effects of IDDS include granuloma formation, hypogonadism, immunosuppression, development of tolerance to medication, and respiratory depression.[33]

If a patient's prognosis is less than 3 months, then the permanent implant of IDDS may not be an option. Instead, a tunneled intraspinal catheter can be placed. The catheter, which can be placed in the epidural or intrathecal space, is tunneled subcutaneously and attached to an external pump. This offers a less invasive and more cost-effective approach compared to an internalized IDDS with a subcutaneous pump.

OTHER THERAPIES

There are several other minimally invasive procedures that can be effectively utilized in pelvic cancer pain particularly in patients where other interventions are insufficient or the patient is not a good surgical candidate.[36] Barriers include cost and availability. Radiofrequency ablation uses a high-frequency current to heat and necrose sites of bone or neurologic involvement. Percutaneous laser ablation works similarly using photons rather than current and has been used successfully for prostate cancer and spinal metastases. Cryoablation induces necrosis with freezing and has been used for prostate cancer and boney lesions of the pelvis. When used for boney metastases, pain scores significantly decreased at 1-, 4-, 8-, and 24-week follow-up with a 2% risk of developing osteonecrosis.[37] Irreversible electroporation uses a current to disrupt cell membranes and trigger apoptosis without the use of extreme temperatures and can be combined with chemotherapy (electrochemotherapy) though research is still needed on its efficacy for pain in pelvic cancers in humans. Microwave ablation was used in a few cases of recurrent prostate cancer and did reduce pain medication requirements in two patients but was complicated by skin necrosis and nerve injury.[38]

Research examining other treatments such as physical therapy specific to pelvic cancer pain is still limited. Among colon cancer survivors, a lumbopelvic stabilization exercise program did show improvement in pressure pain threshold when measured with an electronic algometer, but there was not a significant improvement in a subjective pain questionnaire.[39]

Patients with cancer should be referred to psychosocial support and peer groups early in the process because of the overlap between mood and pain as discussed previously, and because conventional treatments are often inadequate.[40] Cognitive behavior therapy (CBT) is a technique used to train a patient to alter their patterns of thinking and behavior and is effective in treating depression. Although further research is needed, a meta-analysis in breast cancer patients showed an improvement in pain and distress in patients receiving CBT. Similarly, CBT can be applied to patients with malignant pelvic pain. EMG biofeedback has also been discussed as a promising treatment option. In one study among cancer patients in a palliative care unit, patients were given visual or audio EMG displays and used deep breathing techniques to decrease EMG potentials. This resulted in a significant decrease in pain scores.[41]

REFERENCES

1. Rigor BM. Pelvic cancer pain. *J Surg Oncol.* 2000;75(4): 280–300. https://doi.org/10.1002/1096-9098(200012) 75:4<280::AID-JSO13>3.0.CO;2-Q.
2. Rawla P, Sunkara T, Barsouk A. Epidemiology of colorectal cancer: incidence, mortality, survival, and risk factors. *Przegląd Gastroenterol.* 2019;14(2):89–103. https://doi.org/10.5114/pg.2018.81072.
3. Ovarian Cancer Statistics | How Common is Ovarian Cancer. Available from: https://www.cancer.org/cancer/ovarian-cancer/about/key-statistics.html. Accessed 30 May, 2020.
4. Cervical Cancer Statistics | Key Facts About Cervical Cancer. Available from: https://www.cancer.org/cancer/cervical-cancer/about/key-statistics.html. Accessed 30 May, 2020.
5. Rawla P. Epidemiology of prostate cancer. *World J Oncol.* 2019;10(2):63–89. https://doi.org/10.14740/wjon1191.
6. Anekar AA, Cascella M. WHO analgesic ladder. In: *StatPearls.* StatPearls Publishing; 2020. Available from: http://www.ncbi.nlm.nih.gov/books/NBK554435/. Accessed May 30, 2020.
7. Das S, Jeba J, George R. Cancer and treatment related pains in patients with cervical carcinoma. *Indian J Palliat Care.* 2005;11(2):74. https://doi.org/10.4103/0973-1075.19183.
8. IsHak WW, Wen RY, Naghdechi L, et al. Pain and depression: a systematic review. *Harv Rev Psychiatr.* 2018;26(6):352–363. https://doi.org/10.1097/HRP.0000000000000198.
9. Yang SE, Park YG, Han K, Min JA, Kim SY. Association between dental pain and depression in Korean adults using the Korean National Health and Nutrition Examination survey. *J Oral Rehabil.* 2016;43(1):51–58. https://doi.org/10.1111/joor.12343.
10. Fritzsche K, Sandholzer H, Brucks U, et al. Psychosocial care by general practitioners—where are the problems? Results of a demonstration project on quality management in psychosocial primary care. *Int J Psychiatr Med.* 1999; 29(4):395–409. https://doi.org/10.2190/MCGF-CLD4-0FRE-N2UK.
11. Cocksedge KA, Simon C, Shankar R. A difficult combination: chronic physical illness, depression, and pain. *Br J Gen Pract J R Coll Gen Pract.* 2014;64(626):440–441. https://doi.org/10.3399/bjgp14X681241.
12. Urits I, Burshtein A, Sharma M, et al. Low back pain, a comprehensive review: pathophysiology, diagnosis, and treatment. *Curr Pain Headache Rep.* 2019;23(3):23. https://doi.org/10.1007/s11916-019-0757-1.
13. Bamonti PM, Moye J, Naik AD. Pain is associated with continuing depression in cancer survivors. *Psychol Health Med.* 2018;23(10):1182–1195. https://doi.org/10.1080/13548506.2018.1476723.
14. Origoni M, Leone Roberti Maggiore U, Salvatore S, Candiani M. Neurobiological mechanisms of pelvic pain. BioMed Res Int. https://doi.org/10.1155/2014/903848.
15. Büssing A, Ostermann T, Neugebauer EAM, Heusser P. Adaptive coping strategies in patients with chronic pain conditions and their interpretation of disease. *BMC Publ Health.* 2010;10:507. https://doi.org/10.1186/1471-2458-10-507.
16. Temme KE, Pan J. Musculoskeletal approach to pelvic pain. *Phys Med Rehabil Clin N Am.* 2017;28(3):517–537. https://doi.org/10.1016/j.pmr.2017.03.014.
17. Tauben D. Nonopioid medications for pain. *Phys Med Rehabil Clin N Am.* 2015;26(2):219–248. https://doi.org/10.1016/j.pmr.2015.01.005.
18. Vardy J, Agar M. Nonopioid drugs in the treatment of cancer pain. *J Clin Oncol.* 2014;32(16):1677–1690. https://doi.org/10.1200/JCO.2013.52.8356.
19. Leppert W, Buss T. The role of corticosteroids in the treatment of pain in cancer patients. *Curr Pain Headache Rep.* 2012;16(4):307–313. https://doi.org/10.1007/s11916-012-0273-z.
20. Mishra S, Bhatnagar S, Goyal GN, Rana SPS, Upadhya SP. A comparative efficacy of amitriptyline, gabapentin, and pregabalin in neuropathic cancer pain: a prospective randomized double-blind placebo-controlled study. *Am J Hosp Palliat Care.* 2012;29(3):177–182. https://doi.org/10.1177/1049909111412539.
21. Fine PG, Portenoy RK. Establishing "best practices" for opioid rotation: conclusions of an expert panel. *J Pain Symptom Manage.* 2009;38(3):418–425. https://doi.org/10.1016/j.jpainsymman.2009.06.002.
22. Bruera E, Paice JA. Cancer pain management: safe and effective use of opioids. *Am Soc Clin Oncol Educ Book.* 2015:e593–599. https://doi.org/10.14694/EdBook_AM.2015.35.e593.
23. Davila GW, Ghoniem GM, Nasseri Y, eds. *Pelvic Floor Dysfunction: A Multidisciplinary Approach.* Springer-Verlag; 2006. https://doi.org/10.1007/b136174.

24. Lee C-J, Lee S-C. Chapter 10—Sympathetic nerve block and neurolysis. In: Kim DH, Kim Y-C, Kim K-H, eds. *Minimally Invasive Percutaneous Spinal Techniques*. W.B. Saunders; 2010:170−183. https://doi.org/10.1016/B978-0-7020-2913-4.00010-0.

25. Plancarte R, de Leon-Casasola OA, El-Helaly M, Allende S, Lema MJ. Neurolytic superior hypogastric plexus block for chronic pelvic pain associated with cancer. *Reg Anesth*. 1997;22(6):562−568.

26. Ferreira F, Pedro A. Ganglion impar neurolysis in the management of pelvic and perineal cancer-related pain. *Case Rep Oncol*. 2020;13(1):29−34. https://doi.org/10.1159/000505181.

27. Sousa Correia J, Silva M, Castro C, Miranda L, Agrelo A. The efficacy of the ganglion impar block in perineal and pelvic cancer pain. *Support Care Cancer*. 2019;27(11): 4327−4330. https://doi.org/10.1007/s00520-019-04738-9.

28. Flagg A, McGreevy K, Williams K. Spinal cord stimulation in the treatment of cancer-related pain: "back to the origins.". *Curr Pain Headache Rep*. 2012;16(4):343−349. https://doi.org/10.1007/s11916-012-0276-9.

29. Melzack R, Wall PD. Pain mechanisms: a new theory. *Science*. 1965;150(3699):971−979. https://doi.org/10.1126/science.150.3699.971.

30. Bentley WE. Spinal cord stimulation for chronic pelvic pain. In: Sabia M, Sehdev J, Bentley W, eds. *Urogenital Pain: A Clinicians Guide to Diagnosis and Interventional Treatments*. Springer International Publishing; 2017:177−185. https://doi.org/10.1007/978-3-319-45794-9_11.

31. Lihua P, Su M, Zejun Z, Ke W, Bennett MI. Spinal cord stimulation for cancer-related pain in adults. *Cochrane Database Syst Rev*. 2013;(2):CD009389. https://doi.org/10.1002/14651858.CD009389.pub2.

32. Yang CC. Neuromodulation in male chronic pelvic pain syndrome: rationale and practice. *World J Urol*. 2013;31(4): 767−772. https://doi.org/10.1007/s00345-013-1066-7.

33. Xing F, Yong RJ, Kaye AD, Urman RD. Intrathecal drug delivery and spinal cord stimulation for the treatment of cancer pain. *Curr Pain Headache Rep*. 2018;22(2):11. https://doi.org/10.1007/s11916-018-0662-z.

34. Smith TJ, Staats PS, Deer T, et al. Randomized clinical trial of an implantable drug delivery system compared with comprehensive medical management for refractory cancer pain: impact on pain, drug-related toxicity, and survival. *J Clin Oncol*. 2002;20(19):4040−4049. https://doi.org/10.1200/JCO.2002.02.118.

35. Deer TR, Provenzano DA, Hanes M, et al. The Neurostimulation Appropriateness Consensus Committee (NACC) recommendations for infection prevention and management. *Neuromodulation*. 2017;20(1):31−50. https://doi.org/10.1111/ner.12565.

36. Cascella M, Muzio MR, Viscardi D, Cuomo A. Features and role of minimally invasive palliative procedures for pain management in malignant pelvic diseases: a review. *Am J Hospice Palliat Med*. 2017;34(6):524−531. https://doi.org/10.1177/1049909116636374.

37. Callstrom MR, Dupuy DE, Solomon SB, et al. Percutaneous image-guided cryoablation of painful metastases involving bone: multicenter trial. *Cancer*. 2013;119(5): 1033−1041. https://doi.org/10.1002/cncr.27793.

38. Shimizu T, Endo Y, Mekata E, et al. Real-time magnetic resonance-guided microwave coagulation therapy for pelvic recurrence of rectal cancer: initial clinical experience using a 0.5 T open magnetic resonance system. *Dis Colon Rectum*. 2010;53(11):1555−1562. https://doi.org/10.1007/DCR.0b013e3181e8f4b6.

39. Changes in Pain and Muscle Architecture in Colon Cancer Survivors After a Lumbopelvic Exercise Program: A Secondary Analysis of a Randomized Controlled Trial | Pain Medicine | Oxford Academic. Available from: https://academic.oup.com/painmedicine/article/18/7/1366/3062399. Accessed 30 May, 2020.

40. Tatrow K, Montgomery GH. Cognitive behavioral therapy techniques for distress and pain in breast cancer patients: a meta-analysis. *J Behav Med*. 2006;29(1):17−27. https://doi.org/10.1007/s10865-005-9036-1.

41. Tsai P-S, Chen P-L, Lai Y-L, Lee M-B, Lin C-C. Effects of electromyography biofeedback-assisted relaxation on pain in patients with advanced cancer in a palliative care unit. *Cancer Nurs*. 2007;30(5):347−353. https://doi.org/10.1097/01.NCC.0000290805.38335.7b.

42. Singh V. *Male Genital Organs*. In: *Textbook of Anatomy Abdomen and Lower Limb*. Vol. II. Elsevier Health Sciences; 2014.

43. Hunter CW, Yang A. Dorsal root ganglion stimulation for chronic pelvic pain: a case series and technical report on a novel lead configuration. *Neuromodulation*. 2019;22(1): 87−95. https://doi.org/10.1111/ner.12801.

44. Lin C-P, Lin W-Y, Lin F-S, Lee Y-S, Jeng C-S, Sun W-Z. Efficacy of intrathecal drug delivery system for refractory cancer pain patients: a single tertiary medical center experience. *J Formos Med Assoc*. 2012;111(5):253−257. https://doi.org/10.1016/j.jfma.2011.03.005.

CHAPTER 5

Chronic Prostatitis

NEWAJ ABDULLAH, MD • KRISHNA B. SHAH, MD

INTRODUCTION

Prostatitis presents as a pattern of symptoms characterized by pelvic pain, dysuria, urgency, frequency, sensation of incomplete voiding, and, in some cases, fever.[1] Prostatitis is the most common urologic condition affecting men under 50 years old and is the third most common urologic condition affecting men older than 50 years old.[2] Worldwide the prevalence of prostatitis ranges from 2.2% to 16%.[1,3] In North America, the mean prevalence of prostatitis is 6.9%.[3] With myriads of symptomology, prostatitis is often difficult to diagnose and can result in a large number of physician visits. The Urologic Disease in America study estimated the annual physician visit rate to be 1798 per 100,000 population for prostatitis.[4] In the year 2000, the United States spent 84 million dollars solely on diagnosis and management of this condition.[4] Therefore, this condition can pose a tremendous personal and economic burden to individuals and society.

ETIOLOGY AND PATHOGENESIS

Prostatitis is traditionally thought to be caused by bacterial infections; however, recent developments suggest the etiology of this condition to be complex and multifactorial.[1] Acute and chronic bacterial prostatitis makes up a small subset of the population affected by this condition.[1] The most common bacterial agents implicated are from the *Enterobacteriaceae* family, which originate in the gastrointestinal flora.[5] Other infectious agents include *Enterococci* family, *Corynebacterium* species, *Chlamydia* trachomatis, *Ureaplasma* urealyticum, and *Candia* species.[1,5−9] There are certain host factors that increase the risks of developing prostatitis by allowing infectious agents to transcend into the prostatic tissue, including dysfunctional voiding syndrome and intraprostatic ductal reflux.[1,10]

Interestingly, approximately 95% of prostatitis cases are noninfectious. Inflammatory nonbacterial prostatitis is thought to be immunologically mediated and caused by unknown antigens or even an autoimmune process.[1] This is supported by numerous studies demonstrating elevated levels of IgA and IgM antibodies (not microorganism specific), cytokines, and complement factors in the prostatic tissue.[1]

In a large number of patients presenting with prostatitis, no infectious source or inflammation can be found. Emerging evidence suggests that these patients have a dissociation between their central nervous system and pelvic floor where they are unable to voluntarily the striated muscles of the pelvis in a coordinated fashion.[11] This may lead to some of the urinary symptoms associated with prostatitis. Studies have also shown that many patients with prostatitis have myofascial trigger points and autonomic nervous system changes in the pelvis that explain the associated pelvic pain.[12,13] The pathogenesis of noninfectious noninflammatory prostatitis is continuously evolving; however, current evidence suggests that pelvic floor dysfunction and neural sensitization are some of the major driving factors in this condition.[11,13]

CLINICAL FEATURES

The National Institute of Health (NIH) classifies prostatitis in four different categories as shown in Table 5.1.[1,14] Category I is acute bacterial prostatitis.[1,14,15] Category II is chronic bacterial prostatitis where patients have chronic lower urinary tract infection from a prostatic nidus.[1,14,15] Category III is nonbacterial prostatitis. Category III is further subdivided into category IIIA and IIIB.[1,14,15] Category IIIA is nonbacterial inflammatory prostatitis as evidenced by the presence of leukocytes in postprostatic massage urine or semen samples. Category IIIB is nonbacterial noninflammatory prostatitis due to a lack of leukocytes in the postprostatic massage. Finally, category IV is asymptomatic inflammatory prostatitis. Patients are

Interventional Management of Chronic Visceral Pain Syndromes. https://doi.org/10.1016/B978-0-323-75775-1.00021-0

TABLE 5.1
Classification and Clinical Features of Prostatitis.

National Institute of Health Classification	Traditional Classification	Description	Clinical Features
Category I	Acute bacterial prostatitis	Acute infection of the prostate gland	Fever, chills, malaise, nausea/vomiting, dysuria, urgency, frequency, hesitancy and sensation of incomplete emptying, pain in suprapubic region/perineum
Category II	Chronic bacterial prostatitis	Chronic infection of the prostate gland	Pelvic pain, dysuria, urgency, frequency, hesitancy, and sensation of incomplete emptying
Category IIIA	Nonbacterial inflammatory prostatitis	Large number of leukocytes in prostatic secretions, postprostatic massage urine or semen	Pain in the perineum, suprapubic region, and penis
Category IIIB	Nonbacterial noninflammatory prostatitis	Minimal number of leukocytes in prostatic secretions, postprostatic massage urine or semen	Pain in the perineum, suprapubic region, and penis
Category IV	Asymptomatic	Presence of leukocytes and/or bacterial in prostatic secretions, postprostatic massage urine or semen	Asymptomatic

classified as having category IV prostatitis by the presence of significant leukocytes (or bacteria or both) in prostate-specific specimens (semen, tissue biopsy) in the absence of typical chronic pelvic pain.[1,14,15]

Patients with category I prostatitis will present with dysuria, urgency, frequency, hesitancy, and sensation of incomplete emptying.[1,15] Patients will also report pain in the suprapubic region and perineum.[1,15] Occasionally, patients may have discomfort in their external genitalia. Category I prostatitis manifests with significant systemic symptoms including fever, chills, malaise, nausea, or vomiting.[1] In several cases, the patient may present with florid septicemia.[1] With timely diagnosis and appropriate treatment, most acute bacterial prostatitis resolve; however, 5% of acute bacterial prostatitis may progress to chronic bacterial prostatitis.[16]

The hallmarks of category II prostatitis are recurrent urinary tract infections.[1,15] These patients may have multiple acute episodes spaced by asymptomatic periods.[1,15] Each of these episodes are characterized by irritative and obstructive urinary symptoms.[1,15] Almost all of these patients will have a long history of pelvic pain. Systemic symptoms such as fever, chills, malaise, nausea, and vomiting are uncommon.[1,15]

Category IIIA and IIIB prostatitis have similar clinical symptoms. The predominant feature of category III prostatitis is a pain in the perineum, suprapubic region, and penis.[17] The NIH Chronic Prostatitis Cohort Study is one of the largest population-based studies that characterize category III prostatitis. Based on this study, perineal pain is the most prevalent pain symptom (63%), following by testicular pain (58%), pain in the pubic region (42%), and pain in the penis (32%).[18] One of the most prominent and important symptoms of this condition is pain during or after ejaculation.[18] In addition to pain, patients may or may not have urinary urgency, frequency, hesitancy, or sensation of incomplete voiding.[1] Many patients with category III prostatitis have severely diminished quality of life; and therefore, may have concurrent psychiatric conditions such as depression or maladaptive coping skills.[19]

Category IV prostatitis is a condition that presents without symptoms.[1] These patients are incidentally discovered during the evaluation of benign prostatic hyperplasia, elevated prostate-specific antigen, prostate malignancy, or infertility. Evaluation for these conditions may reveal the presence of bacteria or leukocytes in the postprostate massage urine specimen or inflammatory infiltrate in the prostate biopsy specimen.[1]

DIAGNOSIS

Diagnosis of prostatitis requires a comprehensive history, physical exam, and appropriate laboratory testing. With regards to laboratory testing, the gold standard for evaluation of prostatitis is the Meares–Stamey Test (also known as 4-Glass Test).[1] This diagnostic test involves four glass test tubes. Test tube 1 contains the first 10 mL of urine and represents the urethral specimen. Test tube 2 contains midstream urine and represents urine from the bladder. Test tube 3 contains expressed prostatic specimens after a prostate massage. Test tube 4 contains the first 10 mL of urine after prostate massage and represents a prostatic specimen. All of these specimens undergo cytologic evaluation and culture. Table 5.2 shows the cytologic and culture results from these specimens depending on the etiology of prostatitis.

The Meares–Stamey test can be time consuming. Many clinicians use a 2-Glass Test where the urine sample is collected before and after a prostate massage.[20] These urine specimens are used for cytologic evaluation and culture. This technique is fast and cost effective. The 2-Glass Test has 91% sensitivity and specificity compared with the gold standard Meares–Stamey test.[20] Table 5.3 shows the interpretation of a 2-Glass Test.

Additional diagnostic tests may be needed to rule out other pathologies. In the setting of hematuria, clinicians may perform a cystoscopy to rule out urothelial carcinoma.[1] Many patients may have elevated prostate-specific antigen, and depending on the level

of this marker, the patient may need to undergo a transrectal ultrasound-guided prostate biopsy to rule out prostate cancer.[1] Pelvic pain is an important component of prostatitis. However, pelvic pain can originate from other pathologies in the pelvis. The cystometric evaluation may be needed in these cases to rule out hyperactive detrusor muscle or detrusor sphincter dyssynergia as the source of pelvic pain.[21]

PHYSICAL EXAM FINDINGS

The NIH Chronic Prostatitis Collaborative Research Network (NIH CPCRN) developed a validated symptom and quality of life assessment tool called NIH-Chronic Prostatitis Symptom Index (NIH–CPSI; Fig. 5.1).[1,22] All patients should complete this evaluation to establish a baseline and assess improvement after intervention.[1] All patients with a suspected

TABLE 5.3
Technique and Interpretation of the Pre- and Post-Massage Two-Glass Test for Symptomatic Prostatitis.

Classification	Specimen	Pre-M	Post-M
CAT I	WBC	+	+
	Culture	+	+
CAT II	WBC	+/−	+
	Culture	+/−	+
CAT IIIA	WBC	−	+
	Culture	−	−
CAT IIIB	WBC	−	−
	Culture	−	−

CAT, category; Pre-M, preprostate massage; Post-M, postprostate massage; WBC, white blood cell.

TABLE 5.2
Technique and Interpretation of the Meares–Stamey Four-Glass Test for Symptomatic Prostatitis.

Classification	Specimen	TT1	TT2	EPS	TT3
CAT I	WBC	+	+	+	+
	Culture	+	+	+	+
CAT II	WBC	−	+/−	+	+
	Culture	−	+/−	+	+
CAT IIIA	WBC	−	−	+	+
	Culture	−	−	−	−
CAT IIIB	WBC	−	−	−	−
	Culture	−	−	−	−

CAT, category; EPS, expressed prostatic secretion; TT, test tube; WBC, white blood cell.

Male Genitourinary Pain Index

1. In the last week, have you experienced any pain or discomfort in the following areas?

a. Area between rectum and testicles (perineum)   ☐$_1$ Yes   ☐$_0$ No
b. Testicles   ☐$_1$ Yes   ☐$_0$ No
c. Tip of penis (not related to urination)   ☐$_1$ Yes   ☐$_0$ No
d. Below your waist, in your pubic or bladder area   ☐$_1$ Yes   ☐$_0$ No

2. In the last week, have you experienced:

a. Pain or burning during urination?   ☐$_1$ Yes   ☐$_0$ No
b. Pain or discomfort during or after sexual climax (ejaculation)? ☐$_1$ Yes   ☐$_0$ No
c. Pain or discomfort as your bladder fills?   ☐$_1$ Yes   ☐$_0$ No
d. Pain or discomfort relieved by voiding?   ☐$_1$ Yes   ☐$_0$ No

3. How often have you had pain or discomfort in any of these areas over the last week?

☐$_0$ Never   ☐$_1$ Rarely   ☐$_2$ Sometimes   ☐$_3$ Often   ☐$_4$ Usually   ☐$_5$ Always

4. Which number best describes your AVERAGE pain or discomfort on the days you had it, over the last week?

☐ ☐ ☐ ☐ ☐ ☐ ☐ ☐ ☐ ☐ ☐
0   1   2   3   4   5   6   7   8   9   10

No   Pain as bad as you
Pain   can imagine

5. How often have you had a sensation of not emptying your bladder completely after you finished urinating, over the last week?

☐$_0$ Not at all   ☐$_1$ Less than 1   ☐$_2$ Less than half the   ☐$_3$ About half   ☐$_4$ More than   ☐$_5$ Almost
                    time in 5   time   the time   half the time   always

6. How often have you had to urinate again less than two hours after you finished urinating, over the last week?

☐$_0$ Not at all   ☐$_1$ Less than 1   ☐$_2$ Less than half the   ☐$_3$ About half   ☐$_4$ More than   ☐$_5$ Almost
                    time in 5   time   the time   half the time   always

7. How often have your symptoms kept you from doing the kinds of things you would usually do, over the last week?

☐$_0$ None   ☐$_1$ Only a little   ☐$_2$ Some   ☐$_3$ A lot

8. How much did you think about your symptoms, over the last week?

☐$_0$ None   ☐$_1$ Only a little   ☐$_2$ Some   ☐$_3$ A lot

9. If you were to spend the rest of your life with your symptoms just the way they have been during the last week, how would you feel about that?

☐$_0$ Delighted
☐$_1$ Pleased
☐$_2$ Mostly satisfied
☐$_3$ Mixed (about equally satisfied and dissatisfied)
☐$_4$ Mostly dissatisfied
☐$_5$ Unhappy
☐$_6$ Terrible

FIG. 5.1 NIH chronic prostatitis symptom index.

diagnosis of prostatitis should undergo a thorough physical exam. In category I prostatitis, patients may appear flushed, febrile, tachycardic, tachypneic, and even hypotensive.[1] Patients will also have suprapubic pain or may show urinary retention on a bladder scan. The prostate exam will demonstrate a hot, boggy, and tender prostate.[1] In category II and III prostatitis, a physical exam may be unremarkable. Digital rectal exam and palpation of the perineum may demonstrate tender points in the external genitalia, perineum, coccyx, external anal sphincter, and internal pelvic floor/side wall.[1,12]

TREATMENT

Prostatitis is a complex disease process with multiple etiologies and diverse symptomology. Patients with prostatitis can present with features ranging from voiding dysfunction to chronic pelvic pain. Treatments for prostatitis vary based on symptoms and include antibiotics, α-adrenergic blockers, antiinflammatory agents, hormonal therapy, extracorporeal shockwave therapy, transurethral microwave therapy, neuroablative procedures, and neuromodulation. Most of these treatment modalities can be provided by primary care providers and urologists. Patients with prostatitis will interface with a pain specialist for the treatment of chronic pelvic pain. Therefore, we focus on various treatment modalities for the management of chronic pelvic pain in this chapter.

Lifestyle Modification and Conservative Therapies: Lifestyle modifications should be considered as the first approach for management of chronic pelvic pain.[23−26] All patients should be educated on his pelvic pain syndrome.[23] Many of these patients have underlying triggers (i.e., food, drink, activities) for their pelvic pain that should be avoided.[24] Patients are encouraged to engage in low impact activities such as walking, yoga, swimming, and stretching.[25] Some patients can benefit from local heat therapy to the pelvis using a hot water bottle, heating pad, or hot bath. None of these interventions have been proven in clinical trials for chronic pelvic pain; however, they have shown benefit in some patients in clinical practice.[25,26]

Pelvic Floor Physiotherapy and Biofeedback: Chronic pain from prostatitis can be associated with myofascial trigger points.[12] These myofascial trigger points are painful and add to the pain from the underlying chronic pelvic pain syndrome. Pelvic floor physiotherapy and biofeedback techniques are helpful in providing pain relief in this patient population. Anderson and colleagues studied the effect of myofascial trigger-point

release and paradoxical relaxation techniques in 138 males with chronic pelvic pain syndrome and noted that 77% reported marked improvement in symptoms.[27] Cornel and colleagues studied the effect of biofeedback in 33 males with chronic prostatitis and pelvic pain, and found the CPSI score to decrease from 23.6 to 11.4.[28]

Medications: Patients with chronic prostatitis and chronic pelvic pain have attributes of neuropathic pain.[1] Gabapentinoids are helpful in ameliorating this type of pain. In 2010, the NIH CPCRN conducted a randomized placebo-controlled trial to evaluate the effect of pregabalin in men with long-standing, treatment-refractory chronic pelvic pain syndrome.[29] Forty-seven percent of the treatment group reported a 6-point decrease in total NIH−CPSI score at 6 weeks compared to 35.8% in the placebo group. Although this improvement in NIH−CPSI pain score is not statistically significant, it demonstrates that many patients benefit from gabapentanoids in clinical practice. Tricyclic antidepressants are another class of drugs that can be considered for the treatment of chronic pelvic pain syndromes. These are widely used in the treatment of neuropathic pain and has shown to be beneficial for pelvic pain in prostatitis.[30]

Superior Hypogastric Plexus Block, Neurolysis: The superior hypogastric plexus (SHP) is part of the abdominal and pelvic autonomic nervous system.[31,32] Like the celiac plexus, it is located in the retroperitoneum and situated bilaterally along the anterior surface of the L5 vertebral body.[31,32] The superior hypogastric plexus is responsible for transmitting sympathetically mediated visceral pain from the descending colon, rectum, and internal genitalia.[31,33] Superior hypogastric plexus blocks have been performed for various types of pelvic pain such as endometriosis and pelvic malignancy pain syndromes.[31] In addition, case reports have demonstrated therapeutic benefits for patients with chronic prostatitis and postprostatectomy penile/urethral pain.[34,35] The technical details of this procedure are beyond the scope of this chapter; however, the SHP is typically targeted from a posterior approach at the level of the lower one-third of the fifth lumbar vertebral body and upper one-third of the first sacral vertebral body in the retroperitoneum as shown in Fig. 5.2.[31] A vast majority of these blocks are done under fluoroscopic guidance, but the use of computer tomography (CT) and ultrasound have been reported as well.[31] This block can be initially performed using local anesthetic and if successful, chemical neurolysis is achieved using phenol or ethanol.[31] De Leon-Casasola and colleagues reported a 69% success rate using neurolytic SHP block for pain

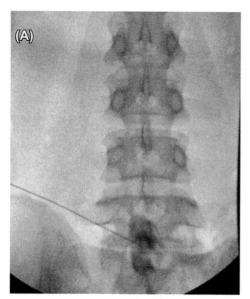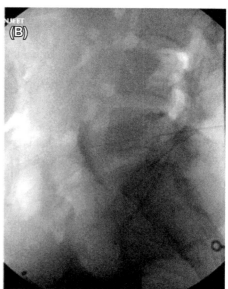

FIG. 5.2 Single needle superior hypogastric plexus neurolysis under fluoroscopic guidance. Final needle position is shown in the **(A)** anteroposterior and **(B)** lateral views. Contrast medium outlining the plexus is shown by the arrow.

originating from pelvic cancer. These patients also demonstrated decreased oral opioid intake after the block.[36]

Inferior Hypogastric Plexus Block: The inferior hypogastric plexus (IHP) is located presacrally and on the lateral aspects of the rectum ventral to the S2–S4 vertebrae.[31,37] It is composed of sympathetic fibers from the hypogastric and pelvic splanchnic nerves, preganglionic parasympathetic fibers from pelvic splanchnic nerves, and afferent fibers from the pelvic viscera.[31,37] This block can theoretically treat pain secondary to chronic prostatitis. Shultz and colleagues were the first group to fluoroscopically perform this block via a transsacral approach in a group of 11 females with pelvic pain.[37] Their study reported a 73% success rate. Mohamed et al. also describes neurolytic IHP block in pelvic cancer patients. Patients from this study reported a 43% reduction in pain 1 week after the block.[38] IHP block has not been studied in the chronic prostatitis population.

Ganglion Impar Block: The sympathetic chains from both sides of the sacral vertebrae fuse together and terminate in a single ganglion called the ganglion impar.[31] It is located anterior to the sacrococcygeal ligament.[31,32] The ganglion impar provides sympathetic innervation to pelvic viscera as well as carry both sympathetic and nociceptive fibers to the perineum, distal rectum, perianal region, and distal urethra.[31]

Fluoroscopically guided ganglion impar blocks were originally used to treat sympathetically mediated pelvic cancer pain. They are now used for a wide array of pelvic pain syndromes, including chronic prostatitis.[31] The transcoccygeal approach is the most popular technique because it allows the shortest needle trajectory while avoiding surrounding structures. The patient is positioned prone and the needle is advanced through the sacrococcygeal ligament until the tip is just posterior to the rectum. Most commonly local with or without steroid is used for this block.[39] In contrast, chemical neurolysis is generally reserved for cancer pain as this technique tends to cause neuritis and neuralgia.[31,39] In the setting of refractory pain from chronic prostatitis, and after successful diagnostic ganglion impar block, one may consider neurolysis using radiofrequency ablation or cryoablation.[31,40,41] Both of these techniques offer fewer complications compared to chemical neurolysis with ethanol or phenol.[40,41] Radiofrequency and cryoablation also cause less surrounding tissue damage, leading to less motor, sexual, bladder and bowel dysfunctions.[40,41]

Pudendal Nerve Block: The pudendal nerve originates from the ventral rami of the S2–S4 nerve roots.[31,32] It courses around the sacrospinous ligament and attaches to the medial portion of the ischial tuberosity. The nerve terminates after passing through the urogenital diaphragm to reach the external genitalia.[31] This nerve

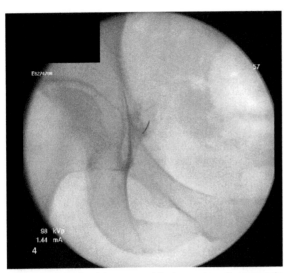

FIG. 5.3 Pudendal nerve block under fluoroscopic guidance. Final needle position is shown at the tip of the ischial spine (white arrow), which is where the pudendal nerve leaves the pelvis.

innervates the penis, bulbospongiosus muscle, ischiocavernosus muscles, perineum, and anus.[31] Pudendal nerve blocks are useful for treating various pelvic and perineal pain syndromes, including chronic prostatitis. In the male population, the pudendal nerve is blocked in the prone position either blindly using anatomic landmark, or more commonly, using fluoroscopic guidance. When done under fluoroscopy, the nerve is targeted at the level of the ischial spine (Fig. 5.3). The nerve is generally blocked with local anesthetic with or without corticosteroid.[42] Cryoablation and radiofrequency ablation may also be performed for longer analgesic relief. In addition to fluoroscopy, CT and ultrasound guidance have also been reported.[31,42]

Neuromodulation: Neuromodulators have been used for various chronic pain conditions for decades.[43] The use of neuromodulation has been documented in pelvic pain caused by interstitial cystitis and bladder pain syndrome in women.[44] Presently, more studies are needed to determine the efficacy of neuromodulation in the management of chronic prostatitis and chronic pelvic pain syndromes in males.[44] However, paresthesia mapping can be conducted during a spinal cord stimulator trial to determine a patient's individualized response.

The exact mechanism by which spinal cord stimulators work has not been definitively established. Traditionally based on the "gate control" theory of pain, it is thought that the application of nonpainful sensory

inputs via electrical pulses to the dorsal column of the spinal cord, nerve root, or peripheral nerve effectively "gate" off ascending pain signals.[44-46] The pelvis is innervated by sensory and motor neurons from the S1—S4 nerve roots, parasympathetic neuron from S1—S4, and sympathetic nerve fibers from T10—L1 levels.[44] Therefore, the treatment of chronic pelvic pain is aimed at these critical sites. Sacral nerve stimulation (SNS), percutaneous tibial nerve stimulation (PTNS), and pudendal nerve stimulations are used for the treatment of pelvic pain.[1,44]

Sacral nerve stimulation: In SNS, a multipolar lead is placed through the sacral foramen to stimulate the sacral nerve root.[44] The electrical stimulus is produced by a generator that is connected to the lead and is implanted nearby. Sacral nerve stimulation is commonly used for the treatment of interstitial cystitis and bladder pain syndrome in women.[44,47] Numerous studies have shown its effectiveness in the management of pelvic pain. Siegal and colleagues published a case series with 10 patients treated with SNS for chronic pelvic pain.[48] Eight cases had leads placed in the S3 foramens while two cases had leads placed in the S4 foramens. Nine patients responded positively with SNS, and of these, six patients reported substantial improvement in their pelvic pain at 19-week follow-up.

Zabihi and colleagues studied 23 patients with intractable pelvic pain from both bladder pain syndrome and chronic pelvic pain syndrome from prostatitis.[49] All of these patients underwent bilateral lead placement for sacral nerve stimulation, but the leads were placed in the caudal epidural space for S2—4 sacral neuromodulation instead of a transforaminal approach; percutaneous access was achieved by gaining epidural access at the sacral hiatus. Ten out of the 23 patients reported improvement in their pain (defined as >50% improvement). Although there is robust evidence supporting the role of sacral nerve stimulation in interstitial cystitis and bladder pain syndrome, few studies have specifically looked at its role in chronic pelvic pain syndrome from prostatitis. However, as the pattern of pain in chronic pelvic pain syndrome secondary to prostatitis is similar to that of interstitial cystitis and bladder pain syndrome, this treatment modality can be considered.

Percutaneous tibial nerve stimulation: The posterior tibial nerve is one of the terminal branches of the sciatic nerve. Percutaneous stimulation of the posterior tibial nerve can send electrical signals to the L4—S3 spinal level via the sciatic nerve and alter pain signals transmitted via this circuitry.[43] Presently, PTNS is FDA approved to be used as a therapeutic approach for overactive bladder but numerous studies have shown that PTNS can help to mediate pelvic pain.[44,50,51] For overactive bladder symptoms, the posterior tibial nerve is stimulated for 30 min every week for 12 weeks.[44] Kabay and colleagues used this regimen in their study of 89 patients with refractory NIH category III pelvic pain, and found that those individuals treated with PTNS have significant improvement in their pain score after 12 weeks of treatment.[52] Although its success rate may lag behind SNS, PTNS is an attractive option due to its noninvasive nature and significant reduced cost compared to SNS.

Pudendal nerve stimulation: The pudendal nerve contains fibers from the sacral nerve roots. Stimulation of the pudendal nerve is a potential alternative avenue for the management of pelvic pain. In a prospective, single-blinded, randomized, cross-over trial, Peter and colleagues subjected 22 patients with interstitial cystitis to SNS followed by pudendal nerve stimulation.[53] Patients had 44% improvement in their symptoms after SNS, and of all patients who underwent subsequent pudendal nerve stimulation, 17 of them showed 59% improvement in their symptoms. Although there is a theoretical benefit of pudendal nerve stimulation, there is a paucity of robust studies evaluating the role of pudendal nerve stimulation for the management of pelvic pain.

REFERENCES

1. Nickel JC. Inflammatory and pain condition of the male genitourinary tract: prostatitis and related pain conditions, orchitis, and epididymitis. In: Partin A, ed. *Campbell-Walsh Urology 11th Edition Review E-Book.* 11th ed. Vol. 1. Elsevier; 2015:304–333.
2. Collins MM, Stafford RS, O'Leary MP, Barry MJ. How common is prostatitis? A national survey of physician visits. *J Urol.* 1998;159(4):1224–1228.
3. Nickel JC, Wagenlehner FME, Pontari M. Male chronic pelvic pain syndrome (CPPS). In: Chapple C, Abrams P, eds. *Male Lower Urinary Tract Symptoms (LUTS). An International Consultation on Male LUTS.* Société Internationale d'Urologie (SIU); 2013:331–372.
4. Pontari MA, Joyce GF, Wise M, McNaughton-Collins M. Urologic diseases in America project. *Prostatitis J Urol.* 2007;177(6):2050–2057. https://doi.org/10.1016/j.juro.2007.01.128.
5. Schneider H, Ludwig M, Hossain HM, Diemer T, Weidner W. The 2001 Giessen Cohort Study on patients with prostatitis syndrome–an evaluation of inflammatory status and search for microorganisms 10 years after a first analysis. *Andrologia.* 2003;35(5):258–262.
6. Bergman B. On the relevance of gram-positive bacteria in prostatitis. *Infection.* 1994;22(Suppl 1):S22. https://doi.org/10.1007/BF01716032.
7. Domingue GJ. Cryptic bacterial infection in chronic prostatitis: diagnostic and therapeutic implications. *Curr Opin Urol.*

8. 1998;8(1):45–49. https://doi.org/10.1097/00042307-199801000-00009.
8. Shurbaji MS, Gupta PK, Myers J. Immunohistochemical demonstration of Chlamydial antigens in association with prostatitis. *Mod Pathol.* 1988;1(5):348–351.
9. Weidner W, Diemer T, Huwe P, Rainer H, Ludwig M. The role of *Chlamydia trachomatis* in prostatitis. *Int J Antimicrob Agents.* 2002;19(6):466–470. https://doi.org/10.1016/s0924-8579(02)00094-8.
10. Dellabella M, Milanese G, Muzzonigro G. Correlation between ultrasound alterations of the preprostatic sphincter and symptoms in patients with chronic prostatitis-chronic pelvic pain syndrome. *J Urol.* 2006;176(1):112–118. https://doi.org/10.1016/S0022-5347(06)00567-2.
11. Zermann D-H, Schmidt RA. Neurophysiology of the pelvic floor: its role in prostate and pelvic pain. In: Nickel JC, ed. *Textbook of Prostatitis.* 1st ed. ISIS Medical Media Ltd; 1999:95–105.
12. Anderson RU, Sawyer T, Wise D, Morey A, Nathanson BH. Painful myofascial trigger points and pain sites in men with chronic prostatitis/chronic pelvic pain syndrome. *J Urol.* 2009;182(6):2753–2758. https://doi.org/10.1016/j.juro.2009.08.033.
13. Yilmaz U, Liu Y-W, Berger RE, Yang CC. Autonomic nervous system changes in men with chronic pelvic pain syndrome. *J Urol.* 2007;177(6):2170–2174. https://doi.org/10.1016/j.juro.2007.01.144. discussion 2174.
14. Krieger JN, Nyberg L, Nickel JC. NIH consensus definition and classification of prostatitis. *J Am Med Assoc.* 1999;282(3):236–237. https://doi.org/10.1001/jama.282.3.236.
15. Schaeffer A. Chronic prostatitis and chronic pelvic pain syndrome. *N Engl J Med.* 2006;355:1690–1698.
16. Cho IR, Lee KC, Lee SE, et al. Clinical outcome of acute bacterial prostatistis, a multicenter study. *Korean J Urol.* 2005;46(10):1034–1039.
17. Shoskes DA, Landis JR, Wang Y, et al. Impact of post-ejaculatory pain in men with category III chronic prostatitis/chronic pelvic pain syndrome. *J Urol.* 2004;172(2):542–547. https://doi.org/10.1097/01.ju.0000132798.48067.23.
18. Wagenlehner FME, van Till JWO, Magri V, et al. National Institutes of Health Chronic Prostatitis Symptom Index (NIH-CPSI) symptom evaluation in multinational cohorts of patients with chronic prostatitis/chronic pelvic pain syndrome. *Eur Urol.* 2013;63(5):953–959. https://doi.org/10.1016/j.eururo.2012.10.042.
19. Nickel JC, Tripp DA, Chuai S, et al. Psychosocial variables affect the quality of life of men diagnosed with chronic prostatitis/chronic pelvic pain syndrome. *BJU Int.* 2008;101(1):59–64. https://doi.org/10.1111/j.1464-410X.2007.07196.x.
20. Nickel JC. The pre and post massage test (PPMT): a simple screen for prostatitis. *Tech Urol.* 1997;3(1):38–43.
21. Theodorou C, Konidaris D, Moutzouris G, Becopoulos T. The urodynamic profile of prostatodynia. *BJU Int.* 1999;84(4):461–463. https://doi.org/10.1046/j.1464-410x.1999.00167.x.
22. Litwin MS, McNaughton-Collins M, Fowler FJ, et al. The National Institutes of Health chronic prostatitis symptom index: development and validation of a new outcome measure. Chronic Prostatitis Collaborative Research

Network. *J Urol.* 1999;162(2):369–375. https://doi.org/10.1016/s0022-5347(05)68562-x.

23. Turner JA, Ciol MA, Von Korff M, Liu Y-W, Berger R. Men with pelvic pain: perceived helpfulness of medical and self-management strategies. *Clin J Pain.* 2006;22(1):19–24. https://doi.org/10.1097/01.ajp.0000148630.15369.79.

24. Herati AS, Moldwin RM. Alternative therapies in the management of chronic prostatitis/chronic pelvic pain syndrome. *World J Urol.* 2013;31(4):761–766. https://doi.org/10.1007/s00345-013-1097-0.

25. Herati AS, Shorter B, Srinivasan AK, et al. Effects of foods and beverages on the symptoms of chronic prostatitis/chronic pelvic pain syndrome. *Urology.* 2013;82(6):1376–1380. https://doi.org/10.1016/j.urology.2013.07.015.

26. Giubilei G, Mondaini N, Minervini A, et al. Physical activity of men with chronic prostatitis/chronic pelvic pain syndrome not satisfied with conventional treatments–could it represent a valid option? The physical activity and male pelvic pain trial: a double-blind, randomized study. *J Urol.* 2007;177(1):159–165. https://doi.org/10.1016/j.juro.2006.08.107.

27. Anderson RU, Wise D, Sawyer T, Chan C. Integration of myofascial trigger point release and paradoxical relaxation training treatment of chronic pelvic pain in men. *J Urol.* 2005;174(1):155–160. https://doi.org/10.1097/01.ju.0000161609.31185.d5.

28. Cornel EB, van Haarst EP, Schaarsberg RWMB-G, Geels J. The effect of biofeedback physical therapy in men with Chronic Pelvic Pain Syndrome Type III. *Eur Urol.* 2005;47(5):607–611. https://doi.org/10.1016/j.eururo.2004.12.014.

29. Pontari MA, Krieger JN, Litwin MS, et al. Pregabalin for the treatment of men with chronic prostatitis/chronic pelvic pain syndrome: a randomized controlled trial. *Arch Intern Med.* 2010;170(17):1586–1593. https://doi.org/10.1001/archinternmed.2010.319.

30. Curtis Nickel J, Baranowski AP, Pontari M, Berger RE, Tripp DA. Management of men diagnosed with chronic prostatitis/chronic pelvic pain syndrome who have failed traditional management. *Rev Urol.* 2007;9(2):63–72.

31. Nagpal AS, Moody EL. Interventional management for pelvic pain. *Phys Med Rehabil Clin.* 2017;28(3):621–646. https://doi.org/10.1016/j.pmr.2017.03.011.

32. Willard FH, Schuenke MD. The neuroanatomy of female pelvic pain. In: Bailey A, Bernstein C, eds. *Pain in Women: A Clinical Guide.* Springer; 2013:17–55. https://doi.org/10.1007/978-1-4419-7113-5.

33. Kanazi GE, Perkins FM, Thakur R, Dotson E. New technique for superior hypogastric plexus block. *Reg Anesth Pain Med.* 1999;24(5):473–476. https://doi.org/10.1016/s1098-7339(99)90018-4.

34. Gofeld M. Peripheral and visceral sympathetic blocks. In: Benzon HT, Rathmell J, Wu CL, Turk DC, Argoff CE, Hurley RW, eds. *Practical Management of Pain.* 5 edition. Slsevier Mosby; 2014:755–767.

35. Rosenberg SK, Tewari R, Boswell MV, Thompson GA, Seftel AD. Superior hypogastric plexus block successfully treats severe penile pain after transurethral resection of the prostate. *Reg Anesth Pain Med.* 1998;23(6):618–620. https://doi.org/10.1016/s1098-7339(98)90092-x.

36. de Leon-Casasola OA, Kent E, Lema MJ. Neurolytic superior hypogastric plexus block for chronic pelvic pain associated with cancer. *Pain.* 1993;54(2):145–151. https://doi.org/10.1016/0304-3959(93)90202-z.

37. Schultz DM. Inferior hypogastric plexus blockade: a transsacral approach. *Pain Physician.* 2007;10(6):757–763.

38. Mohamed SA-E, Ahmed DG, Mohamad MF. Chemical neurolysis of the inferior hypogastric plexus for the treatment of cancer-related pelvic and perineal pain. *Pain Res Manag.* 2013;18(5):249–252. https://doi.org/10.1155/2013/196561.

39. Toshniwal GR, Dureja GP, Prashanth SM. Transsacrococcygeal approach to ganglion impar block for management of chronic perineal pain: a prospective observational study. *Pain Physician.* 2007;10(5):661–666.

40. Wemm K, Saberski L. Modified approach to block the ganglion impar (ganglion of Walther). *Reg Anesth.* 1995;20(6):544–545.

41. Kırcelli A, Demirçay E, Özel Ö, et al. Radiofrequency thermocoagulation of the ganglion impar for coccydynia management: long-term effects. *Pain Pract.* 2019;19(1):9–15. https://doi.org/10.1111/papr.12698.

42. Waldman SD. Pudendal nerve block. In: *Atlas of Interventional Pain Management.* 4 edition. Elsevier Saunders; 2014:638–646.

43. Landau B, Levy RM. Neuromodulation techniques for medically refractory chronic pain. *Annu Rev Med.* 1993;44:279–287. https://doi.org/10.1146/annurev.me.44.020193.001431.

44. Yang CC. Neuromodulation in male chronic pelvic pain syndrome: rationale and practice. *World J Urol.* 2013;31(4):767–772. https://doi.org/10.1007/s00345-013-1066-7.

45. Melzack R, Wall PD. Pain mechanisms: a new theory. *Science.* 1965;150(3699):971–979. https://doi.org/10.1126/science.150.3699.971.

46. Dasgupta R, Critchley HD, Dolan RJ, Fowler CJ. Changes in brain activity following sacral neuromodulation for urinary retention. *J Urol.* 2005;174(6):2268–2272. https://doi.org/10.1097/01.ju.0000181806.59363.d1.

47. Feler CA, Whitworth LA, Fernandez J. Sacral neuromodulation for chronic pain conditions. *Anesthesiol Clin.* 2003;21(4):785–795. https://doi.org/10.1016/s0889-8537(03)00085-3.

48. Siegel S, Paszkiewicz E, Kirkpatrick C, Hinkel B, Oleson K. Sacral nerve stimulation in patients with chronic intractable pelvic pain. *J Urol.* 2001;166(5):1742–1745.

49. Zabihi N, Mourtzinos A, Maher MG, Raz S, Rodríguez LV. Short-term results of bilateral S$_2$-S$_4$ sacral neuromodulation for the treatment of refractory interstitial cystitis, painful bladder syndrome, and chronic pelvic pain. *Int UrogynEcol J Pelvic Floor Dysfunct.* 2008;19(4):553–557. https://doi.org/10.1007/s00192-007-0466-x.

50. Kim SW, Paick J-S, Ku JH. Percutaneous posterior tibial nerve stimulation in patients with chronic pelvic pain: a preliminary study. *Urol Int.* 2007;78(1):58–62. https://doi.org/10.1159/000096936.

51. Biemans JMAE, van Balken MR. Efficacy and effectiveness of percutaneous tibial nerve stimulation in the treatment of pelvic organ disorders: a systematic review. *Neuromodul J Int Neuromodul Soc.* 2013;16(1):25–33. https://doi.org/10.1111/j.1525-1403.2012.00504.x. discussion 33.

52. Kabay S, Kabay SC, Yucel M, Ozden H. Efficiency of posterior tibial nerve stimulation in category IIIB chronic prostatitis/chronic pelvic pain: a Sham-Controlled Comparative Study. *Urol Int.* 2009;83(1):33–38. https://doi.org/10.1159/000224865.

53. Peters KM, Feber KM, Bennett RC. A prospective, single-blind, randomized crossover trial of sacral vs pudendal nerve stimulation for interstitial cystitis. *BJU Int.* 2007;100(4):835–839. https://doi.org/10.1111/j.1464-410X.2007.07082.x.

CHAPTER 6

Coccydynia

RANA AL-JUMAH, MD • KRISHNA B. SHAH, MD

INTRODUCTION

Coccydynia is defined as pain located at the coccyx in the area commonly known as the tailbone.[1] The pain can also extend to the lower sacrum, adjacent muscles, and surrounding soft tissues. The coccyx is composed of one to four segments joined with the distal sacrum by the sacrococcygeal joint. The first and second segments can be mobile and predispose patients to pathological hypermobility. The anatomical structure of the coccyx is also a contributing factor to coccydynia.[2,3] The coccyx is curved forward, contains a bony spicule, and is more anteriorly subluxed, thereby placing it at higher risk for external injury. The coccygeal plexus, which has contributions from the S4—S5 nerve roots and coccygeal nerves, provides somatic and autonomic innervation to the perineum, genitals and anus.[3-5]

The treatment of coccydynia can be challenging. However, a large percentage of patients' pain resolve within weeks to months. Unfortunately, a small number of these patients will go on to develop chronic pain.[5]

ETIOLOGY AND PATHOGENESIS

The majority of coccydynia cases are caused by a traumatic event. Female and obese patients have a higher prevalence. The female coccyx is more posteriorly located and larger compared to males, which can leave it more vulnerable to injury during a traumatic fall or vaginal childbirth.[5-7] Many cases are also idiopathic in nature and ultimately do not have an identifiable cause. Children are less likely to present with coccydynia than adolescents and adults.[1,2,8]

The innervation of the coccyx is complex. Most of the coccyx receives its innervation from the lower sacral spinal nerves and the coccygeal nerves.[9] The anterior portion of the coccyx is innervated predominantly by the sacrococcygeal plexus, which receives contributions from the ventral rami of the S4 and S5 spinal nerves as well as the coccygeal nerves.[9] The sacrococcygeal plexus also innervates the coccygeal ligaments, periosteum, sacrococcygeal joint, soft tissue overlying the ventral coccyx, anterior musculature of the coccyx, and external anal sphincter. The skin and soft tissue overlying the posterior portion of the coccyx is innervated by the coccygeal nerves and posterior rami of S4 and S5. Additionally, the ganglion impar, which sits at the anterior surface of the coccyx, carries visceral afferent fibers from pelvic structures, including the rectum. Therefore, coccygeal pain can actually be referred pain from nearby viscera.[10,11]

Coccydynia pain can be divided into nociceptive or neuropathic pain. Nociceptive pain can be secondary to tissue injury, inflammation, or structural changes that can trigger a primary afferent sensory neuron. Nociceptive pain can further be divided into visceral or somatic pain. Visceral pain originates from nearby viscera and somatic pain originates from skin, muscles, and tissue. Common causes are listed in Table 6.1.[2]

Neuropathic pain results from nerve damage in the central or peripheral nervous system. Pain is characterized by burning, persistent numbness, and tingling sensations. Causes of neuropathic pain are also listed in Table 6.1 and include dural irritation from disc herniation, neoplasms and cysts located along the sacral nerve roots or at the tip of the coccyx.[2,12]

CLINICAL FEATURES

The most common clinical presentation of patients with coccydynia includes point tenderness or generalized pain over the coccyx.[13] The pain is usually described as dull and aching with sharp stabbing pains associated with increased physical movement. Other classic symptoms include pain with prolonged sitting or standing and an exacerbation of pain when going from a seated to a standing position.[7] The pain can become worse with a reclining angle of the spine due to additional weight bearing pressure on the coccyx, which causes hypermobility of the coccygeal bones.[14,15] It is also common for patients to feel the urge to defecate,

Interventional Management of Chronic Visceral Pain Syndromes. https://doi.org/10.1016/B978-0-323-75775-1.00019-2

TABLE 6.1
Etiologies of Coccydynia.

Somatic (Nociceptive) Pain	Neuropathic Pain
• Obstetrical trauma	
• Coccyx fracture	
• Myofascial pain	
• Pelvic floor muscle spasm	• Ganglion impar
• Sacrococcygeal arthritis	stimulation
• Infection (abscess or cyst)	• Disc herniation
• Hypermobility of	• Neoplasms
sacrococcygeal joint	• Cysts
• Coccyx subluxation	
• Psychological conditions	
• Obesity	

Based on, De Andrés J, Chaves S. Coccygodynia: a proposal for an algorithm for treatment. *J Pain*. 2003;4(5):257–266.

have dyschezia, or even experience pain with bowel movements. Female patients with coccydynia may experience dyspareunia and dysmenorrhea.[7,16,17]

Patients typically respond to the pain by attempting the following alleviating maneuvers: leaning forward with the hips flexed, sitting on one buttock or leg to decrease weight bearing on the coccyx, or by avoiding prolonged sitting. It is important to note, however, that these maneuvers can also lead to increased pelvic muscle tension, resulting in pelvic floor dysfunction.[14,18] Patients tend to limit their own functional capacity by avoiding contact sports, such as cycling, due to the pain.[7,14]

DIAGNOSIS

Coccydynia is diagnosed predominantly based on clinical manifestations. A focused physical exam and medical history should be obtained from the patient including history of any recent trauma, vaginal delivery, and malignancy. Upon physical assessment of the patient, it is important to note the patient's BMI. A research study has shown that a BMI greater than 27.4 in women and 29.4 in men increases the risk of developing coccydynia due to a reduction in the degree of pelvic rotation while sitting. The coccyx in obese patients is susceptible to subluxation due to increases in intrapelvic pressures that occur with falls and repetitive sitting.[3,15,19] A detailed psychiatric history should also be completed to assess for anxiety or depression as an underlying cause or exacerbation of coccydynia.[20]

Dynamic radiographs may be able to demonstrate coccygeal mobility, fusion of the sacrococcygeal and superior intercoccygeal joints, osteolytic lesions, fractures,

osteoarthritis, subluxation, and pelvic rotation. A dynamic series of films include lateral and oblique views while the patient is in the sitting and standing positions.[6,7,21] Further testing should be based on the patient's clinical presentation and may include lumbar radiographs, complete blood count (rule out infectious process), stool guaiac to detect occult blood, and magnetic resonance imaging (MRI) or ultrasound to exclude occult pelvic mass or tumor.[1,7] MRI may provide better visualization of the coccyx tip where possible cysts, abscesses, bursitis, or tumors may be noted.[1,2] MRI may also be useful in showing edema or inflammation around the areas of subluxation or hypermobility.[22]

PHYSICAL EXAM FINDINGS

A focused physical exam is used to confirm the diagnosis of coccydynia as well as to rule out other causes of pain. Physical examination should include visual inspection of the spine, sacroiliac joint, anus, and hips for general deformities. Inspection should also include surrounding skin and soft tissues to identify possible cysts, pelvic masses, fistulas, external hemorrhoids or fissures that could be the source of pain. General neurologic assessment should include lower extremity muscle strength, sensory testing of sacral dermatomes, and lower extremity reflexes. Patient with coccydynia should not present with focal neurologic deficits.[7,14]

Moreover, patients will often exhibit point tenderness over the coccyx, sacrococcygeal ligaments, and pubococcygeal ligaments. Having the patient go from a sitting to a standing position can exacerbate the pain over the coccyx. Sharp paresthesias into the rectum with any movement of the coccyx may be noted as well.[1,7,16,17]

For patients exhibiting postpartum coccydynia, the pain in the coccyx may radiate to the hip and lumbar regions especially after prolonged sitting or standing.[23] When performing a digital rectal exam, the coccyx can be manipulated with the forefinger and thumb to elicit pain and coccyges muscle spasms. During manipulation, hypermotility or hypomotility of the sacrococcygeal joint may be noted. Palpation of pelvic floor muscles, including the levator ani and obturator internus, may demonstrate pelvic floor overactivity and hypertonia.[1,3,16] It is also important to note any rectal fissures that may be a cause of referred pain.

TREATMENT

Unaddressed, coccydynia can cause a decline in quality of life due to worsening functional status. The majority of patients respond well to conservative treatments,

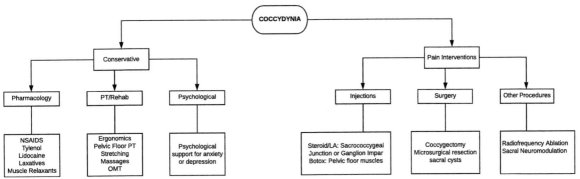

FIG. 6.1 Coccydynia treatment options. *LA*, Local Anesthetic; *OMT*, Osteopathic Manipulative Treatment; *PT*, Physical Therapy.

particularly during the early onset of its course. When conservative treatments fail, various pain interventions are then sought out (Fig. 6.1).

Medication Management

First-line therapy for coccydynia includes the use of nonsteroidal antiinflammatory (NSAIDs) agents such as ibuprofen, celecoxib, and meloxicam. If there is suspicion for acute fracture, these medications should be avoided until it is ruled out due to the risks of impaired periosteal healing. If NSAIDs are contraindicated, then acetaminophen is recommended. Topical lidocaine cream or gel is also often utilized in the area of pain. Muscle relaxants as well as laxatives or stool softeners can be considered to ease dyschezia.[1,5,7] Although opioids may be considered for patients with acute pain from an injury, in general, we do not recommend the use of chronic opioids for the treatment of chronic nonmalignancy pain syndromes.

Physiotherapy/Rehabilitation

To supplement pharmacologic therapies, patients can utilize ergonomic adaptations including a foam donut or wedge-shaped cushion to alleviate pressure off of the coccyx.[16] Patients can also participate in various forms of physiotherapy and rehabilitation. These treatments may provide symptomatic relief and allow the associated pelvic muscles and ligaments to heal.[2,3]

Overactive pelvic floor muscles that result in pelvic floor myofascial pain have been shown to be one of the causes of coccydynia. A published study used down training and relaxation of overactive pelvic floor muscles to provide symptomatic relief of myofascial pain. The patients in this study showed a mean improvement of 62% in their average pain scores. Many of the patients also had improvement in their dyspareunia symptoms as the hypertonia resolved.

Patients have also reported pain relief through various stretching exercises, pelvic massage, and manipulation for pelvic muscle spasms.[17,19]

Coccydynia can be caused by hypermobility of the sacrococcygeal joint. Osteopathic manipulative treatment (OMT) focuses on improving functionality and mobility by normalization of the abdomen-pelvic fascia tendons through fascial unwinding techniques in association with direct mobilization of the sacrococcygeal joint. OMT was found to improve myofascial pain that many patients with coccydynia experience.[24]

Injection Therapy

Coccygeal injections with steroids and local anesthetics are primarily used after medication and rehabilitation therapies have failed. A steroid and local anesthetic administered at the sacrococcygeal joint can be done with ultrasound or fluoroscopic guidance. The patient is placed in the prone position and the sacrococcygeal joint is identified at the base of the sacrum. A mixture of steroid and local anesthetic is injected into the joint. Many patients tend to find relief with this technique, especially if the origin of their coccydynia is caused by arthritis or trauma.[2,5,25]

Coccygeal block, ablation: If a patient's pain is suspected to originate from the soft tissue of the posterior portion of the coccyx (i.e., tender to palpation, pain with sitting), a block may be performed at the sacrococcygeal junction to target the coccygeal nerves, which would serve as a diagnostic and treatment tool. Pain arising from structures innervated by the sacrococcygeal plexus (i.e., the respective pelvic musculature or ligaments), which lies on the anterior surface of the coccyx, would not be expected to respond to these blocks.[9] Radiofrequency lesions using conventional or pulse ablation settings can be considered for patients with a positive block who desire longer relief. Multiple lesions can be done starting from the sacrococcygeal junction down to the lower third of the coccyx.[9] Cooled radiofrequency ablation, where larger lesions can be created by at 60°C, can also be utilized to maximize the chances of ablating the nerves.

Ganglion Impar block, ablation: The ganglion impar can also be blocked for symptomatic pain relief of coccydynia. It represents the termination of the paired paravertebral sympathetic chains and sits anterior to the sacrococcygeal junction.[26,27] Although it is not believed to have significant innervation for the periosteum of the coccyx, it receives afferent nerve fibers from the distal rectum and anus, among other pelvic visceral organs. Patients may experience referred pain to the coccyx, and therefore ganglion impar injection may serve as a useful diagnostic and treatment tool.[26,27]

The transcoccygeal approach under fluoroscopy is the most popular technique because it allows the shortest needle trajectory while avoiding surrounding structures. The patient is positioned prone, and the needle is advanced through the sacrococcygeal ligament until the tip is just posterior to the rectum.[26,28,29] Contrast is used to confirm appropriate needle placement, and then a local anesthetic with corticosteroid is injected (Fig. 6.2). A small case series found that patients had 20%–75% relief after undergoing ganglion impar blocks with 0.5% bupivacaine, lasting anywhere from a few hours to 3 months.[30] Much like for the coccygeal nerves, radiofrequency ablation can be performed at the ganglion impar for patients with a positive block. In a study of coccydynia patients who underwent conventional radiofrequency ablation at 80°C for 90 s, 90.2% reported pain relief at 6 months following the procedure.[26]

Botox: Additionally, a study found Botulinum Toxin A injected into the pelvic floor muscles (puborectalis, pubococcygeus, iliococcygeus, and coccygeus) using electromyography was beneficial for women with high tone pelvic floor dysfunction who had tried conservative therapy without any relief.[31,32]

Neuromodulation

There are few published studies on the use of neuromodulation for coccydynia, particularly sacral nerve stimulation. Lee et al. described a caudal approach for the treatment of chronic coccydynia.[33] A needle entrance point caudal to the sacral hiatus was used. Two Tuohy needles were advanced into the sacral hiatus using fluoroscopic guidance in the lateral view. Two percutaneous leads were advanced into the posterior sacral epidural space and perioperative testing was performed to confirm appropriate coverage[33] (Fig. 6.3). Burst stimulation was found to be most effective compared to traditional tonic stimulation.[33]

Although dorsal root ganglion (DRG) stimulation has been approved by the US Food and Drug Administration for complex regional pain syndrome, it has recently increased in popularity for the treatment of many off-label conditions, particularly for the treatment of chronic pain disorders in areas that have been difficult to treat with conventional dorsal column stimulation, such as the foot, abdomen, and groin. A case

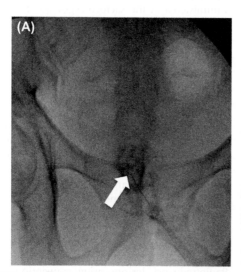
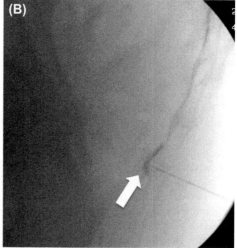

FIG. 6.2 Transcoccygeal approach for ganglion impar block under fluoroscopic guidance. Final needle position is shown in the **(A)** lateral and **(B)** anteroposterior views. Contrast medium outlining the structure is shown by the *arrows*.

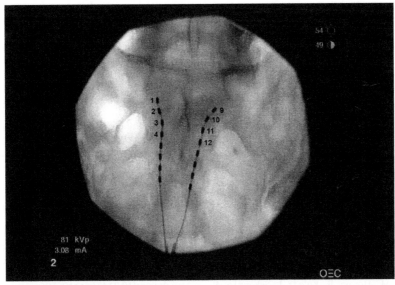

FIG. 6.3 Bilateral spinal cord stimulator leads for sacral stimulation for coccydynia seen on a posterior-anterior (PA) view of the sacrum. (Credit: Lee DW, Lai A. Sacral burst neuromodulation via caudal approach as a treatment for chronic coccydynia. *Neuromodulation*. 2018, 10.1111/ner.12808.)

report describing the success of DRG stimulation for coccydynia has been described; stimulator leads were placed at the bilateral L1 and S2 DRG with nearly 100% coverage of pain (Fig. 6.4).[27]

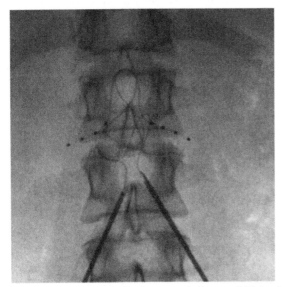

FIG. 6.4 Anterior-posterior fluoroscopic image of bilateral dorsal root ganglion stimulation leads on the L1 level. (Credit: Giordano NL, Helmond NV, Chapman KB. Coccydynia treated with dorsal root Ganglion stimulation. *Case Rep Anesthesiol*. 2018:1–4.)

Currently, there are no large clinical trials examining the efficacy of spinal cord stimulation for the treatment of coccydynia. However, it is reasonable to trial patients if conservative treatment and injections have not provided adequate pain relief.[27,33]

Coccygectomy

Surgical procedures for the treatment of coccydynia is usually reserved when all conservative measures have failed to provide adequate pain relief. The most common surgery performed is a partial coccygectomy where the coccyx immediately proximal to the sacrococcygeal junction is amputated. The efficacy of this surgical procedure is not fully understood and it carries a high complication and failure rate. However, success with a partial coccygectomy is usually seen with abnormal coccygeal hypermobility or deformity. If the pain is due to perineural cysts, microsurgical resection has been shown to improve coccygeal pain.[5,7,17,34]

REFERENCES

1. Waldman SD. Coccydynia. In: Waldman SD, ed. *Atlas of Common Pain Syndromes*. Vol. 97. Philadelphia, PA: Elsevier; 2012:378–382.
2. De Andrés J, Chaves S. Coccygodynia: a proposal for an algorithm for treatment. *J Pain*. 2003;4(5):257–266.
3. Maigne JY, Doursounian L, Chatellier G. Causes and Mechanisms of common coccydynia: role of Body mass index and coccygeal trauma. *Spine*. 2000;25:3072–3079.

4. Moore KL, Delley AF. *Clinically Oriented Anatomy*. 4th ed. Philadelphia, PA: Lippincott Williams & Wilkins; 1999.

5. Lirette LS, Chaiban G, Tolba R, Eissa H. Coccydynia: an overview of the anatomy, etiology, and treatment of coccyx pain. *Ochsner J*. 2014;14(1):84−87.

6. Yamashita K. Radiological study of 1500 coccyces. *Nippon Seikeigeka Gakkai Zasshi*. 1988;62:23−36.

7. Vora A, Chan S. Coccydynia. In: Frontera WR, Rizzo TD, Silver JK, eds. *Essentials of Physical Medicine and Rehabilitation: Musculoskeletal Disorders, Pain, and Rehabilitation*. Vol. 99. Philadelphia, PA: Elsevier; 2018:538−542.

8. Maigne JY, Pigeau I, Aguer N, Doursounian L, Chatellier G. Chronic coccydynia in adolescents. A series of 53 patients. *Eur J Phys Rehabil Med*. 2011;47(2):245−251.

9. Chen Y, Huang-Lionnet JHY, Cohen SP. Radiofrequency ablation in coccydynia: a case series and comprehensive, evidence-based review. *Pain Med*. 2016. https://doi.org/10.1093/pm/pnw268.

10. Malec MM, Horosz B, Koleda I, et al. Neurolytic Block of ganglion of Walter for the management of chronic pelvic pain. *Wideochir Inne Tech Maloinwazyjne*. 2014;9(3):458−462.

11. Malec-Milewska M, Horosz B, Koleda I, Sekowska A, Kucia H, Kosson D, et al. Neurolytic block of ganglion of walther for the management of chronic pelvic pain. *Videosurg Other Miniinvasive Tech*. 2014;3:458−462. https://doi.org/10.5114/wiitm.2014.43079.

12. Ferrell BA. Pain. In: Osterwall D, Brummel-Smith K, Beck JC, eds. *Comprehensive Geriatric Assessment*. New York: McGraw-Hill; 2000:381−397.

13. Nelson DA. Coccydynia and lumbar disk disease: historical Correlations and clinical cautions. *Perspect Biol Med*. 1991;34:229−238.

14. Foye PM. Coccydynia: tailbone pain. *Phys Med Rehabil Clin*. 2017; 28(3):539−549. https://doi.org/10.1016/j.pmr.2017.03.006.

15. Maigne J-Y, Lagauche D, Doursounian L. Instability of the coccyx in coccydynia. *J Bone Joint Surg*. 2000;82(7):1038−1041. https://doi.org/10.1302/0301-620x.82b7.10596.

16. Nathan ST, Fisher BE, Roberts CS. Coccydynia: a review of pathoanatomy, aetiology, treatment and outcome. *J Bone Jt Surg Br*. 2010;92(12):1622−1627.

17. Scott KM, Fisher LW, Bernstein IH, Bradley MH. The treatment of chronic coccydynia and post coccygectomy pain with pelvic floor physical therapy. *Pharm Manag*. 2017; 9(4):367−376.

18. Foye PM, Buttaci CJ, Stitik TP, Yonclas PP. Successful injection for coccyx pain. *Am J Phys Med Rehabil*. 2006;85(9): 783−784.

19. Maigne JY, Chatellier G. Comparison of three manual coccydynia treatments: a pilot study. *Spine*. 2001;26(20): E479−E483. discussion E484.

20. Maroy B. Spontaneous and evoked coccygeal pain in depression. *Dis Colon Rectum*. 1988;31(3):210−215. https://doi.org/10.1007/bf02552548.

21. Maigne JY, Guedj S, Straus C. Idiopathic Coccygodynia: lateral Roentgenograms in the sitting position and coccygeal discography. *Spine*. 1994;19:930−934.

22. Fogel GR, Cunningham P, Esses S. Coccygodynia: evaluation and management. *J Am Acad Orthop Surg*. 2004; 12(1):49−54.

23. Embaby H, Elgendy S, Hasanin ME. Effect of muscle energy technique in treating post-partum coccydynia: a randomized control trial. *Phys Ther Rehabil*. 2017;4(1):5. https://doi.org/10.7243/2055-2386-4-5.

24. Origo D, Tarantino A, Nonis A, Vismara L. Osteopathic manipulative treatment in chronic coccydynia: a case series. *J Bodyw Mov Ther*. 2018;22(2):261−265. https://doi.org/10.1016/j.jbmt.2017.06.010.

25. Traycoff RB, Crayton H, Dodson R. Sacrococcygeal pain syndromes: diagnosis and treatment. *Orthopedics*. 1989; 12:1373−1377.

26. Adas C, Ozdemir U, Toman H, Luleci N, Luleci E, Adas H. Transsacrococcygeal approach to ganglion impar: radiofrequency application for the treatment of chronic intractable coccydynia. *J Pain Res*. 2016;9:1173−1177. https://doi.org/10.2147/jpr.s105506.

27. Giordano NL, Helmond NV, Chapman KB. Coccydynia treated with dorsal root ganglion stimulation. *Case Rep Anesthesiol*. 2018;2018:1−4.

28. Sagir A, Ozasalan S, Koroglu A. Application of ganglion impar block in patient with coccyx dislocation. *Agri*. 2011;23(3):129−133.

29. Reig E, Abejon D, del Pozo C, Insausti J, Contreas R. Thermocoagulation of the ganglion impar or ganglion of Walther: description of a modified approach. Preliminary result in chronic, nononcological pain. *Pain Pract*. 2005; 5(2):103−110.

30. Haider N. Coccydynia treated with spinal cord stimulation: a case report. In: *Proceedings of the American Academy of Pain Medicine 24th Annual Meeting*. 2008.

31. Morrissey D, El-Kawand D, Ginzburg N, Wehbe S, O'Hare P, Whitmore K. Botulinum toxin A injections into pelvic floor muscles under electromyographic guidance for women with refractory high-tone pelvic floor dysfunction. *Female Pelvic Med Reconstr Surg*. 2015;21(5):277−282.

32. Abbot JA, Jarvis SK, Lyons SD, et al. Botulinum toxin type A for chronic pain and pelvic floor spasms in women: a randomized controlled trial. *Ostet Gynecol*. 2006;108(4): 915−923.

33. Lee DW, Lai A. Sacral burst neuromodulation via caudal approach as a treatment for chronic coccydynia. *Neuromodulation*. 2018. https://doi.org/10.1111/ner.12808.

34. Kerr EE, Benson D, Schrot RJ. Coccygectomy for chronic refractory coccygodynia: clinical case series and literature review. *J Neurosurg Spine*. 2011;14(5):654−663.

CHAPTER 7

Pudendal Neuralgia

RANA AL-JUMAH, MD • KRISHNA B. SHAH, MD

INTRODUCTION

Pudendal neuralgia was first described in 1987 by Amarenco et al.[1] Also known as Alcock's canal syndrome, cyclist syndrome, or pudendal nerve entrapment syndrome, it affects both men and women and presents as pain in the dermatomal distribution of the pudendal nerve, including the penis, scrotum, vulva, clitoris, perineum, and rectum.[2] This condition is often misdiagnosed or unrecognized by the vast majority of physicians, including pelvic pain specialists. The prevalence of pudendal neuralgia is unknown, but Spinosa et al. state an incidence rate as high as 1% of the general population, with women being more affected than men.[3]

ETIOLOGY AND PATHOGENESIS

The pudendal nerve is derived from the ventral rami of the second, third, and fourth sacral spinal nerves.[4,5] The nerve passes through the piriformis muscle, where it is joined with the pudendal artery and vein. This neurovascular bundle travels together between the sacrospinous and sacrotuberous ligaments (Fig. 7.1).[6] As the pudendal nerve exits and reenters the pelvis, it is contained within the pudendal canal.[5] The pudendal nerve divides into multiple branches including the inferior anal nerve, perineal nerve, and dorsal nerve of the penis.[2,7]

The pudendal nerve carries sensory, motor, and sympathetic fibers.[5] The inferior anal nerve provides innervation to the external anal sphincter, distal anal canal, and the anal skin. The perineal nerve divides into posterior labial (female), scrotal (male), and muscular branches. The muscular branch provides innervation to the superficial transverse perineal muscle, bulbospongiosus, ischiocavernosus, deep transverse perineal muscle, sphincter urethrae, anterior portion of the external anal sphincter, and levator ani.[2] The dorsal nerve of the penis/clitoris is the terminal branch of the pudendal nerve and provides sensory innervation to the respective male and female genitalia.[2,8]

Pudendal neuralgia can arise from multiple mechanisms (Table 7.1).[2] Compression is the most common cause of nerve injury and may be transient or permanent. The degree of injury is mainly affected by the duration of pressure applied to the perineum and can occur at several locations along its course.[9−11] Prolonged sitting or repetitive impact often leads to mechanical compression, causing entrapment at the sacrospinous or sacrotuberous ligaments. Pelvic floor muscle spasms or scar tissue from trauma may also result in nerve entrapment.[12−14]

Direct nerve injury can occur from excessive stretching or transection of the nerve, as seen during vaginal deliveries, pelvic surgeries, and traumatic falls.[15] Pudendal nerve injury is often observed after corrective procedures for pelvic organ prolapse, with many patients reporting symptoms of pudendal neuralgia immediately postoperatively.[7,15−18] Less common causes of pudendal neuralgia include infection, tumor growth, pelvic radiation, or immunological processes.[15−18] Herpes zoster has been shown to cause pudendal neuralgia due to herpetic inflammation.[19]

Lastly, severe pudendal neuralgia can develop into complex regional pain syndrome (CRPS), which is a dysfunction of the peripheral and central nervous systems that are manifested by sensory and motor signs/symptoms such as burning pains, swelling, muscle spasms, and trophic changes among others.[2,8,20] Traditionally, thought of as a dysfunction that occurs predominantly in the extremities, it is believed that pudendal neuralgia may progress in its symptomatology and develop into CRPS.[2] This may lead to a more complex treatment course, given that many of the signs and symptoms are irreversible if left untreated.

CLINICAL FEATURES

Patients with pudendal neuralgia typically complain of perineal and rectal pain, often describing a foreign body sensation as if they are continuously sitting on an object.[21,22] Moreover, the pain may be unilateral or

Interventional Management of Chronic Visceral Pain Syndromes. https://doi.org/10.1016/B978-0-323-75775-1.00007-6

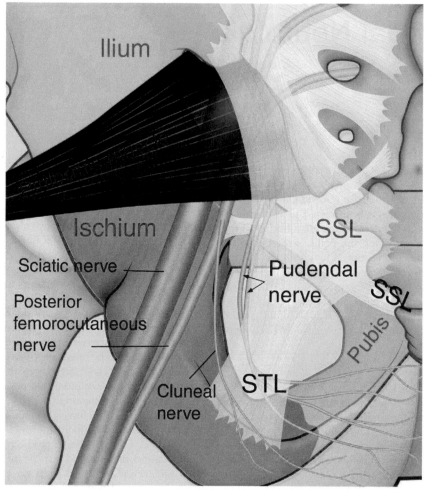

Rev Colomb Anestesiol. 2017;45:200–9

FIG. 7.1 The pudendal is shown coursing under the sacrospinous (SSL) and sacrotuberous (STL) ligaments, where entrapment can occur. (From Rojas-Gómez MF, Blanco-Dávila R, Tobar Roa V, Gómez González AM, Ortiz Zableh AM, Ortiz Azuero A. Anestesia regional guiada por ultrasonido en territorio del nervio pudendo. *Rev Colomb Anestesiol* 2017;45:200–209.)

bilateral in nature. They may also have symptoms at the urogenital or anal regions depending on where along the course in the pelvis the nerve is affected. In females, these areas include the vulva, vagina, clitoris, and labia. For males, the glans penis and scrotum (excluding testes) can be affected.[22,23]

Neuropathies are typically described as a burning sensation with associated numbness or a sense of heaviness.[22,23] The pain can also exhibit sharp or aching features. Peripheral and central sensitization, as seen with features of increased sensitivity to painful stimuli (hyperalgesia) or pain with nonpainful stimuli (allodynia), are common among patients.[24,25] Pain is often provoked by movement and sitting, especially while driving or using a bicycle. Patients may report relief with standing and sitting on a toilet or donut cushion, which provides relief by reducing the pressure applied at the ischial tuberosities. As the disease progresses, patients can develop constant chronic pain that is also present in the standing position.[22,26] A small percentage of patients can also exhibit vague neuropathic pain symptoms in the posterior thigh and lower abdomen that is not an area in the pudendal nerve distribution. The pain in these regions is usually due to muscle spasms or referred somatic pain[2,5,8,15,22].

TABLE 7.1 Common Causes of Pudendal Neuralgia.		
Pelvic Surgery	Prolonged Sitting	Infection
Vaginal childbirth	Constipation	Malignancy
Traumatic fall	Excessive masturbation	Anal intercourse
Repetitive cycling	Pelvic radiation	Herpes zoster

NANTES ESSENTIAL DIAGNOSTIC CRITERIA*

Pain in the territory of the pudendal nerve: From the anus to the penis or clitoris: this criteria excludes pain located in the gluteal, sacrum, or coccygeal regions. The pain may be located superficially in vulvovaginal or anorectal regions.

Pain is predominantly experienced while sitting: while sitting the pain is from the increased pressure placed on the nerve. For patients with progressed pudendal neuralgia, the pain can become constant and present even when standing.

Pain does not wake the patient at night: perineal pain does not usually cause patients to wake up at night. Pudendal neuralgia can cause frequent awakenings at night due to the other associated symptoms including increased urinary frequency.

Pain with no objective sensory impairment: if the patient presents with perineal sensory deficit then a lesion of the sacral nerve roots or sacral plexus is possible and may also include sphincter motor disorders. It has been hypothesized that due to anatomic location of many nerves coursing closely together, there can be sensory impairment in areas near the regions innervated by the pudendal nerve.

Pain is relieved by diagnostic pudendal nerve block: local anesthetic infiltration of the pudendal nerve reduces pain dramatically. Even though it is listed as an essential criterion, there is the possibility that it can also relieve pain related to any perineal disease or nerve lesions located distal to the site of infiltration.

*From Hibner M, Castellanos M, et al. *Glob Libr Women's Med*, (ISSN: 1756–2228) 2011; doi:10.3843/GLOWM.10468.

Patients may present with dysuria, dyschezia, dyspareunia, and pain with ejaculation.[8,23,24] A subset of patients may experience restless genital syndrome, causing persistent sexual arousal that is painful.[21,23] Patients can also develop fecal incontinence from decreased sphincter tone. Urinary frequency and urgency have been noted and can mirror symptoms of interstitial cystitis.[8,23,24]

DIAGNOSIS

Pudendal neuralgia is primarily a clinical diagnosis. Developed in 2006, the Nantes criteria describe the diagnostic components for pudendal neuralgia by entrapment (Table 7.2).[23,24] These components have been validated, and patients meeting all the criteria have demonstrated better outcomes from decompression surgery compared to those who partially meet them.[23,24] The criteria were formed to limit the misdiagnosis of pudendal neuralgia. The five essential components are as follows: (1) pain in the distribution of the pudendal nerve, (2) pain predominantly while sitting, (3) pain does not wake up the patient during the night, (4) pain with no objective sensory impairment, (5) pain is relieved with a pudendal nerve block.[23,24]

TABLE 7.2 Features of Pudendal Neuralgia.	
Nantes Diagnostic Criteria for Pudendal Nerve Entrapment[a]	**Exclusion Criteria**
Pain in the anatomical territory of the pudendal nerve	Purely coccygeal, gluteal, hypogastric pain
Pain worsened with sitting	Exclusively paroxysmal pain
Patient is not woken at night from the pain	Exclusive pruritus
No objective sensory loss on physical exam	Imaging abnormalities able to account for the pain
Analgesic relief with pudendal nerve block	

[a] All criteria must be present.
From Labat JJ, Riant T, Robert R, et al. Diagnostic criteria for pudendal neuralgia by pudendal nerve entrapment (Nantes criteria). *Neurourol Urodyn* 2008;27(4):306–310. (Elsevier).

Imaging: Doppler ultrasound is a relatively low-cost diagnostic imaging modality that can be a useful diagnostic tool.[27] As the neurovascular bundle travels together, it is believed that compression of the nerve may lead to compression of the pudendal vein; Doppler technology should be able to assess for any changes in venous flow. High-frequency ultrasound can also assist with identifying other signs of nerve inflammation and compression, such as edema and any flattening of the nerve, respectively. Functional magnetic resonance imaging (MRI) can be performed to assess nerve integrity, though it has not been shown to be accurate enough to diagnose pudendal nerve compression and is viewed as experimental. Nonetheless, MRI can evaluate the spinal cord and nerve roots for any compressive pathologies as well as tumors or cysts that may be the source of pain[23,27].

Nerve conduction studies: Pudendal neuropathy can be measured with sensory-evoked potentials, motor-evoked potentials, and pudendal nerve terminal motor latency testing (PNTML). PNTML involves applying an impulse through the vagina or rectum at the ischial spine. The impulse time is measured as it travels through the perineal muscles, and if latency is present, pudendal neuropathy is likely to be diagnosed.[26,28] PNTML values, however, are subject to high variability in patients who have undergone previous pelvic surgery or have a history of vaginal delivery due to stretching of the pelvic floor muscles.[29] PNTML is also subject to substantial operator variability, which can lead to subject inconsistencies.[2]

Pudendal nerve block, botulinum toxin injections: Diagnostic block not only aids in the diagnosis of the neuralgia, but also serves as a treatment option by injecting local anesthetic and steroid around the pudendal nerve to relieve pain. The block can be performed with or without imaging, which is discussed in the Treatments section.[9,30–32] Diagnostic block should provide pain relief within an hour for local anesthetic administration. To discern whether a patient's symptoms are due to nerve injury or compression from pelvic muscle dysfunction, botulinum toxin injections at the respective pelvic floor muscles may be performed.[2]

PHYSICAL EXAM FINDINGS

Physical exam of the patient should include a detailed examination of the patient's back, abdomen, and pelvic floor muscles with an emphasis on any obvious signs of infection, palpable masses, lacerations, or skin erythema. Natal cleft livedo reticularis or cutis anserine skin changes can be seen in patients who develop CRPS due to pudendal neuralgia.[2,20,24] Other potential signs include changes in skin color/temperature/texture, allodynia, and hyperalgesia.[2]

Palpation of the coccygeal muscles, obturator internus, levator ani, psoas major and abdominal muscles should be assessed for tenderness and muscle spasms. A neurological examination should also be performed to include sensation to touch and pinprick. Painful palpation is common along the distributions of the pudendal nerve, including the clitoris or glans penis, posterior labia or posterior scrotum, and the posterior perianal skin[2,8,29].

The most common physical exam finding is reproducible pain, or a positive Tinel's sign, when pressure is applied to the pudendal canal and ischial spine where the sacrospinous ligament inserts. Tinel's sign is usually described as a numbing or tingling sensation when palpation or percussion of a certain nerve is performed. There can also be a positive Tinel's sign when percussing the dorsal branch of the pudendal nerve affecting the clitoris or glans penis.[2,28,29] In many cases of pudendal neuralgia, patients do not present with neurological deficits.[2,8]

TREATMENT

Along with lifestyle modifications, the mainstay treatment for pudendal neuralgia is conservative management with pharmacologic and physical therapy. When these measures are unable to provide adequate pain relief, an interventional approach with injections and surgery may be considered. A multimodal approach to pudendal neuralgia is often required.[8,9,22]

Lifestyle modifications: Lifestyle modifications should be implemented immediately to avoid additional injury or worsening of symptoms.[8] Provocative exercises or activities that exacerbate pain should be stopped. If pain is present with prolonged sitting, modifying position, or avoidance of sitting should take precedence. If patients are unable to avoid sitting, a cushion should be utilized to support the ischial tuberosities to decrease pressure on the pelvic floor muscles and pudendal nerve. Other modifications that should be employed include avoiding hard surfaces, cycling, hip flexion exercises, and squats focused on the lower body muscles.[8,22]

Physical therapy: When applicable, physical therapy is centered on addressing pelvic floor muscle dysfunction. The majority of patients experience muscle spasms and muscle shortening of the pelvic girdle. Physical therapists work with patients on manual therapies to lengthen the pelvic muscles and work on strengthening exercises, stretching, biofeedback techniques, and trigger point release to relax the pelvic floor muscles.[8,33,34]

Medications: When lifestyle modifications and physical therapy fail to provide adequate relief, medical management can be considered. Neuropathic medications are a staple for the treatment of pudendal neuralgia.[8] Gabapentinoids, such as gabapentin and pregabalin, are anticonvulsants that are used for a variety of other neuropathic pain syndromes and have both been used for the treatment of pudendal neuralgia; neither of these medications has been FDA-approved for this syndrome specifically.[8] Additionally, tricyclic antidepressants and serotonin-norepinephrine reuptake inhibitors are other agents that have been shown to be beneficial in reducing neuropathic symptoms.[35,36] Muscle relaxants, such as cyclobenzaprine, tizanidine, and baclofen, are commonly prescribed for patients with a myofascial component to their pain. Nonsteroidal antiinflammatory drugs and paracetamol should also be used when appropriate.[35]

Botulinum toxin injection: If physical therapy does not improve pelvic floor muscle dysfunction, then botulinum toxin injections into the pelvic floor muscles as an alternative treatment can be considered.[33] Administration of 50–400 units of botulinum toxin have been reported in the literature.[33] A concerning complication is accidental injection into the anal or urinary sphincter, which can lead to transient incontinence.[33] Patient may resume physical therapy after 5–7 days. It is important to note that while effective in up to 67% of patients with pelvic floor dysfunction, the success rate of botulinum toxin injection is 30% when used for pudendal neuralgia specifically.[8]

Pudendal nerve block: Pudendal nerve block injections serve as a diagnostic and therapeutic procedure. Injections can be performed using anatomical landmarks, fluoroscopic guidance, computed tomography (CT), or ultrasound.[8,37–39] Unilateral or bilateral injections are performed depending on the laterality of the patient's pain. A combination of long-acting local anesthetic, such as bupivacaine, and corticosteroids are commonly used for the injectate.[40–42]

When using the landmark technique in female patients, the transvaginal approach requires the patient to be placed in the lithotomy position. The ischial spine is palpated and the needle is guided toward the tip of the ischial spine. The needle is advanced through the vaginal mucosa until it reaches the sacrospinous ligament. With fluoroscopy or CT guidance, the patient is placed in the prone position and the needle is advanced to the tip of the ischial spine (Fig. 7.2). The needle is slightly withdrawn after contact with the ischial spine is made and medication is administered after negative aspiration rules out intravascular injection.[39]

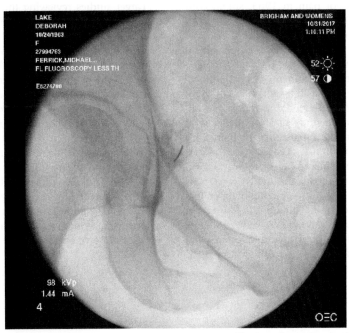

FIG. 7.2 **Pudendal nerve block under fluoroscopic guidance.** Final needle position is shown at the tip of the ischial spine (*white arrow*), which is where the pudendal nerve leaves the pelvis.

Pulsed radiofrequency. Pulse radiofrequency (PRF) is a minimally invasive treatment option for pudendal neuralgia. Particularly in patients with previous positive diagnostic block, PRF is thought to be successful by neural modulation without affecting the motor or sensory nerve fibers.[43–45] PRF avoids the use of high temperatures compared to conventional continuous radiofrequency procedures.[46] One study treated women with chronic pelvic pain from refractory pudendal neuralgia with transvaginal PRF at 42°C for 90 s for four courses of treatment. All of the women had significant decreases in their pain scores after at least one round of PRF.[43]

Cryoneuroablation: Cryoneuroablation involves freezing the pudendal nerve. The identification of the nerve can be done by landmark palpation or under image guidance (CT, fluoroscopy). A 17-gauge cryoablation probe is advanced typically to the distal portion of the pudendal canal. After the nerve is identified, sensory and motor stimulation is used to confirm the placement. Two 8–5 min freeze-thaw intervals can be completed.[47]

Patients treated with cryoneuroablation at the pudendal canal with CT guidance showed a significant decrease in visual analog scale (VAS) pain scores. VAS scores decreased from a baseline score of 7.6–3.1 at the 6 month postprocedure follow up.[47]

Neuromodulation: Based on Melzack and Wall's "Gate Control Theory" of pain in 1965, spinal cord stimulators (SCS) work by the application of nonpainful sensory inputs via electrical pulses to the dorsal column of the spinal cord, nerve root, or peripheral nerve to effectively "gate" off ascending pain signals.[48] Traditionally used for the treatment of postlaminectomy pain syndrome and CRPS, SCS devices have been used successfully for pudendal neuralgia as well. A multicenter prospective study of 27 patients with pudendal neuralgia found a reduction in pain with dorsal column stimulation.[49] Leads were placed with a most caudal lead placed below the caudal extremity of the conus medullaris. This level was determined before the procedure utilizing preoperative MRI. In addition, intraoperative stimulation testing was also done for adequate coverage. Twenty patients proceeded with permanent implant and reported a significant reduction in pain at the 15-month follow-up.[49]

Stimulation of the dorsal roots ganglion (DRG) has also been found to be effective for the treatment of pudendal neuralgia as well and offers some advantages over traditional dorsal column stimulators.[50] DRG stimulation allows focused stimulation of particular dermatomes (Fig. 7.3) with the added benefit of utilizing less overall energy since the cerebrospinal fluid layer at the level of the DRG is relatively thin. There is also less risk of unwanted paresthesias with positional changes compared to dorsal column stimulators.[6,50] In a case series of seven patients for chronic pelvic pain, two of the patients were diagnosed with pudendal neuralgia. Both patients were trialed with leads placed at the L1 and S2 foramens along their respective DRG's on the ipsilateral side of pain. Both patients had greater than 85% reduction in pain during the trial phase and were waiting for permanent implantation at the time of the study's publication.[50] It has been suggested that L1 lead placement modulates the L1 dermatome, which includes the groin, but limited in the genital and perineum region. Similarly, S2 lead placement involves the leg and buttock but is also limited in the pelvic area. However, when both the L1 and S2 roots are stimulated together, appropriate pelvic coverage is obtained.[50] Physicians should also consider appropriate perioperative testing to confirm appropriate pain coverage.

Larger studies reviewing the efficacy of dorsal column and dorsal root ganglion stimulation for pudendal neuralgia are needed.

Decompression surgery: When conservative therapies options fail, pudendal nerve decompression surgery should be considered, particularly if nerve entrapment is suspected. About 40% of patients who receive transgluteal pudendal decompression surgery experience roughly a 40% reduction in overall pain symptoms.[38] The transgluteal approach is the more widely used method compared to transvaginal or transrectal techniques due to greater visualization of the pudendal nerve. An incision through the gluteal muscles is made by exposing the sacrotuberous and sacrospinous ligaments. The pudendal nerve can be found below the ligaments and once visualized neurolysis is completed in cases of nerve entrapment.[1]

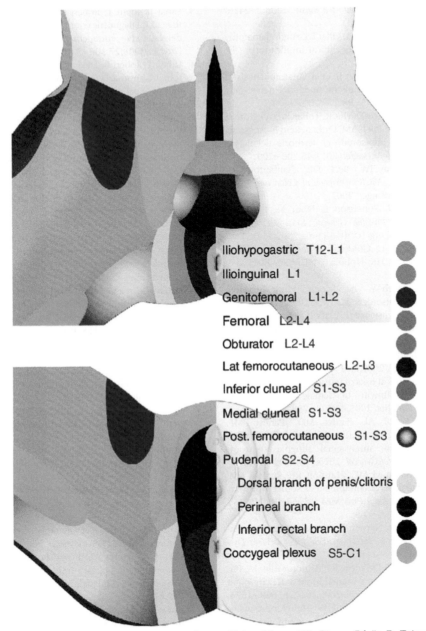

Iliohypogastric T12-L1

Ilioinguinal L1

Genitofemoral L1-L2

Femoral L2-L4

Obturator L2-L4

Lat femorocutaneous L2-L3

Inferior cluneal S1-S3

Medial cluneal S1-S3

Post. femorocutaneous S1-S3

Pudendal S2-S4

Dorsal branch of penis/clitoris

Perineal branch

Inferior rectal branch

Coccygeal plexus S5-C1

FIG. 7.3 Distribution of perineal dermatomes shown. (Rojas-Gómez MF, Blanco-Dávila R, Tobar Roa V, Gómez González AM, Ortiz Zableh AM, Ortiz Azuero A. Anestesia regional guiada por ultrasonido en territorio del nervio pudendo. Rev Colomb Anestesiol 2017;45:200–209.)

REFERENCES

1. Amarenco G, Kerdraon J, Bouju P, Le Budet C, Cocquen AL, Bosc S, et al. Efficacity and safety of different treatments of perineal neuralgia due to compression of the pudendal nerve within the ischio-rectal fossa or by ischiatic spine. *Rev Neurol*. 1997;153:331–334.

2. Hibner M, Castellanos M, Desai N, Balducci J. *Glob Libr Women's Med*. 2011. https://doi.org/10.3843/GLOWM.10468. ISSN: 1756-2228.

3. Spinosa JP, de Bisschop E, Laurencon J, Kuhn G, Dubuisson JB, Riederer BM. Sacral staged reflexes to localize the pudendal compression: an anatomical

validation of the concept. *Rev Med Suisse.* 2006;2, 2416-2418. 2420-2421.

4. Shafik A, el-Sherif M, Youssef A, Olfat ES. Surgical anatomy of the pudendal nerve and its clinical implications. *Clin Anat.* 1995;8(2):110–115.

5. Robert R, Prat-Pradal D, Labat JJ, et al. Anatomic basis of chronic perineal pain: role of the pudendal nerve. *Surg Radiol Anat.* 1998;20(2):93–98.

6. Rojas-Gómez MF, Blanco-Dávila R, Tobar Roa V, Gómez González AM, Ortiz Zableh AM, Ortiz Azuero A. Anestesia regional guiada por ultrasonido en territorio del nervio pudendo. *Rev Colomb Anestesiol.* 2017;45:200–209.

7. Wolff BG, Fleshman JW, Beck DE, Pemberton JH, Wexner SD, eds. *The ASCRS Textbook of Colon and Rectal Surgery.* New York: Springer; 2007.

8. Hibner M, Desai N, Robertson L, Nour M. Pudendal neuralgia. *J Minim Invasive Gynecol.* Mar. 2010;17(2): 148–153. https://doi.org/10.1016/j.jmig.2009.11.003.

9. Goldstein A, Pukall C, Goldstein I. *Female Sexual Pain Disorders.* Chichester, UK; Hoboken, NJ: Wiley-Blackwell; 2009:112–118.

10. Leibovitcha I, Morb Y. The vicious cycling: bicycling related urogenital disorders. *Eur Urol.* 2005;47:277–287.

11. Schrader SM, Breitenstein MJ, Clark JC, et al. Nocturnal penile tumescence and rigidity testing in bicycling patrol officers. *J Androl.* 2002;23:927–934.

12. Shafik A. Pudendal canal syndrome: a cause of chronic pelvic pain. *Urology.* 2002;60:199.

13. Delmas V. Anatomical risks of transobturator suburethral tape in the treatment of female stress urinary incontinence. *Eur Urol.* 2005;48:793–798.

14. Jelovsek JE, Sokol AI, Barber MD, Paraiso MF, Walters MD. Anatomic relationships of infracoccygeal sacropexy (posterior intravaginal slingplasty) trocar insertion. *Am J Obstet Gynecol.* 2005;193:2099–2104.

15. Ramsden CE, McDaniel MC, Harmon RL, Renney KM, Faure A. Pudendal nerve entrapment as source of intractable perineal pain. *Am J Phys Med Rehabil.* 2003;82(6): 479–484.

16. Fisher HW, Lotze PM. Nerve injury locations during retropubic sling procedures. *Int UrogynEcol J Pelvic Floor Dysfunct.* 2011;22(4):439–441.

17. Lien KC, Morgan DM, Delancey JO, Ashton-Miller JA. Pudendal nerve stretch during vaginal birth: a 3D computer simulation. *Am J Obstet Gynecol.* 2005;192(5):1669–1676.

18. Antolak DJ, Hough DM, Pawlina W. The chronic pelvic pain syndrome after brachytherapy for carcinoma of the prostate. *J Urol.* 2002;167:2525.

19. Howard EJ. Postherpetic pudendal neuralgia. *JAMA.* 1985; 253(15):2196.

20. Hsu ES. Practical management of complex regional pain syndrome. *Am J Ther.* 2009;16(2):147–154.

21. Waldinger MD, Venema PL, van Gils AP, Schweitzer DH. New insights into restless genital syndrome: static mechanical hyperesthesia and neuropathy of the nervus dorsalis clitoridis. *J Sex Med.* 2009;6(10):2778–2787.

22. Potts JM, Stanley Jr A. *Genitourinary Pain and Inflammation.* Cleveland, OH: Humana Press; 2008:39–56.

23. Labat JJ, Riant T, Robert R, Amarenco G, Lefaucheur JP, Rigaud J. Diagnostic criteria for pudendal neuralgia by pudendal nerve entrapement (Nantes Criteria). *Neurourol Urodyn.* 2008;27:306–310.

24. Labat JJ, Robert R, Delavierre D, Sibert L, Rigaud J. Symptomatic approach to chronic neuropathic somatic pelvic and perineal pain. *Prog Urol.* 2010;20(12):973–981.

25. Labat JJ, Robert R, Bensignor M, Buzelin JM. Neuralgia of the pudendal nerve. Anatomo-clinical considerations and therapeutic approach. *J Urol.* 1990;96(5):239–244.

26. Byrne PJ, Quill R, Keeling PWN. Pudendal nerve neuropathies are extremely common in chronic constipation and faecal incontinence. *Gastroenterology.* 1998;114(suppl S).

27. Beco J, Mouchel J, Mouchel T, Spinosa JP. Concerns about the use of colour Doppler in the diagnosis of pudendal nerve entrapment. *Pain.* 2009;145(1–2):261. author reply 2.

28. Le Tallec de Certaines H, Veillard D, Dugast J, et al. Comparison between the terminal motor pudendal nerve terminal motor latency, the localization of the perineal neuralgia and the result of infiltrations. Analysis of 53 patients. *Ann Readapt Med Phys.* 2007;50(2):65–69.

29. Olsen AL, Ross M, Stansfield RB, Kreiter C. Pelvic floor nerve conduction studies: establishing clinically relevant normative data. *Am J Obstet Gynecol.* 2003;189(4):1114–1119.

30. Amarenco G, Ismael SS, Bayle B, Denys P, Kerdraon J. Electrophysiological analysis of pudendal neuropathy following traction. *Muscle Nerve.* 2001;24:116–119.

31. Vodusek DB, Light JK, Libby JM. Detrusor inhibition induced by stimulation of pudendal nerve afferents. *Neurourol Urodyn.* 1986;5:381.

32. Ricchiutu VS, Haas CA, Seftel AD, et al. Pudendal nerve injury associated with avid bicycling. *J Urol.* 2000;162: 2099–2100.

33. Abbott J. Gynecological indications for the use of botulinum toxin in women with chronic pelvic pain. *Toxicon.* 2009;54(5):647–653.

34. Prendergast SA, Rummer EH. The role of physical therapy in the treatment of pudendal neuralgia. *Vision.* 2007;15: 1–2.

35. Benson JT, Griffis K. Pudendal neuralgia, a severe pain syndrome. *Am J Obstet Gynecol.* 2005;192(5):1663–1668.

36. Cifu DX, Kaelin D, Kowalske K, Lew H, Miller M, Ragnarsson K, et al. *Braddom's Physical Medicine & Rehabilitation.* Philadelphia, Pa: Elsevier; 2016, 845-849.e3.

37. Fanucci E, Manenti G, Ursone A, et al. Role of interventional radiology in pudendal neuralgia: a description of techniques and review of the literature. *Radiol Med.* 2009; 114(3):425–436.

38. Chowdhury S, Trescot A. *Peripheral Nerve Entrapments: Clinical Diagnosis and Management.* Switzerland: Springer International Publishing; 2016:499–514.

39. Abdi S, Shenouda P, Patel N, Saini B, Bharat Y, Calvillo O. A novel technique for pudendal nerve block. *Pain Physician.* 2004;7(3):319–322.

40. Bellingham GA, Bhatia A, Chan CW, Peng P. Randomized controlled trial comparing pudendal nerve block under ultrasound and fluoroscopic guidance. *Reg Anesth Pain Med.*

2012;37(3):262−266. https://doi.org/10.1097/aap.0b013e318248c51d.

41. Mamlouk MD, van Sonnenberg E, Dehkarghani S. CT-guided nerve block for pudendal neuralgia: diagnostic and therapeutic implications. *AJR Am J Roentgenol.* 2014; 203(1):196−200.

42. Filippiadis DK, Velonakis G, Mazioti A, et al. CT-guided percutaneous infiltration for the treatment of Alcock's neuralgia. *Pain Physician.* 2011;14(2):211−215.

43. Frank CE, Flaxman T, Goddard Y, Chen I, Zhu C, Singh SS. The use of PulsedPulsed radiofrequency for the treatment of pudendal neuralgia: a case series. *J Obstet Gynaecol Can.* 2019;41(11):1558−1563.

44. Rhame EE, Levey KA, Gharibo CG. Successful treatment of refractory pudendal neuralgia with pulsed radiofrequency. *Pain Physician.* 2009;12:633−638.

45. Shi Y, Wu W. Treatment of neuropathic pain using pulsed radiofrequency: a meta-analysis. *Pain Physician.* 2016;19: 429−444.

46. Ozkan D, Akkaya T, Yildiz S, et al. Ultrasound-guided pulsed radiofrequency treatment of the pudendal nerve in chronic pelvic pain. *Anaesthesist.* 2016;65:134−136.

47. Prologo JD, Lin RC, Williams R, Corn D. Percutaneous CT-guided cryoablation for the treatment of refractory pudendal neuralgia. *Skeletal Radiol.* 2015;44(5):709−714.

48. Moore DM, Mccrory C. Spinal cord stimulation. *BJA Educ.* 2016;16(8):258−263. https://doi.org/10.1093/bjaed/mkv072.

49. Buffenoir K, Rioult B, Hamel O, Labat J-J, Riant T, Robert R. Spinal cord stimulation of the conus medullaris for refractory pudendal neuralgia: a prospective study of 27 consecutive cases. *Neurourol Urodyn.* 2013;34(2): 177−182. https://doi.org/10.1002/nau.22525.

50. Hunter CW, Yang A. Dorsal root ganglion stimulation for chronic pelvic pain: a case series and technical report on a novel lead configuration. *Neuromodulation.* 2019;22(1): 87−95. https://doi.org/10.1111/ner.12801. Epub 2018 August 1.

CHAPTER 8

Postsurgical Pelvic Pain

NEWAJ ABDULLAH, MD • KRISHNA B. SHAH, MD

INTRODUCTION

Chronic pelvic pain can originate from various etiologies such as chronic prostatitis, pelvic inflammatory disease, endometriosis, vulvodynia, interstitial cystitis, and surgery in the pelvis. In this chapter, we focus on postsurgical pelvic pain in both men and women.

Chronic Postsurgical Pelvic Pain in Men

Inguinodynia: Inguinal hernia repair is the most common surgery in the United States and worldwide.[1] Each year more than 2 million of these procedures are performed worldwide, and there are over 800,000 cases done in the United States annually.[1,2] Inguinal hernia is more common in males than females.[3] The prevalence of inguinal hernia is 90.8% in males and 9.2% in females.[3] Inguinal hernia repair is the most common identifiable factor that is associated with inguinodynia.[4] Inguinodynia is a form of chronic postsurgical pain defined as persistent groin pain lasting for more than 2 months following surgery.[5] It is estimated that 10%–12% of all inguinal hernia repair patients develop moderate to severe inguinodynia, and of these patients, approximately 6% develop chronic debilitating pain that negatively impacts their activities of daily living and employment.[1,6–8]

Chronic Orchialgia: Chronic orchialgia is described as testicular discomfort that can range from a heavy sensation in the groin to frank pain.[4] A complaint of orchialgia is considered to be chronic when the discomfort lasts for more than 3 months.[4,9,10] Vasectomy is a well-known risk factor for the development of chronic orchialgia. Fifty million men undergo vasectomy procedures annually worldwide, with over 500,000 cases being performed in the United States.[4,9–11] It is estimated that 1%–2% of men who undergo vasectomies will develop chronic orchialgia, with some studies reporting incidence rates as high as 54%.[12–15] Besides vasectomy, surgical repair of the varicose pampiniform plexus can cause nerve damage as well and

lead to chronic orchialgia.[11] Nerve injury from inguinal hernia repairs can also cause chronic orchialgia.[5]

Pelvic Pain from Other Postsurgical Etiology: There is a paucity of data in the literature on the incidence of pelvic pain after other types of pelvic surgeries in men such as radical prostatectomy and cystectomy. These surgeries often require extensive lymph node dissection in the pelvis and dissection around major nerves such as the obturator nerve.[16,17] For instance, nerve-sparing prostatectomies require careful dissection of the neurovascular bundle around the lateral wall of the prostate.[18] These surgical maneuvers can potentially lead to nerve injury and the development of neuropathic pain. Furthermore, postoperative adhesions that develop after these surgeries can lead to visceral or somatic pain in the pelvis.

Chronic Postsurgical Pelvic Pain in Women

Chronic Postsurgical Pain after Cesarean Section: Chronic pain after the cesarean section was not well studied until 2004.[19] Numerous studies have emerged since then, establishing the association between chronic pain and cesarean deliveries.[20,21] Chronic pain after cesarean section persists for 3 months after delivery and can be at the scar site, localized deep in the pelvis, or at the anterior abdominal wall below the umbilicus and buttock.[22] Based on the current literature, the prevalence of chronic pain, either at the scar site or in the pelvis, at 6 months postcesarean section ranges from 12% to 18%.[19–22] The prevalence of disabling pain has ranged from 4% to 7% with an associated decline in the quality of life for the mother and mother–child relationship.[19–22] With rates of cesarean section on the rise, recognizing the importance of prevention and treatment of postoperative pelvic pain is paramount.[23]

Chronic Postsurgical Pain after Hysterectomy: Hysterectomy is a common surgery in women. According to the Center for Disease Control, there are over 600,000 hysterectomies performed every year in the United

Interventional Management of Chronic Visceral Pain Syndromes. https://doi.org/10.1016/B978-0-323-75775-1.00002-7

States.[24] Similar to the cesarean section, hysterectomy is associated with the development of chronic pain in the pelvis and at the scar site.[25] Posthysterectomy pelvic pain in women between the age 18 and 49 is 14% in the United States and 24% in the United Kingdom.[25−27] The prevalence is reported to be higher in other countries. For example, based on Danish Hysterectomy Database, posthysterectomy pelvic pain was reported by 31% of patients 1 year after surgery.[25]

ETIOLOGY AND PATHOGENESIS

The mechanisms underlying the development of chronic postsurgical pelvic pain is complex and poorly understood. Almost all forms of chronic postsurgical pain have attributes of both neuropathic and non-neuropathic pain.[2,28] Neuropathic pain after surgery is thought to be caused by damage to nerves. In the case of inguinodynia and vasectomy-related orchialgia, injury to the iliohypogastric, ilioinguinal, and genitofemoral nerves have been implicated.[2,6,28] In surgeries involving deep pelvic organs such as prostatectomy, cystectomy, hysterectomy, and cesarean section, injury to nerves that course through the pelvis (i.e., obturator nerve) are thought to mediate the development of postsurgical pelvic pain.[16−18,22,25] In animal studies, it has been shown that damage to nerves results in the release of inflammatory chemicals.[29] These inflammatory chemicals alter gene expression and produce a state of continuous noxious signal transmission to the higher brain that results in long-term neuroplastic changes.[29]

Damage to nerves can occur intraoperatively from surgical manipulation, leading to subsequent stretch or crush injuries.[28] The use of electrocautery in the nearby vicinity can also cause thermal injury and accidental transection of the nerves.[28] One common etiology for intraoperative nerve injury is from entrapment of the nerve in suture or tacks used to secure the mesh in the case of hernia repair.[28] Nearby neurovascular structures are vulnerable to injury postoperatively as well. Postoperative changes such as fibrosis, meshoma, seroma formation, and adhesions can entrap and impinge nearby neurovascular bundles.[30]

In addition to neuropathic pain, patients can also experience visceral and somatic pain.[31] Somatic pain can occur with recurrence of the pathology such as recurrence of an inguinal hernia. More commonly, somatic pain arises due to the formation of excessive fibrotic tissue, meshoma, or postoperative adhesion

tissues pulling and distorting nearby structures such as the bowel and ovaries.[32] Surgical changes can also entrap the spermatic cord or impinge on the venous flow of the testicle and spermatic cords. This can lead to orchialgia and pain during sexual intercourse.[33,34] Periostitis pubis is characterized by persistent lower abdominal pain and tenderness over the pubis.[30] This is thought to occur due to periosteal anchoring of the mesh during inguinal hernia repair.[30]

CLINICAL FEATURES

Patients with chronic postsurgical pelvic pain present with a wide array of symptomatology. Neuropathic pain usually manifests as neuralgia, hypo/hyperesthesia, hyperalgesia, paresthesia, and allodynia.[28] Patients commonly describe their symptoms as stabbing, burning, pulling, shooting, and prickling in nature.[35] The duration of these symptoms can range from intermittent to constant.[2,35]

As previously mentioned, depending on the etiology, these symptoms can be localized to the deep pelvis, anterior abdominal wall below the umbilicus, inguinal canal, the scrotum or labium, and anterior thigh.[2] In the case of inguinodynia, patients often find their pain to be worse with ambulation, stretching of the upper body, stooping, hyperextension of the hip, or sexual intercourse.[2,28,32] Pain generally improves with laying down and with flexion of the hip or thigh.[28] In the case of chronic orchialgia, patients present with heaviness in the scrotum, pain involving the testicles, and pain with sexual intercourse.[36] These patients generally report that their scrotal pain is aggravated when sitting down.[36] Pain from other pelvic surgeries can present as neuropathic pain at the incision site or deep in the pelvis. Many patients will also report dull and aching discomfort in the pelvis described as pounding, gnawing or pulling.[32] Patients with periostitis pubis from inguinal hernia repair often have tender points at the level of the pubis and associated abdominal pain.[31]

DIAGNOSIS

Clinical features of chronic postsurgical pelvic pain are nonspecific and are shared by a wide array of pathologies. Therefore, evaluation of a patient with chronic pelvic pain after surgery should begin with a broad differential, and a diagnosis is made after excluding other critical pathologies. Evaluation should begin with a comprehensive clinical history and physician exam, ascertaining any history of recent pelvic surgery. One should be cautious to diagnose chronic postsurgical pelvic pain within the first few months after surgery because wound recovery can take several months even after an external surgical scar has healed, and the perceived pain may emanate from the healing process.

Clinical history should delineate the nature and chronicity of the pain. Chronic postsurgical pelvic pain can be neuropathic or nonneuropathic in nature and can be intermittent or persistent; however, the symptoms must be present for 2—3 months to receive a formal diagnosis of chronic postsurgical pelvic pain. Imaging studies can be helpful to rule out other pathologies and assess the presence of meshoma and excessive fibrotic tissues.[37,38] Ultrasound, computed tomography (CT), and magnetic resonance imaging (MRI) have all been utilized as well.[37,38] MRI has been touted as the superior imaging modality for delineating the cause of pain.[28,37,38] Electromyography can detect and rule out peripheral nerve injury.[39] Diagnostic peripheral nerve blocks can also be helpful to identify the source and nerve distribution of the pain.[2,28]

TREATMENT
Noninterventional Therapies
As previously described, chronic postsurgical pelvic pain is complex, with emotional, cognitive, and social factors playing a large role in the development and evolution of the pain syndrome. Therefore, treatment for this condition should be multimodal in approach and include components of psychotherapy, physiotherapy, acupuncture, and mind-body therapies.[2,9]

Pharmacologic treatment options include nonsteroidal anti-inflammatory drugs and steroids.[2,9,40] These agents work by reducing inflammation, but due to their side effect profile, long-term use is limited. The most commonly used agents for associated neuropathic pain disorders are gabapentinoids (i.e., gabapentin and pregablin), selective serotonin and norepinephrine reuptake inhibitors (SNRIs), and tricyclic antidepressants.[2,9,40] Gabapentinoids act as voltage-gated calcium channel antagonists that decrease the release of glutamate and are used for the treatment of many neuropathic pain syndromes, including fibromyalgia; it has also been shown to decrease the

incidence of chronic pain development when given preoperatively.[2,9] Duloxetine and venlafaxine are SNRIs recommended as first-line agents for neuropathic pain syndromes by the International Association for the Study of Pain.[2,40] These agents are low cost and have the added benefit of treating coexisting mood disorders in addition to neuropathic pain.[2]

Because traditional neuropathic agents take time (up to several weeks) to have an adequate analgesic effect, weak opioids such as tramadol can be utilized for episodic exacerbation during titration of these agents.[2] In general, we do not recommend the use of chronic opioids for the treatment of chronic nonmalignancy pain syndromes. However, when judiciously utilized, the lowest effective dose should be given with regular follow up.[2,40]

Nerve Blocks
Nerve blocks are utilized for diagnostic and therapeutic purposes in the setting of inguinodynia and orchialgia.[2,28] Historically, nerve blocks were performed using anatomic landmarks; however, most blocks are now performed under direct visualization using ultrasound guidance.[2]

Ilioinguinal nerve and iliohypogastric nerve provides overlapping sensory innervation involving the hypogastric region, the inguinal crease, the upper medial thigh, the mons pubis, part of labia, and the anterior aspect of the scrotum.[41,42] Ultrasound-guided ilioinguinal nerve and iliohypogastric nerve blocks are effective for inguinodynia. Fig. 8.1 shows an ultrasound image of these two nerves.[43] In a study by Thomassen and colleagues, the authors demonstrated prolonged pain relief for up to 20 months with ultrasound-guided ilioinguinal and iliohypogastric nerve blocks for inguinodynia.[44] It is important to note that due to the proximity of ilioinguinal and iliohypogastric nerves it is difficult to isolate and block the two nerves separately.[42,43]

Numerous case reports have demonstrated ultrasoundguided genitofemoral nerves block for orchialgia as well as inguinodynia; however, in most of these cases, the needle placement and block were distal to the site of injury or entrapment.[45,46] Genitofemoral nerve courses retroperitoneally before entering the inguinal canal; and therefore, any attempt to block this nerve proximal to the site of injury using anterior approach increases the risk of traversing the peritoneum.[47] Currently, there is no case report that

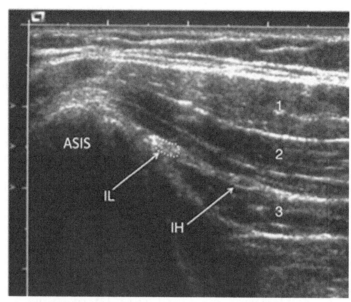

FIG. 8.1 US image shows the ilioinguinal (IL) and iliohypogastric (IH) nerves between the internal oblique (2) and transverse abdominal (3) muscles. To perform this block, a high-frequency US transducer is placed with the inferior end over the ASIS and superior end oriented in an oblique plane toward the umbilicus.   1, external oblique muscle; 2, internal oblique muscle; 3, transverse abdominal muscle; *ASIS*, anterior superior iliac spine.

demonstrates ultrasound-guided technique for selective genitofemoral nerve block proximal to the site of nerve injury. With that said, CT-guided transpsoas genitofemoral nerve block has been demonstrated and is a promising technique to safely block genitofemoral nerve proximal to the site of nerve injury.[47]

While inguinodynia and orchialgia are mediated by the ilioinguinal, iliohypogastric, and genitofemoral nerves, pain from the deep pelvis is mediated by the superior hypogastric plexus, ganglion impar, and pudendal nerve.[48–51] Although less commonly seen, if postoperative pain in the distribution of these nerves is suspected, a block may be done for diagnostic and treatment purposes.

Neurolysis Techniques

Neuroablation with chemical neurolysis, cryoablation, or pulsed radiofrequency can be used to mitigate various forms of chronic postsurgical pelvic pain conditions. Such neurolytic techniques are attempted when nerve blocks have proven to be beneficial and patient desires longer relief.

Cryoablation: Cryoablation involves percutaneously placing a hollow probe near the targeted nerve and applying freezing temperatures, causing nerve destruction via Wallerian degeneration where the axon and myelin sheaths are selectively destroyed leaving behind intact perineurium and epineurium.[2,28,52] This prevents neuroma formation and the subsequent development of deafferentation pain. Numerous studies have demonstrated the efficacy of cryoablation for the treatment of inguinodynia. In a study by Fanelli and colleagues, nine patients with inguinodynia underwent cryoablation of ilioinguinal or genitofemoral nerve under direct surgical visualization and experienced a 77.5% pain reduction from this procedure.[52] In another report by Campos and colleagues, cryoablation of the femoral branch of the genitofemoral nerve was successfully used to treat inguinal pain.[53] Cryoablation can provide up to 1 year of sustained relief.

Radiofrequency ablation: Radiofrequency ablation can also be used to treat inguinodynia and orchialgia. Pulsed radiofrequency ablation uses bursts of high-intensity currents to heat the nerve tissue up to 42°C, thereby inducing thermal destruction of the nerve.[54] The nerve tissue is allowed to cool between the bursts of heat, thereby preventing uncontrolled tissue damage and the subsequent development of neuroma, neuritis, and deafferentation pain.[54] Rozen and colleagues published two reports where pulsed radiofrequency was applied to the T12, L1, and L2 nerve roots for the treatment of inguinodynia.[55,56] Patients experienced 75%−100% pain reduction that lasted for 6−9 months.[55,56] Pulsed radiofrequency ablation has been used to ablate peripheral nerves as well. In their studies, Cohen and Foster successfully treated three patients with inguinodynia by ablating the ilioinguinal nerve and iliohypogastric nerves.[57] To perform the ablation, Cohen and colleagues used anatomic landmark techniques for needle placement and used sensory neurostimulation to confirm the targeted nerve.[57] Patients reported complete pain resolution at 6 months follow-up.[57] In another study by Mitra and colleagues, inguinodynia was treated with pulsed radiofrequency ablation of the ilioinguinal nerve using anatomic landmark and sensory neurostimulation techniques.[58] In their study, the patient reported a significant reduction in visual analog scale (VAS) score from 8/10 to 3/10 at 3-month follow-up.[58]

Chemical neurolysis: Compared to cryoablation and pulsed radiofrequency ablation, chemical neurolysis with phenol or alcohol is less frequently reported in the literature.[2] These neurolytic agents are more prone to cause nearby tissue damage; therefore, their use is typically reserved for cancer-related visceral pelvic pain.[48,49] However, neurolysis of the superior hypogastric plexus and the ganglion impar have been utilized for severe cases of refractory visceral pelvic pain from nonmalignant etiologies.[48]

Neuromodulation

Neuromodulation is an alternative approach for the treatment of chronic postsurgical pelvic pain refractory to pharmacologic and other interventional therapies. Neuromodulation techniques include stimulation of the spinal cord, dorsal root ganglion, and peripheral nerves.[2,48] Traditionally based on the "gate control" theory of pain where nonpainful sensory inputs effectively "gate" off ascending pain signals, stimulation-based therapies deliver electrical impulses to ameliorate pain perception.[2] The mechanisms and details of spinal cord stimulators are discussed in more detail in other chapters of this textbook. Traditionally used for chronic back pain, radicular pain,

and complex regional pain syndrome, neuromodulation therapies are now being applied for the treatment of chronic pelvic pain syndromes as well.

Peripheral Nerve and Dorsal Column Stimulation: Numerous case reports and case series have demonstrated the efficacy of peripheral nerve and dorsal column stimulation for treating inguinodynia and orchialgia. In a case report, Rosendal and colleagues used low-frequency peripheral nerve stimulation of the cutaneous branch of the ilioinguinal nerve and the genital branch of the genitofemoral nerves to treat chronic scrotal pain following a hydrocele repair.[59] The patient's VAS score decreased from 9/10 to 2/10 on the numeric rating scale at a 7-month follow-up.[59] In another report, Banh and colleagues used ilioinguinal nerve stimulation to treat ilioinguinal neuralgia following hernia repair.[60] In this report, patients had minimal pain on 3-months follow-up and were taken off all analgesics, including opioids.[60]

Yakovlev and colleagues used traditional tonic spinal cord stimulation with percutaneous electrode leads placed at the T7−T9 level to successfully treat inguinodynia.[61] In their study, the patient remained pain-free at 1-year follow-up.

Dorsal Root Ganglion Stimulation: Stimulation of the dorsal roots ganglion (DRG) is an alternative treatment modality that has recently increased in popularity, particularly for the treatment of chronic pain disorders in areas that have been difficult to treat with traditional dorsal column stimulation, such as the foot, abdomen, and groin. The DRG is a collection of sensory nerve cell bodies that are located bilaterally at each spinal level and can be accessed percutaneously for focused stimulation of particular dermatomes. Each lead contains four stimulating electrodes that are advanced from the epidural space to the intervertebral foramen where the DRG is located as shown in Fig. 8.2. The number and the respective levels at which the leads are placed is typically dependent on the dermatomal distribution of the patient's pain as shown in Fig. 8.3.[62] Moreover, compared to dorsal column stimulators, DRG stimulation requires less overall energy since the cerebrospinal fluid layer at the level of the DRG is relatively thin. There is also less risk of the patient experiencing unwanted paresthesia with positional changes compared to dorsal column stimulators.

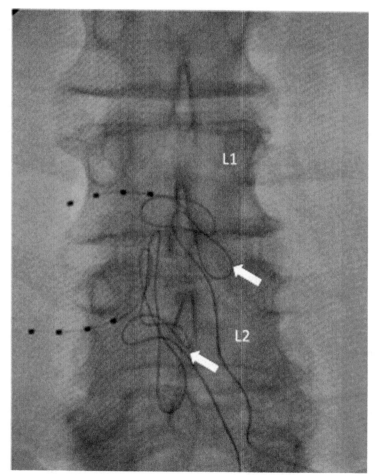

FIG. 8.2 DRG stimulator leads placed under fluoroscopy. Percutaneous DRG lead placement at the left L1 and L2 intervertebral foramens for treatment of pelvic girdle pain. Extraneous strain-relief loops in the epidural space (white arrows) serve to reduce the risk of lead migration.

This technology has been successfully used for the treatment of inguinodynia and chronic pelvic pain. In a case report by Rowland and colleagues, DRG stimulation at the L1 and L2 levels was used for refractory pelvic girdle pain. In this case report, the authors reported that the patient had a 43% reduction in pain at 6 months follow-up.[63] In another multicenter study, Schu and colleagues reported on 29 patients with inguinodynia who underwent dorsal root ganglion implantation between T12 and L4.[64] Nineteen of these patients over 50% pain relief at average follow-up time of 27 weeks.

CONCLUSION
Chronic postsurgical pelvic pain is an unwelcomed consequence that can occur after surgeries in the pelvis or its vicinity. Current approaches for the treatment of this condition include behavioral and pharmacological therapies as well as interventional procedures. Although many of these approaches have shown positive results in the short term, there is a paucity of data on long-term outcomes of available therapies. Future efforts should aim for identifying long-term outcomes of currently available therapies.

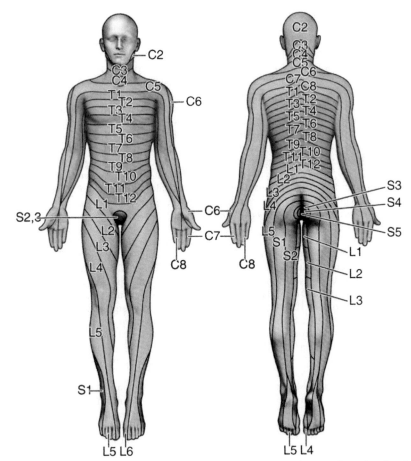

FIG. 8.3 Human dermatome map. (Reproduced from K. Candido, R. Stevens Best Practice & Research Clinical Anaesthesiology, 17:3, 407-428, 2003.)

REFERENCES

1. Alfieri S, Amid PK, Campanelli G, et al. International guidelines for prevention and management of postoperative chronic pain following inguinal hernia surgery. *Hernia J Hernias Abdom Wall Surg.* 2011;15(3):239–249. https://doi.org/10.1007/s10029-011-0798-9.

2. Bjurstrom MF, Nicol AL, Amid PK, Chen DC. Pain control following inguinal herniorrhaphy: current perspectives. *J Pain Res.* 2014;7:277–290. https://doi.org/10.2147/JPR.S47005.

3. Burcharth J, Pedersen M, Bisgaard T, Pedersen C, Rosenberg J. Nationwide prevalence of groin hernia repair. *PLoS One.* 2013;8(1). https://doi.org/10.1371/journal.pone.0054367.

4. Belanger GV, VerLee GT. Diagnosis and surgical management of male pelvic, inguinal, and testicular pain. *Surg Clin N Am.* 2016;96(3):593–613. https://doi.org/10.1016/j.suc.2016.02.014.

5. Macrae W, Devies H. Chronic post-surgical pain. In: Crombie IK, Croft PR, Linton SJ, Leresche L, Korff MV, eds. *Epidemiology of Pain: A Report of the Task Force on Epidemiology of the International Association for the Study of Pain.* 1st ed. IASP Press; 1999.

6. Poobalan AS, Bruce J, Smith WCS, King PM, Krukowski ZH, Chambers WA. A review of chronic pain after inguinal herniorrhaphy. *Clin J Pain.* 2003;19(1):48–54. https://doi.org/10.1097/00002508-200301000-00006.

7. Nienhuijs S, Staal E, Strobbe L, Rosman C, Groenewoud H, Bleichrodt R. Chronic pain after mesh repair of inguinal hernia: a systematic review. *Am J Surg.* 2007;194(3):394–400. https://doi.org/10.1016/j.amjsurg.2007.02.012.

8. Aasvang E, Kehlet H. Chronic postoperative pain: the case of inguinal herniorrhaphy. *Br J Anaesth.* 2005;95(1):69–76. https://doi.org/10.1093/bja/aei019.

9. Tan WP, Levine LA. What can we do for chronic scrotal content pain? *World J Mens Health.* 2017;35(3):146–155. https://doi.org/10.5534/wjmh.17047.

10. Calixte N, Brahmbhatt J, Parekattil S. Chronic testicular and groin pain: pathway to relief. *Curr Urol Rep.* 2017;18(10):83. https://doi.org/10.1007/s11934-017-0722-7.

11. Curran N. Chronic urogenital pain in men. *Rev Pain.* 2008; 2(2):25–28. https://doi.org/10.1177/204946370800200207.

12. Sharlip ID, Belker AM, Honig S, et al. Vasectomy: AUA guideline. *J Urol.* 2012;188(6 Suppl):2482–2491. https://doi.org/10.1016/j.juro.2012.09.080.

13. Leslie TA, Illing RO, Cranston DW, Guillebaud J. The incidence of chronic scrotal pain after vasectomy: a prospective audit. *BJU Int.* 2007;100(6):1330–1333. https://doi.org/10.1111/j.1464-410X.2007.07128.x.

14. Christiansen CG, Sandlow JI. Testicular pain following vasectomy: a review of postvasectomy pain syndrome. *J Androl.* 2003;24(3):293–298. https://doi.org/10.1002/j.1939-4640.2003.tb02675.x.

15. Morris C, Mishra K, Kirkman RJE. A study to assess the prevalence of chronic testicular pain in post-vasectomy men compared to non-vasectomised men. *J Fam Plann Reprod Health Care.* 2002;28(3):142–144. https://doi.org/10.1783/147118902101196298.

16. Fossati N, Willemse P-PM, Van den Broeck T, et al. The benefits and harms of different extents of lymph node dissection during radical prostatectomy for prostate cancer: a systematic review. *Eur Urol.* 2017;72(1):84–109. https://doi.org/10.1016/j.eururo.2016.12.003.

17. Sundi D, Svatek RS, Nielsen ME, Schoenberg MP, Bivalacqua TJ. Extent of pelvic lymph node dissection during radical cystectomy: is bigger better? *Rev Urol.* 2014; 16(4):159–166.

18. Tavukçu HH, Aytac O, Atug F. Nerve-sparing techniques and results in robot-assisted radical prostatectomy. *Investig Clin Urol.* 2016;57(Suppl 2):S172–S184. https://doi.org/10.4111/icu.2016.57.S2.S172.

19. Nikolajsen L, Sørensen HC, Jensen TS, Kehlet H. Chronic pain following caesarean section. *Acta Anaesthesiol Scand.* 2004;48(1):111–116. https://doi.org/10.1111/j.1399-6576.2004.00271.x.

20. Petrou S, Kim SW, McParland P, Boyle EM. Mode of delivery and long-term health-related quality-of-life outcomes: a prospective population-based study. *Birth Berkeley Calif.* 2017;44(2):110–119. https://doi.org/10.1111/birt.12268.

21. Yimer H, Woldie H. Incidence and associated factors of chronic pain after caesarean section: a systematic review. *J Obstet Gynecol Can.* 2019;41(6):840–854. https://doi.org/10.1016/j.jogc.2018.04.006.

22. Lavand'homme P. Long-term problems and chronic pain after cesarean section. In: Capogna G, ed. *Anesthesia for Cesarean Section.* Springer International Publishing; 2018: 169–180. https://doi.org/10.1007/978-3-319-42053-0.

23. Betrán AP, Ye J, Moller A-B, Zhang J, Gülmezoglu AM, Torloni MR. The increasing trend in caesarean section rates: global, regional and national estimates: 1990–2014. *PLoS One.* 2016;11(2):e0148343. https://doi.org/10.1371/journal.pone.0148343.

24. Whiteman MK, Hillis SD, Jamieson DJ, et al. Inpatient hysterectomy surveillance in the United States, 2000-2004. *Am J Obstet Gynecol.* 2008;198(1):34.e1–34.e7. https://doi.org/10.1016/j.ajog.2007.05.039.

25. Brandsborg B, Nikolajsen L, Hansen CT, Kehlet H, Jensen TS. Risk factors for chronic pain after hysterectomy: a nationwide questionnaire and database study. *Anesthesiology.* 2007;106(5):1003–1012. https://doi.org/10.1097/01.anes.0000265161.39932.e8.

26. Hartmann KE, Ma C, Lamvu GM, Langenberg PW, Steege JF, Kjerulff KH. Quality of life and sexual function after hysterectomy in women with preoperative pain and depression. *Obstet Gynecol.* 2004;104(4):701–709. https://doi.org/10.1097/01.AOG.0000140684.37428.48.

27. Gimbel H, Zobbe V, Andersen BM, Filtenborg T, Gluud C, Tabor A. Randomised controlled trial of total compared with subtotal hysterectomy with one-year follow up results. *BJOG Int J Obstet Gynaecol.* 2003;110(12): 1088–1098.

28. Hakeem A, Shanmugam V. Current trends in the diagnosis and management of post-herniorraphy chronic groin pain. *World J Gastrointest Surg.* 2011;3(6):73–81. https://doi.org/10.4240/wjgs.v3.i6.73.

29. Richebé P, Capdevila X, Rivat C. Persistent postsurgical pain: pathophysiology and preventative pharmacologic considerations. *Anesthesiology.* 2018;129(3):590–607. https://doi.org/10.1097/ALN.0000000000002238.

30. Cunningham J, Temple WJ, Mitchell P, Nixon JA, Preshaw RM, Hagen NA. Cooperative hernia study. Pain in the postrepair patient. *Ann Surg.* 1996;224(5): 598–602. https://doi.org/10.1097/00000658-199611000-00003.

31. Loos MJA, Roumen RMH, Scheltinga MRM. Classifying post-herniorrhaphy pain syndromes following elective inguinal hernia repair. *World J Surg.* 2007;31(9): 1760–1765. https://doi.org/10.1007/s00268-007-9121-4. discussion 1766-1767.

32. Heise CP, Starling JR. Mesh inguinodynia: a new clinical syndrome after inguinal herniorrhaphy? *J Am Coll Surg.* 1998;187(5):514–518. https://doi.org/10.1016/s1072-7515(98)00215-4.

33. Delikoukos S, Fafoulakis F, Christodoulidis G, Theodoropoulos T, Hatzitheofilou C. Re-operation due to severe late-onset persisting groin pain following anterior inguinal hernia repair with mesh. *Hernia J Hernias Abdom Wall Surg.* 2008;12(6):593–595. https://doi.org/10.1007/s10029-008-0392-y.

34. Wantz GE. Testicular atrophy and chronic residual neuralgia as risks of inguinal hernioplasty. *Surg Clin N Am.* 1993; 73(3):571–581. https://doi.org/10.1016/s0039-6109(16)46038-x.

35. Vuilleumier H, Hübner M, Demartines N. Neuropathy after herniorrhaphy: indication for surgical treatment and outcome. *World J Surg.* 2009;33(4):841–845. https://doi.org/10.1007/s00268-008-9869-1.

36. Aasvang EK, Møhl B, Kehlet H. Ejaculatory pain: a specific postherniotomy pain syndrome? *Anesthesiology.* 2007; 107(2):298–304. https://doi.org/10.1097/01.anes.00002 70736.28324.61.

37. Amid PK, Hiatt JR. New understanding of the causes and surgical treatment of postherniorrhaphy inguinodynia

and orchalgia. *J Am Coll Surg*. 2007;205(2):381–385. https://doi.org/10.1016/j.jamcollsurg.2007.04.001.

38. Amid PK. Radiologic images of meshoma: a new phenomenon causing chronic pain after prosthetic repair of abdominal wall hernias. *Arch Surg Chic Ill 1960*. 2004;139(12):1297–1298. https://doi.org/10.1001/archsurg.139.12.1297.

39. Kim DH, Murovic JA, Tiel RL, Kline DG. Surgical management of 33 ilioinguinal and iliohypogastric neuralgias at Louisiana State University Health Sciences Center. *Neurosurgery*. 2005;56(5):1013–1020. discussion 1013-1020.

40. Dworkin RH, O'Connor AB, Backonja M, et al. Pharmacologic management of neuropathic pain: evidence-based recommendations. *Pain*. 2007;132(3):237–251. https://doi.org/10.1016/j.pain.2007.08.033.

41. *Truncal and Cutaneous Blocks*. NYSORA; September 20, 2013. https://www.nysora.com/techniques/truncal-and-cutaneous-blocks/truncal-and-cutaneous-blocks/. Accessed May 9, 2020.

42. Hoppenfeld JD. *Fundamentals of Pain Medicine: How to Diagnose and Treat Your Patients*. Wolters Kluwer Health; 2014.

43. Schmutz M, Schumacher PM, Luyet C, Curatolo M, Eichenberger U. Ilioinguinal and iliohypogastric nerves cannot be selectively blocked by using ultrasound guidance: a volunteer study. *Br J Anaesth*. 2013;111(2):264–270. https://doi.org/10.1093/bja/aet028.

44. Thomassen I, van Suijlekom JA, van de Gaag A, Ponten JEH, Nienhuijs SW. Ultrasound-guided ilioinguinal/iliohypogastric nerve blocks for chronic pain after inguinal hernia repair. *Hernia J Hernias Abdom Wall Surg*. 2013;17(3):329–332. https://doi.org/10.1007/s10029-012-0998-y.

45. Peng PWH, Tumber PS. Ultrasound-guided interventional procedures for patients with chronic pelvic pain — a description of techniques and review of literature. *Pain Physician*. 2008;11(2):215–224.

46. Bischoff JM, Koscielniak-Nielsen ZJ, Kehlet H, Werner MU. Ultrasound-guided ilioinguinal/iliohypogastric nerve blocks for persistent inguinal postherniorrhaphy pain: a randomized, double-blind, placebo-controlled, crossover trial. *Anesth Analg*. 2012;114(6):1323–1329. https://doi.org/10.1213/ANE.0b013e31824d6168.

47. Parris D, Fischbein N, Mackey S, Carroll I. A novel CT-guided transpsoas approach to diagnostic genitofemoral nerve block and ablation. *Pain Med Malden Mass*. 2010;11(5):785–789. https://doi.org/10.1111/j.1526-4637.2010.00835.x.

48. Smith SE, Eckert JM. Interventional pain management and female pelvic pain: considerations for diagnosis and treatment. *Semin Reprod Med*. 2018;36(2):159–163. https://doi.org/10.1055/s-0038-1676104.

49. Green IC, Cohen SL, Finkenzeller D, Christo PJ. Interventional therapies for controlling pelvic pain: what is the evidence? *Curr Pain Headache Rep*. 2010;14(1):22–32. https://doi.org/10.1007/s11916-009-0089-7.

50. Plancarte R, Amescua C, Patt RB, Aldrete JA. Superior hypogastric plexus block for pelvic cancer pain. *Anesthesiology*. 1990;73(2):236–239. https://doi.org/10.1097/00000542-199008000-00008.

51. Scott-Warren JT, Hill V, Rajasekaran A. Ganglion impar blockade: a review. *Curr Pain Headache Rep*. 2013;17(1):306. https://doi.org/10.1007/s11916-012-0306-7.

52. Fanelli RD, DiSiena MR, Lui FY, Gersin KS. Cryoanalgesic ablation for the treatment of chronic postherniorrhaphy neuropathic pain. *Surg Endosc*. 2003;17(2):196–200. https://doi.org/10.1007/s00464-002-8840-8.

53. Campos NA, Chiles JH, Plunkett AR. Ultrasound-guided cryoablation of genitofemoral nerve for chronic inguinal pain. *Pain Physician*. 2009;12(6):997–1000.

54. Byrd D, Mackey S. Pulsed radiofrequency for chronic pain. *Curr Pain Headache Rep*. 2008;12(1):37–41. https://doi.org/10.1007/s11916-008-0008-3.

55. Rozen D, Ahn J. Pulsed radiofrequency for the treatment of ilioinguinal neuralgia after inguinal herniorrhaphy. *Mt Sinai J Med N Y*. 2006;73(4):716–718.

56. Rozen D, Parvez U. Pulsed radiofrequency of lumbar nerve roots for treatment of chronic inguinal herniorraphy pain. *Pain Physician*. 2006;9(2):153–156.

57. Cohen SP, Foster A. Pulsed radiofrequency as a treatment for groin pain and orchialgia. *Urology*. 2003;61(3):645. https://doi.org/10.1016/s0090-4295(02)02423-8.

58. Mitra R, Zeighami A, Mackey S. Pulsed radiofrequency for the treatment of chronic ilioinguinal neuropathy. *Hernia J Hernias Abdom Wall Surg*. 2007;11(4):369–371. https://doi.org/10.1007/s10029-007-0191-x.

59. Rosendal F, Moir L, de Pennington N, Green AL, Aziz TZ. Successful treatment of testicular pain with peripheral nerve stimulation of the cutaneous branch of the ilioinguinal and genital branch of the genitofemoral nerves. *Neuromodulation*. 2013;16(2):121–124. https://doi.org/10.1111/j.1525-1403.2011.00421.x.

60. Banh DPT, Moujan PM, Haque Q, Han T-H. Permanent implantation of peripheral nerve stimulator for combat injury-related ilioinguinal neuralgia. *Pain Physician*. 2013;16(6):E789–E791.

61. Yakovlev AE, Al Tamimi M, Barolat G, et al. Spinal cord stimulation as alternative treatment for chronic post-herniorrhaphy pain. *Neuromodulation*. 2010;13(4):288–290. https://doi.org/10.1111/j.1525-1403.2010.00276.x. discussion 291.

62. Patel S. Human dermatomes. In: Tubbs RS, ed. *Nerves and Nerve Injuries*. Elsevier/AP, Academic Press is an imprint of Elsevier; 2015.

63. Rowland DCL, Wright D, Moir L, FitzGerald JJ, Green AL. Successful treatment of pelvic girdle pain with dorsal root ganglion stimulation. *Br J Neurosurg*. 2016;30(6):685–686. https://doi.org/10.1080/02688697.2016.1208810.

64. Schu S, Gulve A, ElDabe S, et al. Spinal cord stimulation of the dorsal root ganglion for groin pain-a retrospective review. *Pain Pract Off J World Inst Pain*. 2015;15(4):293–299. https://doi.org/10.1111/papr.12194.

CHAPTER 9

Functional Anorectal Pain

MARK ABUMOUSSA, MD • M. GABRIEL HILLEGASS, MD • MERON SELASSIE, MD

INTRODUCTION

Rectal pain has been described in the medical literature for over a century. It is a frustrating medical condition for patients for a variety of reasons. Patients with rectal pain are often embarrassed and hesitant to discuss their pain with their physicians leading to a delay in care. To further compound the problem, rectal pain is often underdiagnosed and not well understood by clinicians.[1] Patients are treated by a variety of specialists including psychiatrists, urologists, gynecologists, gastroenterologists, and proctologists. In the majority of cases, no specific etiology is found. This chapter aims to discuss the clinical features and treatment options for proctalgia fugax and levator ani syndrome, collectively known as functional anorectal pain disorders. Due to patients' reticence on this topic, healthcare providers should welcome and encourage open discussion with their patients experiencing rectal pain.

ETIOLOGY AND PATHOGENESIS

The rectum begins at the S3 level as a continuation of the sigmoid colon and has two major flexures: the sacral flexure and the anorectal flexure. The sacral flexure is an anteroposterior curve that concaves anteriorly while the anorectal flexure is an anteroposterior curve with convexity posteriorly. It is the latter flexure that is the main contributor to fecal incontinence as its tone is provided by the puborectalis muscle.[2] The rectum ends in an expanded section called the ampulla which temporarily stores feces until defecation can occur through the anal canal.

The rectum receives both sensory and autonomic innervations. Autonomic innervation originates via lumbar splanchnic nerves that ultimately terminate in the superior and inferior hypogastric plexuses. Rectal branches from the inferior hypogastric plexus accompany rectal vessels to their destination in the rectum. Somatic afferent and efferent innervation of the rectum involves sacral nerve roots originating from S2—S4. The pudendal nerve primarily provides sensation to the anal canal as well as other structures in the perineal area. Furthermore, S4—S5 nerve roots in the form of the coccygeal plexus distribute afferent and efferent nerve fibers to perianal and perineal skin.[3] It is important to note that when presented with complaints of perianal/rectal pain, clinicians must rule out structural causes that may have a coinciding symptom of rectal pain, such as tumors of the gastrointestinal tract and pelvis. This chapter will focus on proctalgia fugax and levator ani syndrome. They are diagnoses of exclusion and consequently are often misdiagnosed.

CLINICAL FEATURES

Proctalgia fugax (PF) is a nonmalignant syndrome that causes sharp, severe, intermittent pain that is localized to the anus and lower rectum.[4] This syndrome is characterized by paroxysms of rectal pain with pain-free periods lasting seconds to minutes in between attacks. Patients often report that suppositories or a digit in the rectum can abort an attack. The origin of this pain is unknown; however, it is hypothesized that spasms of the levator ani muscle, anal sphincter, and sigmoid colon may play a role.[5]

PF has equal prevalence in males and females. It is seen more frequently in patients who suffer from other bowel disorders such as irritable bowel syndrome. PF typically does not present before puberty and does not usually have an identifiable trigger, which can be a source of anxiety and depression for patients. Precipitants of pain include sexual activity, stress, constipation, defecation, and menstruation.[3] It has also been associated with sclerotherapy for hemorrhoids and after vaginal hysterectomies.[6]

Levator ani syndrome (LAS) is characterized by frequent, dull, and relatively constant anorectal pain that is unexplained by an organic cause. Frequently, patients are tender to palpation over the levator ani muscle. Other names for this syndrome include levator spasm, puborectalis syndrome, chronic proctalgia, and pelvic tension myalgia. Observations of this syndrome

Interventional Management of Chronic Visceral Pain Syndromes. https://doi.org/10.1016/B978-0-323-75775-1.00022-2

suggest that patients have increased anal pressures measured by increased electromyogram activity.[7] It is unclear if the higher anal pressures are a result of increased external or internal anal sphincter tone. It has also been suggested that the observed inability to relax pelvic floor muscles in this syndrome implicates an underlying pelvic floor dysfunction.[8]

DIAGNOSIS

The diagnosis of PF is based on characteristic symptoms in the absence of pelvic and anorectal pathology. Criteria are 12 weeks of characteristic symptoms accompanied by the following[9]:

- Recurrent episodes of pain localized to anus or lower rectum
- Episodes that last from seconds to minutes
- No anorectal pain in between episodes

Laboratory tests are largely normal in patients with PF and accompany the nonspecific physical exam findings described above. As a result, the diagnosis of PF requires the clinician to rule out other causes of anorectal pain including hemorrhoids, cryptitis, ischemia, abscess, anal fissure, rectocele, and malignant disease such as rectal cancer.[4] Screening tests such as CBC, ESR, and stool occult blood testing are indicated to screen for possible malignant disease or hematologic disorders. Magnetic resonance imaging and computed tomography should be pursued if suspicion of other diagnoses is high.

In LAS, patients often describe the pain as vague, dull, or a pressure sensation high in the rectum. Sitting usually exacerbates the pain and some patients report warm compresses alleviate the pain.[10]

As with PF, it is important to rule out organic anorectal or pelvic pathology (e.g., Crohn's disease, anal fissures, malignancy). Appropriate testing to exclude these diagnoses should be performed (sigmoidoscopy, ultrasound, pelvic MRI, etc.). Diagnosis is based on meeting the following criteria, with these symptoms lasting at least 12 weeks[9]:

- Chronic or recurrent dull rectal pain or aching
- Episodes lasting 20 min or longer
- Other causes of rectal pain ruled out including ischemia, IBD, cryptitis, fissure, hemorrhoids, prostatitis, etc.

Diagnosis is more likely if patients experience the above symptoms with corresponding physical exam findings. The absence of tenderness to levator ani palpation makes the diagnosis less likely. It is important to note that these patients may also have coinciding mood disorders and catastrophizing behavior commonly seen in chronic pain patients.

PHYSICAL EXAM FINDINGS

A physical exam is largely normal in patients suffering from PF. Patients may appear depressed or anxious as a byproduct of their pain. Along with depression and anxiety, patients with PF may exhibit catastrophizing behaviors manifesting as rumination, magnification, or helplessness about their pain condition. Rectal exams are often normal, but deep palpation may trigger an event.

On physical exam of patients with LAS, the provider may palpate contracted levator ani muscles and patients report tenderness with posterior traction of the puborectalis muscle. In the literature, it is reported that tenderness is asymmetric and the left side may be affected more than the right side.[10] If patients meet clinical criteria for LAS but have absent levator muscle tenderness on palpation, then they are said to have unspecified functional anorectal pain.

TREATMENT

Treatment of functional rectal pain disorders is challenging due in part to psychosocial comorbid conditions that may hamper progress. When available, multidisciplinary pain rehabilitation programs should be utilized in these patients that integrate teams of physical, occupational, and cognitive-behavioral therapists in an outpatient setting. These programs aim to improve physical deconditioning and eliminate an overreliance on medication or health care systems to manage symptoms. Efficacy has been demonstrated in functional abdominal pain syndromes and shows promise for management of pelvic pain among other chronic pain conditions.[11]

A. Conservative and Behavioral Treatments: During an attack, patients have reported several methods to abort the pain. Dilation of the rectum, either digitally or via rectal suppository, has been used successfully in the treatment of PF.[12] Studies suggest that electrogalvanic stimulation and sitz baths may be helpful in the management of LAS. The electrical stimulation of the levator ani muscle has been used to break the spastic cycle. Hot sitz baths may alleviate pain by reducing anal pressures. Digital massage of levator ani muscles and targeted pelvic physiotherapy have shown to relieve pain from contracted muscles as well.[12,13]

B. Biofeedback Therapy (BFT): Biofeedback teaches patients control of autonomic body functions such as heart rate and muscle tension to relieve chronic pain, reduce stress, or achieve other predetermined goals.[14,15] A landmark trial compared the efficacy of biofeedback therapy, electrogalvanic stimulation, and digital massage in 157 patients with LAS. Patients were divided into two groups, those with LAS "highly likely" and LAS "possible." The key distinguishing feature was that the latter group did not have tenderness with the traction of the levator ani muscle. Among patients with highly likely LAS, 87% receiving BFT reported adequate pain relief with greater reduction in pain intensity compared to the electrogalvanic stimulation and massage groups. Participants receiving BFT also reported fewer pain days per month compared to the other treatment groups. Clinical improvement was sustained at 12 months. Patients with a "possible" diagnosis of LAS had negligible improvement with any treatment.[16]

C. Pharmacologic Treatment: Initial treatment of proctalgia fugax includes nonsteroidal antiinflammatory agents or cyclooxygenase-2 inhibitors. If initial treatment fails, a tricyclic antidepressant or gabapentin may be added. Selective serotonin reuptake inhibitors have been used to avoid the anticholinergic effects of tricyclic antidepressants but do not confer the same pain relief. Topical treatments such as nitroglycerin suppositories have proven to be successful. Finally, case reports of pain relief using nifedipine, carbamazepine, diltiazem, and salbutamol have been reported in the literature.[3]

D. Local Injections: For patients who continue to have attacks and pain despite medical therapy, injections of local anesthetic into levator ani muscles may be warranted. Local botulinum A toxin has also been injected with success in case studies. The purported mechanism of pain relief is by relaxation of the internal anal sphincter that interrupts the painful spasms. Success rates are higher in LAS compared to PF due to palpable contraction of levator ani muscles in the former condition.[17]

E. Pudendal Nerve Block: Patients who have pudendal nerve compression along with PF have seen relief with pudendal nerve blocks.[18] Pudendal nerve blocks can be approached via a transvaginal or transperineal approach. Both utilize the lithotomy position and the target is the loss of resistance (LOR) after engaging through the sacrospinous ligament. In the transvaginal approach, the iliac spine is palpated through the lateral vaginal wall, and the needle is advanced into the sacrospinous ligament. The needle is passed 1 cm caudally until LOR and a local anesthetic is injected. In the transperineal approach, the iliac spine is identified, and the needle is advanced transperineally in a posterolateral direction until the ischial spine is reached. The sacrospinous ligament is then engaged, and the needle is advanced 1 cm in a medial inferior direction and a local anesthetic is deposited after negative aspiration.[18,19] With fluoroscopy or CT guidance, the patient is placed in the prone position and the needle is advanced to the tip of the ischial spine. The needle is slightly withdrawn after contact with the ischial spine is made, and medication is administered after negative aspiration rules out the intravascular injection.

F. Ganglion Impar Block: The ganglion impar is the fused terminal portion of the sympathetic chain. It is a retroperitoneal structure that lies just anterior to the sacrococcygeal ligament. It innervates the perineum, distal rectum, anus, and portions of the distal urogynecological system as well. Blocking this ganglion may provide benefits for sympathetically mediated rectal and perineal pain. The most common technique used for this block is a transcoccygeal approach with fluoroscopic guidance. With the patient in the prone position, the C-arm is rotated to the lateral position and the coccyx and sacrococcygeal ligament are visualized. The needle is advanced such that the tip reaches the ventral aspect of the sacroccygeal space. Radiopaque contrast injection should show spread along the ventral aspect of the sacrum and coccyx. The injection is then performed with a local anesthetic and steroid mixture.[20] For patients with refractory pain, radiofrequency ablation may be offered.[21] Radiofrequency ablation has been done for coccydynia at 80°C for 90 s, and it is reasonable to consider these parameters when proceeding with this treatment option for functional rectal pain.

G. Superior Hypogastric Plexus Block: The superior hypogastric plexus is part of the abdominal and pelvic autonomic system. Blocking this plexus provides pain relief in patients with perineal pain and may have a role in PF and LAS. Located along the anterior border of the fifth lumbar vertebrae, it carries sympathetic nerve fibers from the rectum, colon, prostate, and other pelvic organs.[22,23] The superior hypogastric plexus is typically performed in the prone position. Under fluoroscopic guidance, the needle is inserted with a paramedian approach and advanced anterolaterally until the tips sit at the anterior margin of the L5–S1 interspace.

H. Sacral Nerve Stimulation: Sacral nerve stimulator systems provide electrical current to sacral nerves to modulate pelvic pain. The neuroelectrode usually exits at the S3 foramen and like other spinal cord stimulators/peripheral nerve stimulator (PNS) systems attaches to an implantable pulse generator. Although used for a variety of GI and urological conditions, there is a paucity of literature utilizing this therapy for the treatment of functional rectal pain disorders. Govaert and colleagues did a retrospective study of patients treated with sacral nerve stimulation between 2005 and 2008 for functional anorectal pain disorders. All patients had test stimulation to assess sacral neuromodulation outcomes before permanent implantation and had to achieve >50% pain improvement during the trial. Of the nine patients included in the study, four had successful test stimulation and went on to receive permanent implantation. All patients had a significant reduction in pain score through a 24-month follow-up period and improved global perceived effect. Although the preliminary evidence is promising, additional studies are needed to validate this therapy for rectal pain disorders.[24]

REFERENCES

1. Ger GC, Wexner SD, Jorge JM, et al. Evaluation and treatment of chronic intractable rectal pain—a frustrating endeavor. *Dis Colon Rectum.* 1993;36:139–145.
2. Theakson V. *The Rectum – Position – Neurovascular Supply.* Anatomy of Rectum; 2019. https://teachmeanatomy.info/abdomen/gi-tract/rectum/.
3. Wesselmann U, Czakanski PP. Pain of urogenital origin. *Curr Rev Pain.* 1999;3:160–171.
4. Whitehead WE, Wald A, Diamant NE, et al. Functional disorders of the anus and rectum. *Gut.* 1999;45(Suppl 2): II55–I59.
5. Waldman SD. Proctalgia fugax. In: *Atlas of Uncommon Pain Syndromes.* 4th ed. Philadelphia, PA: Elsevier; 2019: 258–260.
6. Vincent C. Anorectal pain and irritation: anal fissure, levator syndrome, proctalgia fugax, and pruritus ani. *Prim Care.* 1999;26:53–68.
7. Grimaud JC, Bouvier M, Naudy B, et al. Manometric and radiologic investigations and biofeedback treatment of chronic idiopathic anal pain. *Dis Colon Rectum.* 1991; 34(8):690–695.
8. Tu FF, Holt JJ, Gonzales J, et al. Physical therapy evaluation of patients with chronic pelvic pain: a controlled study. *Am J Obstet Gynecol.* 2008;198(3), 272.e1–7.
9. Bharucha AE, Wald A, Enck P, et al. Functional anorectal disorders. *Gastroenterol.* 2006;130(5):1510–1518.
10. Grant SR, Salvati EP, Rubin RJ. Levator syndrome: an analysis of 316 cases. *Dis Colon Rectum.* 1975;18(2):161–163.
11. Rome JD, Townsend CO, Bruce BK, Sletten CD, Luedtke CA, Hodgson JE. Chronic noncancer pain rehabilitation with opioid withdrawal: comparison of treatment outcomes based on opioid use status at admission. *Mayo Clin Proc.* 2004;79(6):759–768.
12. Thiele GH. Tonic spasm of the levator ani, coccygeus and piriformis muscle: relationship to coccygodynia and pain in the region of the hip and down the leg. *Trans Am Proctol Soc.* 1936;37:145–155.
13. Dodi G, Bogoni F, Infantino A, et al. Hot or cold in anal pain? A study of the changes in internal anal sphincter pressure profiles. *Dis Colon Rectum.* 1986;29(4):248–251.
14. Gilliland R, Heymen JS, Altomare DF, et al. Biofeedback for intractable rectal pain: outcome and predictors of success. *Dis Colon Rectum.* 1997;40(2):190–196.
15. Heah SM, Ho YH, Tan M, et al. Biofeedback is effective treatment for levator ani syndrome. *Dis Colon Rectum.* 1997;40(2):187–189.
16. Chiarioni G, Nardo A, Vantini I, Romito A, Whitehead WE. Biofeedback is superior to electrogalvanic stimulation and massage for treatment of levator ani syndrome. *Gastroenterol.* 2010;138(4):1321–1329.
17. Katsinelos P, Kalomenopoulou M, Christodoulou K, et al. Treatment of proctalgia fugax with botulinum A toxin. *Eur J Gastroenterol Hepatol.* 2001;13(11):1371–1373.
18. Bascom JU. Pudendal canal syndrome and proctalgia fugax: a mechanism creating pain. *Dis Colon Rectum.* 1998;41(3):406.
19. Ghanavatian S, Derian A. Pudendal nerve block. In: *StatPearls.* Treasure Island (FL): StatPearls Publishing; 2020.
20. Scott-Warren JT, Hill V, Rajasekaran A. Ganglion impar blockade: a review. *Curr Pain Headache Rep.* 2013;17(1): 306.
21. Adas C, Ozdemir U, Toman H, et al. Transsacrococcygeal approach to ganglion impar: radiofrequency application for the treatment of chronic intractable coccydynia. *J Pain Res.* 2016;9:1173–1177. https://doi.org/10.2147/jpr.s105506.
22. Choi JW, Kim WH, Lee CJ, Sim WS, Park S, Chae HB. The optimal approach for a superior hypogastric plexus block. *Pain Pract.* 2018;18:314–321.
23. Waldman SD, Wilson WL, Kreps RD. Superior hypogastric plexus block using a single needle and computed tomography guidance: description of a modified technique. *Reg Anesth.* 1991;16(5):286–287.
24. Govaert B, Melenhorst J, van Kleef M, van Gemert WG, Baeten CG. Sacral neuromodulation for the treatment of chronic functional anorectal pain: a single center experience. *Pain Pract.* 2010;10(1):49–53.

CHAPTER 10

Pancreatic Cancer

CHRISTINE S. HADDAD, MD, PHD • DANIEL J. PAK, MD

INTRODUCTION

Pancreatic adenocarcinoma accounts for 56,000 cancer diagnoses in the United States per year and is fourth among cancer-related deaths.[1] Pancreatic cancer has an extremely poor prognosis and the lowest 5-year survival among any cancer.[2] Early-stage disease rarely presents with symptomatology and almost 50% of patients are advanced stage at the time of diagnosis.[2] Currently, surgical resection via Whipple procedure and adjuvant chemoradiotherapy are the only curable treatments. Thus, palliative treatment to reduce pain and improve quality of life is a crucial aspect of management for these patients. Pain affects approximately 80% of patients with pancreatic cancer, which is also associated with decreased quality of life, impaired functional activity, and reduced survival.[3,4]

ETIOLOGY AND PATHOGENESIS

The pancreas is an important organ involved in digestion and has both exocrine and endocrine functions. The afferent nerve fibers of the pancreas are transmitted with the sympathetic and parasympathetic pathways through a complex collection of ganglia and plexuses en route to the spinal cord.[5] These afferent visceral nerve axons almost completely comprise unmyelinated C and thinly myelinated Aδ fibers that transmit both mechanoreceptive and nociceptive information to the central nervous system.[5] The pancreas specifically receives its extrinsic sympathetic innervation from the celiac plexus (with contributions from the thoracic splanchnic nerves) and parasympathetic innervation from the vagus nerve.

There are two principal mechanisms for the generation of pain in pancreatic cancer: pancreatic duct obstruction and pancreatic neuropathy, which activate mechanical and chemical nociceptors, respectively.[3] Pancreatic duct obstruction is provoked by the release of pancreatic enzymes, particularly after eating. Duct obstruction blocks the flow of these enzymes and causes an increase in parenchymal pressure, which subsequently decreases blood flow and generates ischemic pain.[3] Neuropathic pain occurs due to the invasion of nerves by cancer cells. The incidence of perineural invasion is estimated to be around 70%–90%.[4] Cancer cell invasion promotes activation of local immune cells, release of neurotrophic growth factors, and tissue damage due to inflammation.[6] These changes result in neurogenic pain. Additionally, as the tumor progresses, there is growth of new nerve fibers that also exacerbates pain.[3]

CLINICAL FEATURES

Presenting symptoms of pancreatic cancer vary based on the location of the tumor. Weight loss (92%), jaundice (87%), and pain (72%) are the most common symptoms of pancreatic cancer.[7] Other nonspecific findings of pancreatic cancer include anorexia, dyspepsia, nausea, and vomiting.[8] Pain in pancreatic cancer is usually described as epigastric pain that radiates to the back.

The presence of pain at the time of diagnosis was found to be a predictor of poor survival in a case series.[9,10] In an observational study by Ceyhan et al., patients who were undergoing surgical resection were classified preoperatively in three groups based on their pain scores. The median survivals, measured as the time between surgery and cancer-specific death, for patients with no pain, mild pain, and moderate-to-severe pain were 21.5, 15.0, and 10.0 months, respectively ($P = .0015$).

DIAGNOSIS

For patients presenting with nonspecific complaints, abdominal ultrasonography is often the first imaging

Interventional Management of Chronic Visceral Pain Syndromes. https://doi.org/10.1016/B978-0-323-75775-1.00015-5

modality that is performed. However, abdominal computed tomography (CT) scan is the gold standard for diagnosis and staging. Pancreas protocol scans require triphasic cross-sectional imaging (arterial, late, and venous phase), which allows for an enhancement between the pancreas parenchyma and adenocarcinoma.[7] If a pancreatic mass is seen on imaging, then follow-up endoscopic ultrasound and fine-needle aspiration are indicated. If no mass is seen on imaging but there is high suspicion for malignancy, then endoscopic ultrasonography, endoscopic retrograde cholangiopancreatography, magnetic resonance imaging, or magnetic resonance cholangiopancreatography may be performed for further characterization of disease.[7]

Cancer antigen 19-9 (CA 19-9) is one of the tumor markers used to assess pancreatic cancer. It has limited sensitivity (50%−75%) and specificity (80%−85%). Therefore, it is a poor screening tool in asymptomatic patients.[7] It is mainly used to confirm the diagnosis and predict prognosis in symptomatic patients. It may also be used to monitor for recurrent disease.

Typically, when patients are referred to an interventional pain physician, the diagnosis of pancreatic cancer has already been made. A multidisciplinary team approach involving gastroenterology, oncology, and surgical oncology should be involved when treating these complex patients. Diagnosis for pain secondary to pancreatic cancer is mostly clinical with epigastric discomfort radiating to the back.

PHYSICAL EXAM

Physical exam findings in pancreatic cancer can be variable depending on the stage and the location of the tumor. Patients can have normal exams in the early stages of the disease. In advanced stages, general physical exam findings can include jaundice, cachexia, and abdominal tenderness. Courvoisier sign, defined as a nontender, distended, and palpable gallbladder in a patient with jaundice, is 83%−90% specific but is only 26%−55% sensitive for a biliary obstruction from malignancy.[7] Other nonspecific physical exam findings include Trousseau sign (recurring superficial thrombophlebitis) and Virchow node (left supraclavicular lymphadenopathy), both of which can be found in other abdominal malignancies.[7]

TREATMENT

Treatment for pancreatic cancer pain commonly involves both pharmacologic and interventional options. Patients are initially offered conservative therapy based on the analgesic ladder established by the World Health Organization (WHO). As patients often suffer moderate to severe pain, opioids are used as the mainstay treatment. Interventional procedures, such as celiac plexus neurolysis, intrathecal drug delivery systems, and thoracoscopic splanchnicectomy are considered in patients with intractable pain.

Conservative Systemic Therapies

As previously mentioned, conservative treatment of pain in pancreatic cancer is based on the analgesic ladder set by the WHO.[11] For patients with mild-to-moderate pain, the first step of treatment is prescribing nonopioid analgesics, such as paracetamol and nonsteroidal anti-inflammatory drugs (NSAID). These agents may be used alone or in conjunction with opioids. NSAIDs, which have anti-inflammatory and antipyretic properties, are efficacious for both bone and inflammatory pains. The use of these medications may be limited due to their renal, gastrointestinal, hematological, and cardiac toxicity profiles. Oral corticosteroids are also commonly used in late-stage disease for anorexia, analgesia, and nausea. Bisphosphonates are often given in conjunction with glucocorticoids, such as dexamethasone and prednisone, for malignant bone pain. Tricyclic antidepressants and gabapentinoids are effective for neuropathic pain, though their efficacy for malignancy-specific pain syndromes is not well-established.

For patients who receive inadequate relief with nonopioid analgesics, a trial of weak opioids, such as tramadol or codeine, should be done. If these provide inadequate pain relief, then more potent opioids can be prescribed. There is no significant difference in the analgesic efficacy or tolerability of agents such as oxycodone compared to morphine for moderate to severe cancer pain.[12] Moreover, given that individuals have varying responses to different μ-agonists, opioid rotation should be considered when one agent proves to be ineffective or have intolerable side effects. In such cases, the equianalgesic dose of the new opioid should be reduced by 20%−30% to account for incomplete cross-tolerance and prevent an overdose of the new agent. If a patient is unable to tolerate oral medications and a long-acting opioid is desired, then transdermal fentanyl should be considered. Other routes of rapid fentanyl delivery for breakthrough pain include transmucosal lozenge, sublingual tablet, and nasal spray. Methadone has also been used for pain management in pancreatic cancer patients. Also, it is not uncommon for pancreatic cancer patients to be on multiple opioids at once as the disease progresses and the pain becomes more difficult to control.[13]

As previously mentioned, long term opioid use is often accompanied by frequent side effects, including constipation, nausea, vomiting, sweating, anorexia, dyspepsia, and pruritus. As pain control is crucial for maintaining the quality of life, these side effects can be mitigated by adjuvant medications such as stool softeners, laxatives, appetite stimulants, and antiemetics. Additionally, the regular use of high dose opioids can lead to opioid-induced hyperalgesia, which results in worsening pain despite increased doses of opioids.[14] A study by Zech et al. evaluated the efficacy of therapy according to WHO guidelines in cancer patients. The course of treatment of 2118 patients was assessed prospectively over a period of 140,478 treatment days. Over the whole treatment period, inadequate pain relief was reported in 12% of patients.[15]

Celiac Plexus Neurolysis

The celiac plexus is a large visceral plexus located in the retroperitoneal space around the origin of the celiac trunk at the T12—L1 vertebral levels. It has contributions from multiple ganglia (celiac, superior mesenteric, and aorticorenal ganglia) and serves as a relay center for nociceptive signals that originate from the upper abdominal viscera. The nerve fibers of the celiac plexus are predominantly preganglionic sympathetic efferent nerve fibers derived from the greater splanchnic (T5—T9), lesser splanchnic (T10—T11), and least splanchnic (T12) nerves.[16] Contributions to the celiac plexus also come from parasympathetic efferent fibers of the vagus nerve.[16]

Indications

Celiac plexus neurolysis (CPN) is appropriate for patients with intractable abdominal pain caused by pancreatitis and malignancies of much of the gastrointestinal GI tract, starting from the distal esophagus to the distal transverse colon.[16,17] In addition to pain control, CPN has been shown to be effective in controlling severe nausea and vomiting in patients with pancreatic cancer, which is likely secondary to the resulting unopposed parasympathetic activity and increased peristaltic activity.[16]

Contraindications

Although there are no clear absolute contraindications to CPN, relative contradictions exist. These include the presence of coagulopathy, bleeding disorders, thrombocytopenia, intraabdominal infection or sepsis, abdominal aortic aneurysms, and mural thrombosis of the abdominal aorta.[16,17] CPN is also relatively contradicted in patients with small bowel obstruction due to the effects of the block on increasing bowel motility.[16]

Complications

The most common complication of CPN is local pain (96%), diarrhea (44%), and orthostatic hypotension (38%).[18] Orthostatic hypotension results from local vasodilation and pooling of the blood within splanchnic vessels following sympathetic denervation. Elderly and hypovolemic patients are more prone to these hemodynamic effects.[19] Other rare side effects include local anesthetic toxicity, injury to the aorta or IVC, retroperitoneal hematoma, surrounding organ injury, and paraplegia due to damage to the artery of Adamkiewicz.[20,21] In one report by Davies et al., the incidence of major complications (paraplegia, bladder, and bowel dysfunction) has been reported to be 1 per 683 procedures.[22]

Neurolytic agents

The two main agents used for celiac plexus neurolysis are alcohol and phenol (Table 10.1). The preferred concentration of ethanol for neurolysis is usually 50%—100%, as irreversible damage usually occurs at concentrations greater 50%.[16] The mechanism of neurolysis is the extraction of cholesterol and lipoproteins from the nerve axon as well as precipitation of lipoproteins and mucoproteins, which cause irreversible damage to nerve fibers.[16,19]

TABLE 10.1
Commonly Used Neurolytic Agents for Celiac Plexus Neurolysis.[16]

Agent	Concentration	Viscosity	Onset of Action	Nerve Destruction	Pain with Injection	Mechanism of Action
Phenol	3%—20%	High	Slow	+	Minimal	Protein precipitation, necrosis of neural structures
Ethanol	50%—100%	Low	Fast	++	Can be intense	Extraction of cholesterol and lipoproteins

Phenol, at a concentration of 6%–10%, can also be used for neurolysis. Due to the agent's viscosity, dilute 6% phenol is usually preferred to facilitate easier injection. Similar to ethanol, phenol causes protein precipitation and necrosis of the neural structure.[19] There is limited data comparing the efficacies of alcohol and phenol for CPN.

Ethanol is known to cause severe transient pain on injection, while phenol does not. Thus, the injection of a local anesthetic such as lidocaine or bupivacaine is recommended.[16] Despite this, ethanol is the most commonly used agent for CPN due to its faster onset of action and longer duration of action.[16,17]

Imaging

CPN can be performed with fluoroscopy, ultrasound (US), CT, magnetic resonance imaging (MRI), or endoscopic US. The use of modern C-arm fluoroscopy is wide-spread due to portability and lower cost. However, traditional fluoroscopy does not allow for an accurate distinction of the abdominal viscera. Therefore, the use of CT-guidance has gained popularity due to its ability to allow precise localization of the needle tip while providing visualization of the retroperitoneal anatomy, which is particularly important in cases where normal anatomy is distorted due to tumor invasion.[16,18]

Technique

Posterior Approach: Posterior approaches are typically performed with the patient lying prone, most commonly utilizing the antecrural or retrocrural techniques. The antecrural and retrocrural sites are the spaces anterior and posterior, respectively, to the crura of the diaphragm. The antecrural approach is effective for targeting the celiac plexus while the retrocrural approach targets the splanchnic nerves.

For the antecrural technique under fluoroscopy, a single needle is inserted using a left posterior paramedian approach at the level of the L1 transverse process and advanced toward the anterior surface of the L1 vertebral body, ultimately through the posterior wall of the aorta until blood is aspirated. The needle is advanced further until the needle traverses the anterior wall and blood can no longer be aspirated. Fluoroscopy confirms the needle position in the preaortic space and injection of contrast solution should confirm diffusion into the antecrural space (Fig. 10.1). It is important to note that this transaortic approach has an increased risk of retroperitoneal hemorrhage, particularly in patients with coagulation abnormalities.

The retrocrural approach is a reasonable alternative when the antecrural approach cannot be performed due to tumor invasion of the preaortic space. A bilateral paravertebral approach is typically achieved with two needles inserted at the level of the L1 transverse process and advanced until the tips are just past the anterior surface of the T12-L1 vertebral bodies to block the left and right splanchnic nerve fibers. The retrocrural approach is often combined with the antecrural approach to provide better analgesic effects.[16]

As previously mentioned, the use of CT imaging has increasingly come into favor due to the ability to visualize intraabdominal structures. Axial cuts are used to visualize the celiac trunk, major vascular structures, and organs to determine the optimal needle path to the plexus or splanchnic nerves. Both antecrural and retrocrural

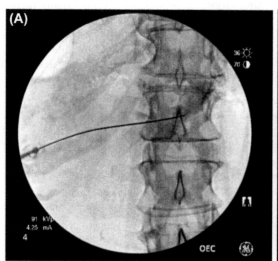 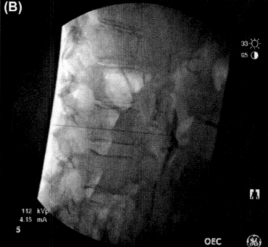

FIG. 10.1 Fluoroscopy-guided transaortic CPN, with AP (**A**) and lateral (**B**) views.

neurolysis can be done under CT guidance with the patient positioned either laterally or prone with a bilateral needle approach. It should be mentioned that the antecrural technique under CT guidance is commonly achieved without traversing any major vessels.

Anterior approach: Due to the high risk of organ perforation, percutaneous anterior approaches are limited to patients where a posterior technique is not feasible and are most often pursued with CT guidance.[16] With the anterior approach, the patient is positioned in the supine position. The needle is introduced through the anterior abdominal wall and advanced perpendicular to the skin until it touches the body of the L1 vertebra. The needle is then pulled back 1–2 cm into the retropancreatic space. The needle tip should be positioned anterior to the aorta and the diaphragmatic crura, between the celiac trunk and the superior mesenteric artery. This procedure is commonly performed on each of the two sides of the celiac plexus.

The anterior approach offers a more comfortable position for the patient. It also has a lower risk of neurologic injury related to the spread of the neurolytic agent into the somatic nerve roots and/or epidural and subarachnoid space. Disadvantages of the anterior approach are secondary to the passage of the needle through the abdominal viscera. Risks include gastric perforation, pancreatic fistula, subcapsular liver hematoma, and chemical peritonitis.

Endoscopic ultrasound-guided approach: This technique combines the modalities of flexible endoscopy with ultrasound to direct the transducer within the upper GI tract to the area of the celiac trunk. Once the desired location is reached, a needle is passed through the scope and advanced past the gastric wall to access the plexus. The advantages of this technique compared to approaches with fluoroscopy and CT imaging is real-time guidance of the needle and the use of color Doppler for identifying major vascular structures. The complication profile is similar to other traditional techniques, with the added issue of gastric perforation and necrosis. Single and bilateral (involving injections on both sides of either celiac axis) needle techniques can be used.[23]

Percutaneous Radiofrequency Ablation

In addition to traditional neurolytic procedures with ethanol and phenol, radiofrequency ablation (RFA) of the splanchnic nerves may also be performed. RFA uses high-frequency alternating current to heat tissues up to 80°C, which results in neurolysis.[4] The procedure was first described by Raj et al. and was shown to be effective in patients with chronic abdominal pain due to chronic pancreatitis, postabdominal surgery pain, and pancreatic and liver cancer.[24] A later study showed

that bilateral splanchnic RFA reduced pain and opioid consumption and improved quality of life in patients with pancreatic cancer.[25]

Intrathecal Drug Delivery Systems

Another effective pain management option for patients with pancreatic cancer is the continuous delivery of medications directly into the cerebrospinal fluid via intrathecal drug delivery systems (IDDS). This requires the surgical implantation of a pump reservoir under the skin of the abdomen. The pump is connected to a tunneled catheter that delivers medication into the CSF. The pump can be refilled sterilely through a subcutaneous access port. The pump can be programmed to deliver a fixed or variable rate with boluses through patient-controlled analgesia programming.

The dorsal horn of the spinal cord plays a crucial role in processing pain signals. Additionally, many of the pain receptors, including opioid (mu, kappa, and delta), GABA, alpha-2, and NMDA receptors, are located within the spinal column. The direct delivery of medications into their site of action provides a more rapid and effective response, and allows the use of smaller doses of medication, thus reducing systemic side effects.[26]

Indications

The use of IDDS is considered in patients with focal pain that is refractory to traditional systemic opioids or those who are unable to tolerate the side effects of opioids. Several factors should be considered when choosing candidates for this therapy, including the patient's life expectancy, support systems, ability to continue regular clinic follow-ups (for refills, dose adjustments), expectations of the therapy, and psychological status.

Medication options

Different classes of medications can be delivered via IDDS. There are currently three medications approved for IDDS by the US Food and Drug Administration: morphine, ziconotide (an N-type calcium channel blocker that acts at the level of the dorsal horn to provide analgesia), and baclofen. Many other agents are commonly used off-label, including hydromorphone, fentanyl, sufentanil, clonidine, and bupivacaine. Drug combinations, typically a combination of an opioid with either bupivacaine or clonidine, are used for mixed nociceptive and neuropathic pain disorders. Recent evidence suggests that intrathecal opioids are superior to oral opioids in managing cancer pain, particularly when oral use is limited by systemic side effects.[26] Additionally, studies have shown that IDDS is effective in providing pain control in ~60%–80% of patient with refractory cancer pain.[26]

Technique

A trial of IDDS is usually performed before implant to determine whether the patient will benefit from permanent implantation. During a trial, the catheter can be placed either into the epidural or intrathecal space. Intrathecal placement provides a closer representation of the actual implant. Epidural placement on the other hand avoids intrathecal entry. Catheter pump trials are usually done for 2–3 days. Alternatively, a single shot spinal injection may be performed for the trial. A trial is typically considered successful if the patient reports >50% in pain scores and function.[27]

Placement of IDDS is a surgical procedure that is performed in the operating room under general anesthesia. The catheter tip is placed according to the corresponding dermatomal distribution of the patient's pain; for abdominal coverage, we suggest that the tip be placed at the level of the T9 or T10 vertebral body (Fig. 10.2).

TABLE 10.2 Adverse Reactions Related to IDDS Medications.	
Medication	**Associated Complications**
Opioids	Respiratory depression, peripheral edema, hormonal changes, immune suppression, hyperalgesia, withdrawal, catheter tip granuloma formation
Baclofen	Respiratory depression, withdrawal, psychosis/suicidality
Ketamine	Demyelination/Necrotizing lesions
Dexmedetomidine	Demyelination/Necrotizing lesions
Local anesthetics	Urinary retention, hypotension, extremity weakness

Complications

According to a retrospective study by Krakovsky, adverse reactions to medications delivered via IDDS were the most common complications.[28] Table 10.2 lists the most common adverse reactions related to medications delivered by IDDS. Serious complications include respiratory depression and anaphylaxis. Other adverse reactions include urinary retention, hypotension, tolerance/withdrawal, and hyperalgesia. In addition to drug-related adverse reactions, device and procedure-related complications can occur. These include infection, postdural puncture headache, bleeding, pocket-site seroma, increased pain, and catheter tip granulomas. Interestingly, hydromorphone and morphine were shown to have a higher incidence of catheter tip granuloma compared to fentanyl.[29] The incidence of infection in all cases reviewed was reported to be 0.7% per year in one study.[30] Adherence to surgical site infection guidelines has been shown to successfully reduce the risk of infection.[26]

Tunneled Intraspinal Catheter Systems

For patients with a terminal prognosis with less than 3 months of life expectancy, one may consider an epidural or intrathecal catheter that is tunneled subcutaneously and attached to an external infusion pump. This is a less invasive and more cost-effective approach compared to an internalized IDDS with a subcutaneous pump. Infection is the most common concern with any chronic indwelling catheter. A systematic review of tunneled intrathecal catheters found an overall infection risk rate of 1.4% for deep infections and 2.3% for superficial infections, which are relatively low and comparable to infection rates with other implanted

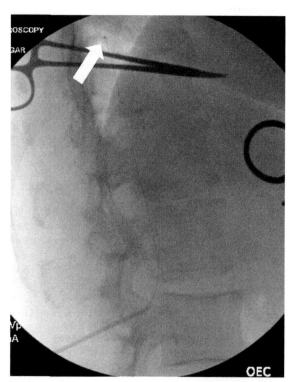

FIG. 10.2 **Catheter placement for intrathecal pump.** Advancement of the intrathecal catheter (tip indicated by the arrow) shown on lateral fluoroscopic imaging.

subcutaneous ports.[31] For patients who are discharged home or to another care facility, it is essential that they have the necessary education and support to manage the external pump device.

Spinal Cord Stimulation

Spinal cord stimulation (SCS) can be considered in patients with chronic abdominal pain resistant to traditional medical and interventional therapies. Based on the "gate control" theory of pain where nonpainful sensory inputs effectively "gate" off ascending pain signals, SCS devices deliver electrical stimulation to the dorsal column of the spinal cord to modulate ascending and descending pain signals. Traditionally used for chronic back pain, radicular pain, and complex regional pain syndrome, there is now limited literature demonstrating analgesic benefit with reduced visual analog scale pain scores and nausea for patients with chronic visceral abdominal pain, including chronic pancreatitis.[32] Stimulation leads are placed in the posterior epidural space between the T4 and T8 vertebral levels for these patients. No studies have specifically examined its efficacy for pancreatic cancer pain. Historically, SCS has a limited role in cancer patients due to the potential need for MRI during the lifetime of the patient, as there are limitations with MRI comptability. When deciding to proceed with SCS, a multidisciplinary team approach should be taken.

As expected with any implantable therapies, SCS devices carry complications including lead migration and associated loss of analgesic therapy, lead fracture, seroma, infection, dural puncture, epidural hematoma, or cord trauma. In addition, these devices also carry the risk of tolerance and a resulting loss of analgesia.[33,34]

Thoracoscopic Splanchnicectomy

An alternative method for the management of pain in pancreatic cancer is thoracoscopic splanchnicectomy (TS). TS is a minimally invasive surgical procedure to dissect the thoracic splanchnic nerves, which normally conduct nociceptive signals from the pancreas to the central nervous system. TS has been shown to lower pain scores and improve quality of life in patients with pancreatic cancer, with minimal effects on pancreatic function.[35,36] TS can be performed unilaterally or bilaterally. Some studies suggest that bilateral TS may yield better pain control compared to unilateral TS, although the data are very limited.[37]

SUMMARY

Pancreatic cancer is a malignant tumor with a very poor prognosis. Pain is one of the most common symptoms of pancreatic cancer, and it often leads to decreased quality of life and impairs functional activity. Conservative management, based on the WHO analgesic ladder, is the most common treatment option. More invasive treatments include celiac plexus block, intrathecal drug delivery systems, spinal cord stimulation, and thoracic splanchnicectomy. These options should be considered at an earlier stage of the disease, to reduce the risk of opioid tolerance and to offer better pain control with improved quality of life.

REFERENCES

1. American Cancer Society. *Cancer Facts and Figures*. Atlanta: American Cancer Society; 2019.
2. Gillen S, Schuster T, Büschenfelde CM, Friess H, Kleeff J. Preoperative/neoadjuvant therapy in pancreatic cancer: a systematic review and meta-analysis of response and resection percentages. *PLoS Med*. April 20, 2010;7(4): e1000267. ISSN 1549-1277.
3. Koulouris AI, Banim P, Hart AR. Pain in patients with pancreatic cancer: prevalence, mechanisms, management and future developments. *Dig Dis Sci*. April 2017;62(4): 861–870. ISSN 0163-2116.
4. Dobosz L, Kaczor M, Stefaniak TJ. Pain in pancreatic cancer: review of medical and surgical remedies. *ANZ J Surg*. October 2016;86(10):756–761. ISSN 1445-1433.
5. Babic T, Travagli RA. *Neural Control of the Pancreas. Pancreapedia: Exocrine Pancreas Knowledge Base*. 2016.
6. Barreto SG, Saccone GT. Pancreatic nociception–revisiting the physiology and pathophysiology. *Pancreatology*. March-April 2012;12(2):104–112. ISSN 1424-3903.
7. De la cruz MS, Young AP, Ruffin MT. Diagnosis and management of pancreatic cancer. *Am Fam Physician*. April 15, 2014;89(8):626–632. ISSN 0002-838x.
8. Krech RL, Walsh D. Symptoms of pancreatic cancer. *J Pain Symptom Manag*. August 1991;6(6):360–367. ISSN 0885-3924 (Print) 0885-3924.
9. Muller MW, Friess H, Köninger J, et al. Factors influencing survival after bypass procedures in patients with advanced pancreatic adenocarcinomas. *Am J Surg*. February 2008; 195(2):221–228. ISSN 0002-9610.
10. Ceyhan GO, Bergmann F, Kadihasanoglu M, et al. Pancreatic neuropathy and neuropathic pain–a comprehensive pathomorphological study of 546 cases, 177-186.e1 *Gastroenterology*. January 2009;136(1). ISSN 0016-5085.
11. World Health Organization. *WHO Guidelines for the Pharmacological and Radiotherapeutic Management of Cancer Pain in Adults and Adolescents*. January 2019.
12. Guo KK, Deng CQ, Lu GJ, Zhao GL. Comparison of analgesic effect of oxycodone and morphine on patients with moderate and advanced cancer pain: a meta-analysis. *BMC Anesthesiol*. September 24, 2018;18(1):132. ISSN 1471-2253.
13. Hameed M, Hameed H, Erdek M. Pain management in pancreatic cancer. *Cancers*. December 24, 2010;3(1): 43–60. ISSN 2072-6694 (Print) 2072-6694.
14. Harris DG. Management of pain in advanced disease. *Br Med Bull*. June 2014;110(1):117–128. ISSN 0007-1420.

15. Zech DF, Grond S, Lynch J, Hertel D, Lehmann KA. Validation of World Health Organization Guidelines for cancer pain relief: a 10-year prospective study. *Pain*. October 1995;63(1):65–76. ISSN 0304-3959 (Print) 0304-3959.

16. Kambadakone A, Thabet A, Gervais D, Mueller PR, Arellano RS. CT-guided celiac plexus neurolysis: a review of anatomy, indications, technique, and tips for successful treatment. *Radiographics*. October 2011;31(6):1599–1621. ISSN 0271-5333.

17. Wang PJ, Shang MY, Qian Z, Shao CW, Wang JH, Zhao XH. CT-guided percutaneous neurolytic celiac plexus block technique. *Abdom Imag*. Nov-Dec 2006;31(6):710–718. ISSN 0942-8925 (Print) 0942-8925.

18. Jain P, Dutta A, Sood J. Coeliac plexus blockade and neurolysis: an overview. *Indian J Anaesth*. 2006;50, 169-177 pp.

19. Mercadante S, Nicosia F. Celiac plexus block: a reappraisal. *Reg Anesth Pain Med*. Jan-Feb 1998;23(1):37–48. ISSN 1098-7339 (Print) 1098-7339.

20. Kaplan R, Schiff-Keren B, Alt E. Aortic dissection as a complication of celiac plexus block. *Anesthesiology*. September 1995;83(3):632–635. ISSN 0003-3022 (Print) 0003-3022.

21. De Conno F, Caraceni A, Aldrighetti L, et al. Paraplegia following coeliac plexus block. *Pain*. December 1993; 55(3):383–385. ISSN 0304-3959 (Print) 0304-3959.

22. Davies DD. Incidence of major complications of neurolytic coeliac plexus block. *J R Soc Med*. May 1993;86(5): 264–266. ISSN 0141-0768 (Print) 0141-0768.

23. Yasuda I, Wang HP. Endoscopic ultrasound-guided celiac plexus block and neurolysis. *Dig Endosc*. May 2017; 29(4):455–462. ISSN 0915-5635.

24. Raj PP, Sahinler B, Lowe M. Radiofrequency lesioning of splanchnic nerves. *Pain Pract*. September 2002;2(3): 241–247. ISSN 1530-7085.

25. Papadopoulos D, Kostopanagiotou G, Batistaki C. Bilateral thoracic splanchnic nerve radiofrequency thermocoagulation for the management of end-stage pancreatic abdominal cancer pain. *Pain Physician*. March-April 2013; 16(2):125–133. ISSN 1533-3159.

26. Bhatia G, Lau ME, Koury KM, Gulur P. Intrathecal Drug Delivery (ITDD) systems for cancer pain. *F1000Res*. 2013;2:96. ISSN 2046-1402 (Print) 2046-1402.

27. Knight KH, Frances B, Mchaourab A, Veneziano G. Implantable intrathecal pumps for chronic pain: highlights and updates. *Croat Med J*. February 2007;48(1): 22–34. ISSN 0353-9504.

28. Krakovsky AA. Complications associated with intrathecal pump drug delivery: a retrospective evaluation. *Am J Pain Manag*. 2007;17(1):4. ISSN 1059-1494.

29. Deer TR, Prager J, Levy R, et al. Polyanalgesic Consensus Conference 2012: recommendations for the management of pain by intrathecal (intraspinal) drug delivery: report of an interdisciplinary expert panel. discussion 464-6 *Neuromodulation*. Sep-Oct 2012;15(5):436–464. ISSN 1094-7159.

30. Fluckiger B, Knecht H, Grossmann S, Felleiter P. Device-related complications of long-term intrathecal drug therapy via implanted pumps. *Spinal Cord*. September 2008; 46(9):639–643. ISSN 1362-4393 (Print) 1362-4393.

31. Aprili D, Bandschapp O, Rochlitz, C, Urwyler A, Ruppen W. Serious complications associated with external intrathecal catheters used in cancer pain patients: a systematic review and meta-analysis. *Anesthesiology*. December 2009;111(6):1346–1355. ISSN 0003-3022.

32. Kapural L, Gupta M, Paicius R, et al. Treatment of chronic abdominal pain with 10-kHz spinal cord stimulation: safety and efficacy results from a 12-month prospective, multicenter, feasibility study. *Clin Transl Gastroenterol*. February 2020;11(2):e00133. ISSN 2155-384x.

33. Bedder MD, Bedder HF. Spinal cord stimulation surgical technique for the nonsurgically trained. *Neuromodulation*. April 2009;12(Suppl 1):1–19. ISSN 1094-7159 (Print) 1094-7159.

34. Kumar K, Hunter G, Demeria D. Spinal cord stimulation in treatment of chronic benign pain: challenges in treatment planning and present status, a 22-year experience. discussion 481-96 *Neurosurgery*. March 2006;58(3):481–496. ISSN 0148-396x.

35. Smigielski J, Piskorz L, Wawrzycki M, Kutwin M, Misiak P, Brocki M. Assessment of quality of life in patients with non-operated pancreatic cancer after videothoracoscopic splanchnicectomy. *Wideochir Inne Tech Maloinwazyjne*. September 2011;6(3):132–137. ISSN 1895-4588 (Print) 1895-4588.

36. Ihse I, Zoucas, E, Gyllstedt E, Lillo-Gil R, Andrén-Sandberg, A. Bilateral thoracoscopic splanchnicectomy: effects on pancreatic pain and function. discussion 790-1 *Ann Surg*. December 1999;230(6):785–790. ISSN 0003-4932 (Print) 0003-4932.

37. Saenz A, Kuriansky J, Salvador L, et al. Thoracoscopic splanchnicectomy for pain control in patients with unresectable carcinoma of the pancreas. *Surg Endosc*. August 2000;14(8):717–720. ISSN 0930-2794 (Print) 0930-2794.

CHAPTER 11

Liver Cancer

DAVID HAO, MD • VWAIRE ORHURHU, MD

INTRODUCTION

Malignancy of the liver is increasingly prevalent and threatening with respect to morbidity and mortality. Hepatocellular carcinoma, the most common primary liver malignancy, is responsible for the third greatest number of cancer-related deaths in the world.[1]

Patients with malignancies of the liver often have multiple symptoms that decrease the quality of life, including chronic fatigue, loss of appetite, gastrointestinal symptoms, and pain. Frequently, the disease may be at an advanced stage such that curative therapies including surgery or transplantation are no longer options. A systematic review and meta-analysis noted that 52% of patients with cancer experienced pain, irrespective of the stage of disease.[2] Pain management is thus one of the most important components of quality of life maintenance in advanced stages of the disease.

ETIOLOGY AND PATHOGENESIS

Pain signals generated by the liver are transmitted by the sympathetic and parasympathetic nervous systems. Nociceptive structures in the liver include the liver capsule, blood vessels, and biliary tract. Afferents travel via the celiac plexus, phrenic nerve, and lower right intercostal nerves.[3]

Abdominal viscera have widely distributed afferents of both sympathetic and parasympathetic innervations. Painful stimuli transmit to the medullary dorsal horn of the spinal cord via unmyelinated C-fibers and lightly myelinated A-delta fibers. The parasympathetic fibers to the viscera are contributed by the vagus and sacral splanchnic nerves that pass through the superior mesenteric plexus into the celiac plexus. The sympathetic fibers are derived from thoracic, lumbar, and sacral splanchnic nerves that pass through the celiac and mesenteric plexus.[4] Although there is substantial variability in the nerve distribution of the liver, it is generally innervated by the hepatic plexus, which is supplied by the celiac plexus and vagal trunks.[5]

Lesions in the liver have the potential to generate pain secondary to stretching of the hepatic capsule, which is termed "hepatic distension syndrome." A similar phenomenon may be seen with distention of the hepatic veins as seen with portal obstruction. Hepatic enlargement also has the potential to cause diaphragmatic irritation, which can manifest as referred pain to the ipsilateral shoulder. This pain is transmitted by the phrenic nerve and is known as *Kehr sign*.[6]

Mechanical irritation and inflammation of the inferior pleura and peritoneum may present as referred liver pain that is somatic and carried by the lower intercostal and subcostal nerves. Compared to visceral pain, somatic pain tends to be sharper and more localized.

CLINICAL FEATURES

Liver malignancies often have a silent clinical course, in part due to the deep position of the liver within the abdominal cavity. Thus, the tumor may be substantial in size and advanced in stage before diagnosis and development of symptomatology. The clinical picture is often variable and presentation is sometimes only seen with liver failure or invasion of the tumor into adjacent structures.[1]

Early satiety, weight loss, and palpable masses in the upper abdomen may be some of the first clinical signs. Pain related to the malignancy, particularly with advanced lesions, may manifest as right upper quadrant pain that is either parietal or visceral in etiology.[7]

Features of the pain tend to be ill-defined, dull, and aching in nature, mild to moderate in severity, and located in the epigastrium or right upper quadrant and back.[8] Severe pain is possible and more commonly related to perihepatitis or infiltration of the diaphragm.[1]

Cancer pain is now increasingly viewed as a distinct entity due to a complex interplay between the immune system and central and peripheral nervous systems and neoplastic cells.[9]

Interventional Management of Chronic Visceral Pain Syndromes. https://doi.org/10.1016/B978-0-323-75775-1.00014-3

DIAGNOSIS

The evaluation of a patient with pain suspected to originate from the liver must start with a comprehensive history and physical exam aimed at identifying the primary liver disease responsible for the pain. Any other potential pathologic processes must be ruled out.[7] An important aspect in narrowing the differential diagnosis is to characterize the quality of the symptoms. Intermittent symptoms with acute bouts of worsening may be suggestive of disease progression (liver failure). Chronic worsening symptoms may suggest a neoplastic or intrinsic cause (chronic hepatitis).[10]

Imaging has an important role, and the choice of modality may be individualized. Modalities such as contrast-enhanced computed tomography, magnetic resonance imaging, and ultrasound all have few false positives as noninvasive diagnostic modalities.[11] These assist with assessing the extent of the primary disease and evaluating for any potential metastatic lesions as well.

Tumor markers, particularly alpha-fetoprotein (AFP) may be helpful adjuncts to the diagnosis of liver malignancy. Although serum AFP, the most commonly used marker, has only mediocre sensitivity and specificity, testing is helpful in increasing the positive predictive value of other diagnostics such as imaging.

DIFFERENTIAL DIAGNOSIS

The differential diagnosis of pain suspected to be hepatic in origin is extremely diverse and span the range of spontaneously resolving aches to surgical emergencies. A careful history and physical exam is necessary to narrow the differential diagnosis and distinguish right upper quadrant pain that is of hepatic origin from pain involving other nearby structures, including the gallbladder, pancreas, and duodenum.[12]

Disorders of the liver may be categorized as infectious or noninfectious. Infectious causes including hepatitis, amebic infections, pyogenic abscesses, and parasitic infections; all of these may also manifest as right upper quadrant pain. Direct toxic injury to the liver from alcohol consumption or medications is an additional consideration. Autoimmune inflammatory disease is a common mimic that may be suspected in the setting of rheumatologic symptoms including myalgias or rashes. Finally, serious disease such as primary or metastatic neoplasm always needs to be considered.[10]

As previously mentioned, the pain of hepatic origin may also be mistaken for pain from the gallbladder or pancreas. Gallstone disease, including acute cholecystitis, cholelithiasis, cholangitis, and choledocholithiasis, may present with varying patterns of abdominal pain. Pancreatic disease including acute pancreatitis, pseudocysts, and abscesses may present in a similar manner.

PHYSICAL EXAM FINDINGS

The physical exam has an important role in narrowing the differential diagnosis of pain suspected to be hepatic in etiology. Vital signs, particularly temperature, are helpful in suggesting infectious processes. Abdominal palpation may help further elucidate the exact location of the pain. Palpation may also suggest the presence or absence of peritoneal signs, masses, or organomegaly. Ascites and abdominal distension may be more suggestive of a hepatic etiology.[10]

TREATMENT

Pharmacologic

Pharmacologic therapy in the management of pain related to liver malignancy is often complicated by coexisting liver disease or cirrhosis. Analgesics are often metabolized by the liver and traditional dosing and frequency may manifest with untoward effects. A comprehensive understanding of pharmacokinetics is necessary due to the potential increased susceptibility to adverse effects.

Nonopioid analgesics

Acetaminophen is safely used in liver malignancy, even with coexisting liver disease, if alcohol is avoided. Although the Food and Drug Administration suggests a maximum daily dose of 4 g, the daily dose may be reduced to 2 g for age greater than 60.[13] Acetaminophen seems to be safe in advanced chronic liver disease or cirrhosis at recommended doses.[14]

Nonsteroidal antiinflammatory drugs (NSAIDs) comprise a diverse group of analgesics that primarily function through reduction of prostaglandins via inhibition of the cyclooxygenase enzyme. A systematic review of NSAIDs in cancer pain from 2019 concluded a paucity of quality data with respect to efficacy but observed that consideration of potential benefits is important.[15] NSAIDs, however, should be used cautiously in the context of coexisting cirrhosis due to the potential for precipitating renal failure, ascites, or gastrointestinal bleeding.

The role of steroids in the modulation of nociceptive pain continues to be investigated as the exact mechanisms remain unclear. It is postulated that the antiinflammatory effects of steroids mediate a reduction in downstream activation of nociceptors. The most commonly prescribed corticosteroid for pain is the long-acting dexamethasone at a starting dose of 4−8 mg. In practice, steroids are prescribed for multiple nonspecific indications in cancer including bone and neuropathic pain, nausea and vomiting, and anorexia.[16]

Extrahepatic spread of liver malignancies, particularly, hepatocellular carcinoma has an estimated rate of 5%−15%. Approximately two-thirds of those patients may experience severe and debilitating skeletal pain. Bisphosphonates are the standard of care for not only preventing, but treating a skeletal-related complications of bone metastases. Clinical trials have established an analgesic benefit to bisphosphonates but additional direct comparisons with randomized trials are needed, including cost−benefit analyses. The analgesic mechanisms continue to be speculative but current opinions center on the reduction of peripheral sensitization.[17]

Opioids

Opioids may be effective for moderate-to-severe pain associated with malignancy of the liver but need to be prescribed cautiously with coexisting hepatic insufficiency. Opioids including tramadol and codeine undergo biotransformation to active metabolites and may be subject to high variability in clinical efficacy.[13]

The original World Health Organization analgesic ladder was proposed in 1986 to improve strategies for cancer pain management. The modern three-step "ladder" for cancer pain in adults notes an escalation of pharmacologic agents to achieve "freedom from cancer pain." The first step comprises nonopioids (aspirin and paracetamol) with or without adjuvants. If pain persists or increases, mild opioids (codeine) with or without adjuvants and nonopioids are trialed. If pain again persists or increases, strong opioids (morphine) with or without adjuvants and nonopioids should be considered.[18] The original ladder was unidirectional with escalation from nonopioids to weaker opioids to stronger opioids. A fourth step to the ladder was later added that integrated nonpharmacologic procedures encompassing interventional and minimally invasive procedures in addition to a bidirectional approach.

Notable elements of the WHO strategy include oral dosing of drugs if possible (preferred to intravenous or rectal) with an around-the-clock schedule as opposed to on-demand. An understanding of the prescribed opioid is imperative as the prescription schedule should ideally follow the pharmacokinetic characteristics of the drugs.

Answering the question of which opioid analgesic to prescribe in the context of the WHO ladder may be challenging for clinicians. Mild or "weak" opioids are often considered for opioid-naïve patients with mild to moderate cancer pain. Examples include codeine, hydrocodone, or tramadol. Available formulations are principally per os (PO) with immediate and sustained release. Escalation to "strong" opioids including oxycodone, hydromorphone, morphine, and fentanyl is considered if pain persists or increases. Oxycodone is formulated PO with immediate and sustained release options. Hydromorphone and morphine have more formulation options including intravenous and subcutaneous. Fentanyl is a rapid-onset potent analgesic with formulations ranging from transdermal to intravenous to transmucosal.[19]

Methadone is a low-cost and highly potent agent that is emerging as an effective analgesic for the management of cancer pain both in opioid-naïve patients and in rotation from other opioids. It is particularly advantageous due to its high oral and rectal absorption and long duration of action. Typical dosing intervals are 8 or 12 h.[19]

The route of administration is important to consider as oral and rectal opioids are directly absorbed from the gastrointestinal tract and undergo significant first-pass metabolism, thus reducing the bioavailability. Hydrophilic opioids including morphine and oxycodone absorb slowly, in contrast to lipophilic opioids including fentanyl and methadone. Other options to enhance adherence or minimize pill-taking behaviors include transdermal and transmucosal opioids.[19]

Opioid rotation is a maneuver to improve the analgesic response by changing the medication, administration route, or both. Equianalgesia tables may be used to guide opioid rotation for reasons ranging from dose-limiting adverse effects to hyperalgesia to inadequate analgesia. A 25%−50% reduction in the calculated dose accounts for incomplete cross-tolerance among opioids. Guidelines for opioid rotation continue to be primarily empirical and close monitoring in this period is crucial.[19]

An additional consideration is the potential to trigger or worsen hepatic encephalopathy. The European Association for the Study of the Liver observes that administering naltrexone with opioids may decrease the risk of hepatic encephalopathy.[14]

Injections
Celiac plexus block

The celiac plexus block is used as a diagnostic and therapeutic intervention that targets afferent nociceptive fibers. It is a frequently utilized technique in the management of intractable abdominal pain from liver malignancy.

TABLE 11.1
Common Imaging Modalities Utilized for Celiac Plexus Neurolysis.

Imaging Modality	Advantages	Disadvantages
Fluoroscopy	Relatively inexpensive, easier access for most providers, relatively simple to perform	Inability to distinguish abdominal viscera and vascular structures
Computed tomography (CT)	Ability to visualize retroperitoneal organs, vascular structures, celiac axis, malignant lesions; great visualization of needle tip and contrast medium; ability to plan needle trajectory in advance of the procedure	Cost, increased radiation exposure, difficult access to CT machine
Ultrasound	No radiation exposure, inexpensive, easier access, identification of vascular structures	Poor visualization of abdominal viscera
Endoscopic ultrasound	Real-time needle guidance, visualization of vascular structures, reduced risk of neurologic complications	Associated risks of endoscopy, risk of gastric perforation/necrosis

CT-guided Celiac Plexus Neurolysis: A Review of Anatomy, Indications, Technique, and Tips for Successful Treatment. Kambadakone et al. (2011).

The celiac plexus consists of three pairs of ganglia including the celiac ganglia, superior mesenteric ganglia, and aorticorenal ganglia that supply autonomic innervation to abdominal organs including the liver. It is located in the retroperitoneum anterolateral to the aorta at the T12-L1 vertebrae and consists of both para-sympathetic and sympathetic nerves.

Multiple approaches to the technique have been described with the most common being the anterior and posterior para-aortic approaches. Imaging guidance is typically utilized, with fluoroscopy and computed to-mography (CT) imaging being the most common modalities (Table 11.1). A diagnostic block with local anesthetic is typically performed before a neurolytic block to confirm efficacy.[20] Common agents such as 3%−6% phenol or 50%−100% alcohol can be used for chemical neurolysis.

The crus of the diaphragm is the anatomical landmark that determines whether the block is a splanchnic or a celiac plexus block. Splanchnic nerves run posterior to the crus (retrocrural) while the celiac plexus runs anterior to the crus (antecrural). Needle positions at the T11 vertebral body will most likely result in a splanchnic nerve block while approaching a T12/L1 vertebral body will more likely result in a celiac plexus block. For the posterior para-aortic approach, the patient is positioned prone with identification of midline spine and vertebral bodies in addition to iliac crests. With imaging guidance, a spinal needle is advanced from posterior to anterior to the ventral surface of the T12-L1 intervertebral space. As the vertebral body is contacted, the spinal needle is advanced roughly 1−2 cm further into the prevertebral fascial plane.

Needle location may be confirmed by the spread of contrast with CT or fluoroscopic imaging.

The anterior approach is particularly advantageous for patients who may be unable to lie in the prone position. Again, the needle trajectory is mapped with imaging guidance, and a spinal needle is inserted toward the abdominal aorta. The needle may encounter abdominal viscera including bowel, stomach, or liver. With the final location anterior to the aorta and diaphragmatic crura, local anesthetic or neurolytic agents may be deposited in the antecrural space. Although the approach may be faster to perform, the use is ultimately limited by the potential for organ injury.[21]

Intercostal nerve block

An intercostal nerve block is a procedure that targets the intercostal nerves, which supply sensory innervation for the back, trunk, and upper abdomen. This technique may be helpful if the pain from the liver malignancy is thought to be somatic in nature as opposed to sympathetically mediated. Pain secondary to hepatic malignancy is mostly located at the right upper quadrant, right infrascapular, right suprascapular, and epigastric/left subcostal region.[22] Pain is usually described as sharp and worse with coughing, deep breathing, and vomiting. Each intercostal nerve originates from spinal nerves. The ventral branch of the divided spinal nerve continues anterolaterally to become the intercostal nerve. Each nerve travels in a neurovascular bundle with an intercostal artery and vein. The target of the block is the deposition of the local anesthetic in the intercostal sulcus outside of the parietal pleura.[23] As the right upper quadrant is the most common presentation for chest wall pain from hepatic lesions, the blockade of right T9–T11 intercostal never and T12 subcostal nerve is recommended. With the insertion site of the intercostal nerve just below the edge of the rib, this block can be performed with the patient sitting, prone, or left lateral decubitus. The insertion site is medial to the posterior axillary line with 5–10 cm lateral to the corresponding vertebral spinous process (Fig. 11.1). This procedure can be performed with the use of ultrasound or radiographic guidance. Using fluoroscopic guidance, a 25 or 22 gauge needle is directed toward the inferior portion of the targeted rib. After contacting the periosteum, the needle can be slowly walked off to slip under the rib. Curving the needle tip can improve steering and placement of the needle tip. With the needle underneath the rib and facing cephalad, the needle tip can be advanced into the intercostal groove where the vein, artery, and intercostal nerve is located from cephalad to caudad. Injection of contrast can be used to confirm the location of the needle tip (Fig. 11.2). After negative aspiration for blood and air, a mixture of lidocaine or bupivacaine with or without corticosteroid is injected. For neurolysis procedures, the intercostal nerve can be blocked with 3–5cc of 0.5% bupivacaine followed by injection of 2–3cc of a neurolytic agent such as 100% alcohol. When patients respond to diagnostic blocks with local anesthetics, the use of radiofrequency ablation techniques have been described in several case reports.[24,25] Incidence of pneumothorax after the procedure is 0.1%.[26,27] It is imperative to monitor vital signs and respiratory status after the procedure.

Intrathecal therapy

Intrathecal therapy (IT) is an option that should be considered for patients with intractable cancer-related pain who have had inadequate relief with systemic opioids or unacceptable side effects from opioids.[21]

By delivering medication directly into the intrathecal space via an indwelling catheter, IT therapy has the

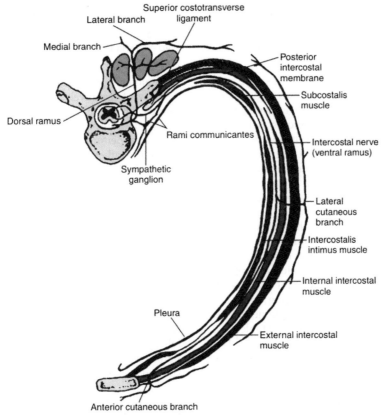

FIG. 11.1 Intercostal nerve anatomy. (Adapted from Ferrante FM, VadeBoncouer TR. *Postoperative Pain Management*. NewYork, Churchill Livingstone: Elsevier; 1993.)

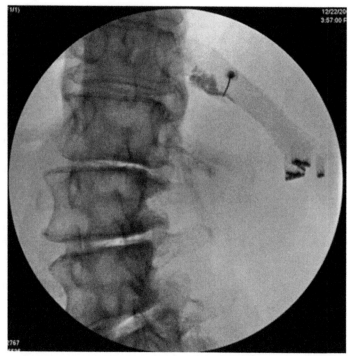

FIG. 11.2 Contrast spread within the right T12 intercostal groove. (Adapted from Lennard TA, Walkowski S, Singla AK, Vivian DG. *Pain Procedures in Clinical Practice*, 3rd ed, Philadelphia, Pennsylvania: Elsevier; 2011.)

distinct advantage of bypassing the blood—brain barrier and delivering medications at low doses. Though previously used as a "last-resort" or salvage therapy for patients unresponsive to high-dose opioids, IT is gaining recognition as an earlier option in the management of malignancy pain syndromes so that pain can be better managed earlier in the disease course before it gets to a point of being uncontrollable.[21] Patients with a defined etiology of pain are recognized as appropriate candidates for IT therapy. In particular, IT opioid therapy is a reasonable strategy for the management of visceral and somatic nociceptive pain such as that experienced with advanced forms of liver cancer.

Currently, morphine, and ziconotide are approved by the Food and Drug Administration for IT analgesia.[28] Multiple additional therapies including local anesthetics, clonidine, baclofen, hydromorphone, and fentanyl are available for administration (Table 11.2). Selection and dosing continue to be ill-defined.[21] However, recent consensus guidelines have been extremely useful for the recommended doses for IT analgesia best practices.[29]

For malignancy of the liver, a trial of intrathecal drug delivery systems (IDDS) before implant is often done to determine the effectiveness of permanent placement.

An epidural or intrathecal catheter is placed for 2—3 days. Alternatively, a single shot spinal may be performed. Greater than 50% reduction of pain is considered a successful trial. Placement of IDDS is a surgical procedure performed under general or spinal anesthesia. The catheter is normally inserted at the L2-3 level and the radio-opaque tip is advanced under fluoroscopy to the desired spinal level. T8 is typically targeted to obtain analgesia for liver malignancy. However, abdominal pain secondary to visceral pathologies have been managed with the tip of the IT catheter located at T1—T9.[30]

If patients have a life expectancy of less than 3 months, then the implant may not be a viable option. Instead, an intraspinal or epidural catheter connected to an external device should be considered for palliative treatment. Risks of infection of indwelling catheters should be weighed against the quality of life and pain relief. Patients and families should be educated on how to use the external device in case the patient is discharged to hospice.

Spinal cord stimulators

Spinal cord stimulation is an attractive nonpharmacologic option for the treatment of patients with

TABLE 11.2
Commonly Used Intrathecal Infusion Agents.

Intrathecal Agent	Maximum Intrathecal Dose Per Day[a]	Notes
Morphine	15 mg/day	Long term infusion associated with catheter tip granuloma. Hydrophilic, can cause respiratory depression, sedation, itching
Hydromorphone	10 mg/day	Can cause respiratory depression, sedation, itching
Fentanyl	1000 mcg/day	Hydrophobic, less risk for respiratory depression
Bupivacaine	15–20 mg/day	Can cause urinary retention, lower extremity weakness, hypotension
Ziconotide	19.2 mcg/day	Can cause fever, hypotension, nausea, confusion, somnolence, urinary retention N-type calcium channel blocker
Clonidine	600 mcg/day	Can cause hypotension, sedation, peripheral edema

The Polyanalgesic Consensus Conference, (PACC): Recommendations on Intrathecal Drug, Infusion Systems Best Practices and Guidelines.
[a] Dose may be increased for end of life care.
Deer et al. (2017).

intractable chronic pain conditions including abdominal pain. The field of neuromodulation continues to advance with novel techniques and waveforms including burst, high frequency, and dorsal root ganglion stimulation.[31] Traditionally used for the treatment of failed back surgery syndrome, complex regional pain syndrome, and peripheral vascular disease, spinal cord stimulator therapy has recently been shown to have therapeutic success in patients with severe visceral abdominal pain. A study from the Cleveland Clinic trialed spinal cord stimulation in 35 patients who were shown to have either visceral or mixed visceral and central pain by retrograde differential epidural block. Moreover, 86% of the patients reported at least 50% pain relief with the completion of the trial.[32] In another study by Kapural et al. patients with chronic abdominal pain secondary to inflammatory, trauma, or functional etiologies were treated with 10-kHz high-frequency spinal cord stimulator implants with leads at T4 through T8. After 12 months of treatment, over 75% of patients endorsed relief of their abdominal pain. Improvement of quality of life as well as mental, physical well-being, sleep quality, and overall satisfaction was also reported. Similarly, a recent case report by Segura et al. revealed that the use of burst spinal cord stimulation improved chronic abdominal pain secondary to chronic pancreatitis.[33] In addition, this study also reported a reduction in opioid consumption and a high degree of patient satisfaction.

Although no case reports to our knowledge describe spinal cord stimulator therapy for hepatocellular carcinoma or other malignancies of the liver, several case reports comment on successful trials for abdominal visceral pain conditions. The largest group was five clinical cases of chronic pancreatitis in which the target was T5–T6 with more than 50% reduction in VAS scores observed 6–8 months postimplant.[34] Successful spinal cord stimulator therapy has also been described in debilitating postprandial pain in the context of extensive intraabdominal surgeries and adhesions.[35]

The mechanism of spinal cord neuromodulation continues to be unclear. Original mechanisms suggested included spinal gating theory in which stimulation of larger afferents may minimize the transmission of visceral pain signals.[36] New animal studies suggest an additional possible mechanism in the antidromic activation of primary efferent fibers in the dorsal columns.[37] The contributions of sympathetic suppression, spinal gating, supraspinal activation, and antidromic activation of neuromodulatory substances continue to be subject to speculation.[35]

Dorsal root ganglion (DRG) stimulation is a promising new modality in the field of neuromodulation as a viable option for the management of chronic intractable pain, particularly for areas that are have been traditionally difficult to treat with traditional spinal cord stimulation (SCS) such as hand, foot, abdomen, and chest. The DRG is integral to sensory transduction and modulation including pain transmission and is implicated in the maintenance of neuropathic pain.[38] It has been suggested that the DRG neurons may be sensitized and hyperexcitable in the setting of injury, thus manifested in altered gene regulations and neuropathic pain.[39] DRG therapy has been described in the treatment of a 49-year old woman with persistent epigastric abdominal pain years after a Roux-en-Y gastric bypass surgery.[40] In this case report, the patient's visceral abdominal pain was successfully managed with SCS leads placed bilaterally at the T-11 dorsal root ganglion.

When considering neuromodulation for these patients, future MRI surveillance should be considered. Often these patients may require repeat MRI to assess the disease course and these devices may not be full-body MRI compatible. This would explain the limited use and studies on the use of spinal cord stimulation in malignant liver patients.

Electroacupuncture

Electroacupunture and multiple acupoint stimulation has been described and studied as a pain management strategy in cancer patients, including advanced hepatocellular carcinoma.[41] A study of electroacupuncture in 65 cases of advanced hepatocellular carcinoma with cancer pain suggested that the onset of the pain relief was slow but may be a viable adjunct for improving analgesia. In addition, a systematic review of 15 randomized controlled trials suggested that acupuncture was an effective adjunct in cancer pain management with pain relief superior to drug therapy alone. The mechanism by which pain relief is attained continues to be unclear.[42]

REFERENCES

1. Attwa MH, El-Etreby SA. Guide for diagnosis and treatment of hepatocellular carcinoma. *World J Hepatol.* 2015;7(12): 1632–1651. https://doi.org/10.4254/wjh.v7.i12.1632.
2. van den Beuken-van Everdingen M, de Rijke J, Kessels A, Schouten H, van Kleef M, Patijn J. Prevalence of pain in patients with cancer: a systematic review of the past 40 years. *Ann Oncol.* 2007;18(9):1437–1449. https://doi.org/10.1093/annonc/mdm056.
3. Atsawarungruangkit A, Pongprasobchai S. Current understanding of the neuropathophysiology of pain in chronic pancreatitis. *World J Gastrointest Pathophysiol.* 2015;6(4): 193–202. https://doi.org/10.4291/wjgp.v6.i4.193.
4. Khan YN, Raza SS, Khan EA. Spinal cord stimulation in visceral pathologies: table 1. *Pain Med.* 2006;7(suppl 1): S121–S125. https://doi.org/10.1111/j.1526-4637.2006.00127.x.
5. Lautt W. *Morgan & Claypool Life Sciences;* 2009. San Rafael (CA): Available from: https://www.ncbi.nlm.nih.gov/books/NBK53061/.
6. Klimpel V. Does Kehr's sign derive from Hans Kehr? A critical commentary on its documentation? *Chirurg.* 2004;75(1): 80–83. https://doi.org/10.1007/s00104-003-0796-2.
7. Kew MC, Dos Santos HA, Sherlock S. Diagnosis of primary cancer of the liver. *Br Med J.* 1971;4(5784):408–411. https://doi.org/10.1136/bmj.4.5784.408.
8. Sun VC-Y, Sarna L. Symptom management in hepatocellular carcinoma. *Clin J Oncol Nurs.* 2008;12(5):759–766. https://doi.org/10.1188/08.CJON.759-766.
9. Chwistek M. Recent advances in understanding and managing cancer pain. *F1000Research.* 2017;6:945. https://doi.org/10.12688/f1000research.10817.1.
10. Avegno J, Carlisle M. Evaluating the patient with right upper quadrant abdominal pain. *Emerg Med Clin.* 2016;34(2): 211–228. https://doi.org/10.1016/j.emc.2015.12.011.
11. Yu NC, Chaudhari V, Raman SS, et al. CT and MRI improve detection of hepatocellular carcinoma, compared with ultrasound alone, in patients with cirrhosis. *Clin Gastroenterol Hepatol.* 2011;9(2):161–167. https://doi.org/10.1016/j.cgh.2010.09.017.
12. Imani F, Motavaf M, Safari S, Alavian SM. The therapeutic use of analgesics in patients with liver cirrhosis: a literature review and evidence-based Recommendations. *Hepat Mon.* 2014;14(10). https://doi.org/10.5812/hepatmon.23539.
13. Tauben D. Nonopioid medications for pain. *Phys Med Rehabil Clin.* 2015;26(2):219–248. https://doi.org/10.1016/j.pmr.2015.01.005.
14. Christian-Miller N, Frenette C. Hepatocellular cancer pain: impact and management challenges. *J Hepatocell Carcinoma.* 2018;5:75–80. https://doi.org/10.2147/JHC.S145450.
15. Magee DJ, Jhanji S, Poulogiannis G, Farquhar-Smith P, Brown MRD. Nonsteroidal anti-inflammatory drugs and pain in cancer patients: a systematic review and reappraisal of the evidence. *Br J Anaesth.* 2019;123(2):e412–e423. https://doi.org/10.1016/j.bja.2019.02.028.
16. Leppert W, Buss T. The role of corticosteroids in the treatment of pain in cancer patients. *Curr Pain Headache Rep.* 2012;16(4):307–313. https://doi.org/10.1007/s11916-012-0273-z.
17. Gralow J, Tripathy D. Managing metastatic bone pain: the role of bisphosphonates. *J Pain Symptom Manag.* 2007; 33(4):462–472. https://doi.org/10.1016/j.jpainsymman.2007.01.001.
18. Ventafridda V, Saita L, Ripamonti C, De Conno F. WHO guidelines for the use of analgesics in cancer pain. *Int J Tissue React.* 1985;7(1):93–96.
19. Wickham RJ. Cancer pain management: opioid analgesics, Part 2. *J Adv Pract Oncol.* 2017;8(6):588–607.
20. Sachdev A, Gress F. Celiac plexus block and neurolysis: a review. *Gastrointestinal Endoscopy Clinics of North America.* 2008;28(4):579–586.
21. Bruel BM, Burton AW. Intrathecal therapy for cancer-related pain. *Pain Med.* 2016;17(12):2404–2421. https://doi.org/10.1093/pm/pnw060.
22. Waldman SD, Feldstein GS, Donohoe CD, Waldman KA. The relief of body wall pain secondary to malignant hepatic metastases by intercostal nerve block with bupivicaine and methylprednisolone. *J Pain Symptom Manag.* 1988;3(1): 39–43. https://doi.org/10.1016/0885-3924(88)90136-4.

23. Matchett G. Intercostal nerve block and neurolysis for intractable cancer pain. *J Pain Palliat Care Pharmacother.* 2016;30(2).

24. Abd-Elsayed A, Lee S, Jackson M. Radiofrequency ablation for treating resistant intercostal neuralgia. *Ochsner J.* 2018; 18(1):91−93.

25. Tewari S, Agarwal A, Gautam SK, Madabushi R. Intercostal neuralgia occurring as a complication of splanchnic nerve radiofrequency ablation in a patient with chronic pancreatitis. *Pain Physician.* 2017;20(5):E747−E750.

26. Moore DC, Bridenbaugh LD. Intercostal nerve block in 4333 patients: indications, technique, and complications. *Anesth Analg.* 1962;41:1−11.

27. Moore DC. Intercostal nerve block for postoperative somatic pain following surgery of thorax and upper abdomen. *Br J Anaesth.* 1975;47(suppl):284−286.

28. Deer TR, Pope JE, Hanes MC, McDowell GC. Intrathecal therapy for chronic pain: a review of morphine and ziconotide as firstline options. *Pain Med.* 2019;20(4): 784−798. https://doi.org/10.1093/pm/pny132.

29. The polyanalgesic consensus conference (PACC): Recommendations on intrathecal drug infusion systems best practices and guidelines. *Neuromodulation.* 2017;20(4): 405−406. https://doi.org/10.1111/ner.12618.

30. Kongkam P, Wagner DL, Sherman S, et al. Intrathecal narcotic infusion pumps for intractable pain of chronic pancreatitis: a pilot series. *Am J Gastroenterol.* 2009; 104(5):1249−1255. https://doi.org/10.1038/ajg.2009.54.

31. Caylor J, Reddy R, Yin S, et al. Spinal cord stimulation in chronic pain: evidence and theory for mechanisms of action. *Bioelectron Med.* 2019;5. https://doi.org/10.1186/s42234-019-0023-1.

32. Kapural L, Nagem H, Tlucek H, Sessler DI. Spinal cord stimulation for chronic visceral abdominal pain. *Pain Med.* 2010; 11(3):347−355. https://doi.org/10.1111/j.1526-4637.2009.00785.x.

33. Delange Segura L, Rodríguez Padilla M, Palomino Jiménez MT, Fernández Baena M, Rodríguez Staff JF. Salvage therapy with burst spinal cord stimulation for chronic pancreatitis: a case report. *Pain Pract.* 2019;19(5):530−535. https://doi.org/10.1111/papr.12771.

34. Kapural L, Rakic M. Spinal cord stimulation for chronic visceral pain secondary to chronic non-alcoholic pancreatitis. *J Clin Gastroenterol.* 2008;42(6):750−751. https://doi.org/10.1097/01.mcg.0000225647.77437.45.

35. Tiede JM, Ghazi SM, Lamer TJ, Obray JB. The use of spinal cord stimulation in refractory abdominal visceral pain: case reports and literature review. *Pain Pract.* 2006;6(3): 197−202. https://doi.org/10.1111/j.1533-2500.2006.00085.x.

36. Melzack R, Wall PD. Pain mechanisms: a new theory. *Science.* 1965;150(3699):971−979. https://doi.org/10.1126/science.150.3699.971.

37. Qin C, Lehew RT, Khan KA, Wienecke GM, Foreman RD. Spinal cord stimulation modulates intraspinal colorectal visceroreceptive transmission in rats. *Neurosci Res.* 2007; 58(1):58−66. https://doi.org/10.1016/j.neures.2007.01.014.

38. Esposito MF, Malayil R, Hanes M, Deer T. Unique characteristics of the dorsal root ganglion as a target for neuromodulation. *Pain Med.* 2019;20(Suppl 1):S23−S30. https://doi.org/10.1093/pm/pnz012.

39. Liem L, van Dongen E, Huygen FJ, Staats P, Kramer J. The dorsal root ganglion as a therapeutic target for chronic pain. *Reg Anesth Pain Med.* 2016;41(4):511−519. https://doi.org/10.1097/AAP.0000000000000408.

40. Kloosterman JR, Yang A, van Helmond N, Chapman KB. Dorsal root ganglion stimulation to treat persistent abdominal pain after bypass surgery. *Pain Med.* August 24, 2019. https://doi.org/10.1093/pm/pnz193. pnz193.

41. Choi T-Y, Lee MS, Kim T-H, Zaslawski C, Ernst E. Acupuncture for the treatment of cancer pain: a systematic review of randomised clinical trials. *Support Care Canc.* 2012;20(6):1147−1158. https://doi.org/10.1007/s00520-012-1432-9.

42. Xu L. Clinical analysis of electroacupuncture and multiple acupoint stimulation in relieving cancer pain in patients with advanced hepatocellular carcinoma. *J Cancer Res Ther.* 2018;14(1):99−102.

FURTHER READING

1. Chandok N, Watt KDS. Pain management in the cirrhotic patient: the clinical challenge. *Mayo Clin Proc.* 2010; 85(5):451−458. https://doi.org/10.4065/mcp.2009.0534.

CHAPTER 12

Gastric Cancer Pain

RONNIE M. IBRAHIM, MD • DANIEL J. PAK, MD

INTRODUCTION

Gastric cancers are organized based on histologic morphology, with the adenocarcinoma subtype being the most common.[3] Gastric cancers also include gastrointestinal lymphomas. Interestingly, there is a dichotomous distribution of gastric cancer subtypes related to geography. As of 2019, an estimated 27,510 annual new cases and 11,140 annual deaths occur in the United States due to gastric cancers.[4] In Asian countries, distal gastric cancers are more common, and in some countries like South Korea are prevalent enough to mandate screening programs. In the West, proximal tumors are more common and present later at more advanced stages.[4]

Risk factors include *H. pylori* infection and associated chronic mucosal inflammation, pernicious anemia, smoking, genetic mutations in cell adhesion proteins, and diets high in salted or smoked foods. The pain associated with advanced gastric cancer is visceral in character and in the epigastric region, owing to the stomach's location. It is often chronic and lifelong in the case of an advanced cancer diagnosis. In addition, due to the mechanical effects of the tumor, symptoms of obstruction can be seen including nausea, vomiting, early satiety, and preclusion of enteral feeding in severe cases. Medical management of gastric cancer pain is guided by the World Health Organization (WHO) pain ladder (Fig. 12.1), which serves as a framework for the escalation of opioids.[5] Consideration should be given to coexisting gastritis, and caution should be taken when considering the use of nonsteroidal antiinflammatory drugs (NSAIDs) for pain. For associated refractory chronic pain syndromes where the pain is poorly controlled with opioids and nonopioid adjuvants, celiac plexus blocks are often performed. Additionally, interventions such as spinal cord stimulators or intrathecal drug delivery systems or epidural devices can be used to reduce pain, improve function, and lower opioid consumption.

ETIOLOGY AND PATHOGENESIS

The afferent nerve fibers of the gastrointestinal tract (GI) travel with sympathetic and parasympathetic nerve fibers via a complex collection of ganglia and plexuses en route to the spinal cord. These visceral nerve axons are almost completely comprised of unmyelinated C and thinly myelinated Aδ fibers. The stomach specifically receives its sympathetic innervation from the celiac plexus via the greater thoracic splanchnic nerves (T5−T9) and parasympathetic innervation from the anterior and posterior trunks of the vagus nerve. Sympathetic communication with the enteric nervous system can be bidirectional, suggesting the role of sympathetic plexus blockade on enteric nociception.[6] The GI tract's sensory innervation involves the mucosa, muscularis mucosa, and the serosa. Several nociceptors have been identified, including mechanoreceptors of varying thresholds, and silent nociceptors, which respond to chemical tissue insult and may be critical in the development of peripheral sensitization and the development of chronic visceral pain.[7]

Biochemical messengers seen in elevated amounts in gastric neoplasms, including cancer-associated trypsins, have been implicated in the activation of primary afferent nociceptors.[8] These species are important to the maintenance of the neoplastic cell matrix and have a secondary effect of inducing substance P and calcitonin gene-related protein from peripheral C fibers. In addition, these molecules can induce hyperalgesia to mechanical stimuli.[9,10] The inflammatory milieu seen in carcinomatous proliferation likely contributes to silent nociceptor-induced peripheral and central sensitization.[11] As seen with many other cancer pain syndromes, perineural invasion of gastric cancers portends a poorer prognosis and is a significant source of neuropathic pain.[12]

Thus, it is expected that gastric neoplasms, like many other enteric neoplasms, cause pain through visceral mechanical afferents, inflammatory-mediated pain and associated hyperalgesia, and sympathetically mediated

Interventional Management of Chronic Visceral Pain Syndromes. https://doi.org/10.1016/B978-0-323-75775-1.00001-5

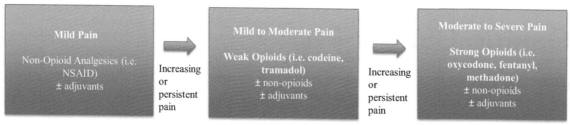

FIG. 12.1 **WHO guidelines for cancer pain relief.** For patients with moderate-to-severe pain, opioids should be considered from the start of therapy.

mechanisms given the communication between the enteric nervous system and sympathetic plexuses. Unfortunately, sympathetically mediated pain remains a poorly understood topic in the realm of pain management, but the benefits of interventional sympathectomy in managing gastric cancer pain are apparent.[13]

CLINICAL FEATURES

The presentation of pain associated with gastric cancer depends on the individual patient's tumor burden with respect to tumor size, perineural invasion, and the presence or absence of obstructive symptoms. The associated pain is generally visceral in nature and can result both from primary tumor burden and from metastatic disease. Mechanical stimuli, such as torsion or distension, stretching of serosal and mucosal surfaces, and compression of nearby nerve structures produce pain.[14] Pain is often constant and epigastric due to the mechanical nociceptive stimulus from a fixed neoplastic mass. Breakthrough abdominal pain has also been characterized as a worsening of background visceral pain secondary to acute changes in visceral lumen distention, commonly observed with food intake. As with any visceral pain, the character is described as "deep," "crampy," and "gnawing," among other terms. It is important to note that the severity of pain does not always reflect the severity of inciting cancer.[3]

Visceral breakthrough pain is worsened by undertreatment or underoptimization of one's antinociceptive regimen. In addition, visceral abdominal breakthrough pain is quite common, with a cited rate of 55% of patients experiencing breakthrough pain, even with well-controlled background pain.[14,15] Breakthrough pain may afflict patients several times per day, with episodes varying in both onset and duration.

Attention should also be given to pain induced by therapeutics as well. Chemotherapy agents including the microtubule inhibitors (docetaxel, paclitaxel) have been linked to myalgias, arthralgias, and neuropathic pain syndromes, as have other agents such as anthracyclines.[16] Radiation therapy can cause mucosal irritation when applied to gastrointestinal organs and is a source of chronic enteropathy and neuropathy.

DIAGNOSIS

Many of the signs and symptoms of gastric malignancy are indolent or mimic other less serious pathologies. Typically, patients remain asymptomatic until they develop more advanced disease, often experiencing weight loss, anorexia, nausea, early satiety, and dysphagia. As often seen with the hypercoagulable state of other malignancies, migratory phlebitis (Trousseau's syndrome) can also be seen. Occult upper GI bleeding may accompany symptoms. Pain, if even present during the early stages of the disease, is typically epigastric, vague, and mild early in the disease course. Diagnosis is made definitively with upper endoscopy and tissue biopsies with adjunct barium contrast imaging. When the diagnosis of a gastric malignancy is confirmed, computed tomography (CT) imaging and positron emission tomography (PET) CT are frequently utilized for staging and to assess for distant metastatic disease. Genetic screening is also useful in cases of familial subtypes of gastric cancer.[17]

DIFFERENTIAL DIAGNOSIS

Many of the symptoms of gastric cancer are both vague and indolent, and are seen in other GI pathologies including acute gastritis, peptic ulcer disease, atrophic gastritis, gastroenteritis, esophagitis, and esophageal cancer.[18] In addition, many of these conditions can mimic the endoscopic appearance of gastric cancer and are excluded after biopsy.[19] Other primary GI malignancies, such as pancreatic cancer and colorectal cancer, can also present with similar symptomatology and should be considered.

PHYSICAL EXAM FINDINGS

Physical exam is usually unrevealing except in cases of advanced disease. Melena, especially in combination with anemia or weight loss, should raise one's clinical suspicion for neoplasm.[18] Physical palpation of an abdominal mass is occasionally seen, as are signs of lymph nodal spread (Virchow node), or from paraneoplastic syndromes including acanthosis nigricans and diffuse seborrheic keratoses.[20]

TREATMENT

As one could expect in the treatment of any malignancy pain syndrome, the psychological aspects of a gastric cancer diagnosis interplay with a patient's management and expectations of his or her pain. As our understanding of the precise mechanisms and development of chronic visceral pain improve, novel pharmacologic agents and their mechanisms remain a topic of significant interest. The optimal treatment of chronic gastric cancer pain involves multimodal pharmacologic therapy including opioid and nonopioid adjuvants and the use of more invasive interventions when appropriate.[21]

Many different agents have been used to treat chronic abdominal visceral pain. However, given the often advanced and terminal nature of many gastric cancer diagnoses, opioids remain the staple pharmacologic choice. Other nonopioid options include NSAIDs, acetaminophen, and neuropathic agents.[5,22,23]

Nonopioid Analgesics

Acetaminophen is a nonopioid analgesic that can be dosed 325–1000 mg by mouth every 4–6 h as needed, up to a maximum of 4000 mg/day. Care should be taken not to exceed this maximum dose due to the risk of hepatotoxicity. Acetaminophen is a common first step analgesic for mild-to-moderate pain and is almost universally tolerated.

NSAIDs are part of the WHO approach to cancer-pain management and are a staple in the management of both acute and chronic pain.[21] In patients with gastric cancer, the use of NSAIDs may be complicated by the exacerbation of comorbid gastritis, chronic GI bleeding, or ulcerative disease. Individual clinical judgment should be taken regarding the use of chronic NSAID therapy in these patients, including the consideration of patients' renal function. Examples of nonselective cyclooxygenase (COX) inhibitors include ibuprofen, naproxen, indomethacin, and ketorolac. These agents have a ceiling effect that limits their utility in controlling cancer pain.[21] COX-2 inhibitors remain an option due to their improved safety profile with regard to GI side effects and thus make them better options for GI cancer pain. Examples include rofecoxib and celecoxib. Celecoxib can be started typically at 200 mg by mouth, twice daily.[24]

Adjuvant analgesics have varying degrees of data supporting their use for chronic cancer pain. These agents include antidepressants, muscle relaxants, antiepileptics, and steroids. They have several advantages including reducing the opioid burden and addressing pain less amenable to opioid pharmacotherapy.[25]

Tricyclic antidepressants (TCAs) can be effective in the treatment of neuropathic pain. Cancer pain syndromes often have neuropathic components due to neural invasion. Although TCAs have been less rigorously studied in the treatment of chronic cancer pain, small studies and clinical experiences have shown them to be beneficial.[23] Common agents include amitriptyline, nortriptyline, and desipramine, which can be started at 10–25 mg, by mouth, nightly. Care should be taken with the significant side effects of cardiotoxicity and anticholinergic effects.[26]

Other antidepressants, including selective serotonin reuptake inhibitors and serotonin-norepinephrine reuptake inhibitors, have less rigorous data supporting their use in neuropathic and cancer pain syndromes but can be considered in the holistic treatment of the cancer patient with psychiatric comorbidities.[27,28]

Low dose steroids can be used for the pain caused by GI tract distention from gastric cancer, and a typical regimen is dexamethasone, 2–4 mg orally, once or twice daily. Adverse effects including mood disturbances, cushingoid changes, fluid retention, and immunosuppression should be weighed against the benefits, which can include a reduction in nausea and improved appetite.[29]

Ketamine administered by monitored intravenous (IV) infusion is effective for allaying cancer pain.[30,31] This is a medical approach to refractory pain, and if administered under regularly scheduled intervals, can reduce basal opioid requirements for patients. Ketamine has been given IV or through 3–5-day continuous intramuscular infusions of 100–500 mg/24 h in monitored palliative care units, and has been shown to reduce opioid requirements and baseline pain scores.[32] Chung and Pharo showed that IV ketamine at 0.2–0.65 mg/kg/h for 30 days in a palliative home care setting resulted in significant improvements in pain with concurrent opioid-sparing effects.[33] Care should be taken to note side effects including hallucinations or dysphoria, nausea, and vomiting, and an increase in oral secretions.

As an outpatient, intranasal ketamine can be considered to reduce oral opioid requirements. The nares and sinus cavities have increased vascular supple and great absorption. In addition, the intranasal route has greater bioavailability compared to the oral route due to the absence of the first-pass metabolism. The data is limited to intranasal ketamine for cancer pain. Intranasal ketamine will have to be made from a compound pharmacy with a specially prepared nasal spray to deliver a mist of atomized medication. Dosing can be used with 100 mg ketamine per ml with 10 mg or 0.1 mL administered per puff with three times per day or four times per day.[34]

Opioids

Opioids are still considered the mainstay treatment for chronic malignant visceral pain, and the WHO analgesic ladder (Fig. 12.1) is the conventionally accepted approach for opioid treatment.[34] Although they carry many adverse effects, opioids are effective if the appropriate regimen is tailored to the individual patient.[35] There is no evidence to suggest the therapeutic superiority of one opioid over another for cancer pain[36]; therefore, given that individuals may have varying responses to different μ-agonists, the opioid rotation should be considered to identify the most effective agent. Sustained-release formulations should be used when appropriate for patients with inadequate pain control with as needed usage of immediate-release (IR) formulations. If oral medications are not well-tolerated and long-acting agents are needed, transdermal fentanyl should be considered.[36]

Less emphasized side effects of chronic opioid use include impairments to fertility and libido, and immunosuppression.[37,38] Doses of commonly used agents are shown in Table 12.1, and both extended-release and immediate-release formulations should be appropriately tailored to the individual patient to provide basal and breakthrough pain relief.[39,40]

Opioid use in cancer survivors is controversial, and it is important to note that the psychosocial hardships associated with cancer treatment, including depression and anxiety, may put these patients at risk for dependency and misuse.

Celiac Plexus Block, Neurolysis

Celiac plexus block and neurolysis remain a staple intervention for patients with refractory abdominal pain secondary to gastric cancer. There are multiple approaches to celiac plexus blockade, with most being performed percutaneously from either an anterior or posterior approach.[41–43] Blockade can be achieved with CT, fluoroscopy, or ultrasound guidance.

Posterior approaches for celiac blocks are typically performed utilizing the antecrural or retrocrural techniques, which refer to the site of injection. The antecrural and retrocrural sites are the spaces anterior and posterior, respectively, to the crura of the diaphragm. The antecrural approach is effective for targeting the celiac plexus (Fig. 12.2) while the retrocrural approach targets the splanchnic nerves. Multiple studies have shown persistent benefit after long term follow-up for up to 3 months in those with pancreatic cancer and other intraabdominal cancers.

A diagnostic block using a small volume of a shorter-acting local anesthetic (such as 9 cc of 2% lidocaine) can be followed with neurolysis using either alcohol or phenol. Bilateral posterior injections of 25–30 mL of 50%–100% ethanol constitute a common approach.[41] Pain relief can be immediate, and the magnitude of visual analog scale (VAS) score reduction is often significant, with some patients reporting scores of <2 following the procedure. In addition, for patients on chronic opioids, reductions of up to 69 mg of morphine equivalents have been seen at 3 months postneurolysis.[42,43] The most common adverse effects of celiac plexus neurolysis include injection site pain, diarrhea, and hypotension due to functional celiac sympathectomy.[43–45]

Spinal Cord Stimulation

Spinal cord stimulators have many uses for chronic pain, including neuropathic pain, ischemic pain, complex regional pain syndrome, and failed back surgery syndrome.[46] Additionally, evidence has shown benefit in reducing both baseline VAS scores and opioid consumption in patients with chronic visceral abdominal pain. A review of case reports demonstrates that optimal placement for patients suffering from pancreatitis, chronic gastroparesis pain, or postsurgical gastric pain involved octrode leads placed at the T5–6 levels. Furthermore, about a third of patients experienced optimal relief at the T2–T4 levels and the T8–T11 levels, indicating the obvious need for individualized mapping.[46] In those patients undergoing permanent stimulator implantation, VAS scores were reduced from a mean of 8 to 2.5, with a morphine equivalent dose reduction ranging from 36 to 160 mg. Given the demonstrated efficacy of spinal cord stimulators for visceral abdominal pain, stimulator implantation remains a long-term management option to consider alongside neurolysis.

TABLE 12.1
Commonly Used Opioids for the Treatment of Gastric Cancer Pain.

Medication	Initial Dosing	Comments
Codeine	15–60 mg every 4–6 h	CYP2D6 metabolism. Not recommended in renal failure.
Tramadol	50–100 mg every 4–6 h	Weak inhibitor of norepinephrine and serotonin reuptake
Hydrocodone	5–10 mg every 4–6 h,	Combined with 300–325 mg acetaminophen depending on formulation
Morphine	15–30 mg every 4–6 h	Available in immediate-release tablet, suppository, oral liquid, IV, and subcutaneous use Metabolites morphine-3 and morphine-6-gluconoride may accumulate in renal failure and alter reliable kinetics
Oxycodone	5–15 mg every 4–6 h	Available in combination with acetaminophen or standalone
Methadone	2–5 mg every 8 h	Unpredictable half-life requires patient individualization in titration. QTc prolonging. NMDA antagonism confers multifactorial analgesia and theoretical protection against opioid-induced hyperalgesia. Relatively safe in renal failure.
Hydromorphone	2–4 mg every 4–6 h	Safer than morphine in renal insufficiency.
Buprenorphine	Buccal film: 75 mcg daily Transdermal patch: 5 mcg/h	Partial mu agonism confers the analgesic ceiling effect. Limited experience in cancer pain.
Fentanyl	Individualized based on daily morphine consumption, mostly used in cancer pain in transdermal formulations. Transdermal fentanyl dose typically starts at 12–25 mcg/h	Intranasal formulations, buccal, and sublingual tablets and lozenges exist for breakthrough cancer pain. Safe for use in renal failure.

Furthermore, the recent development of high frequency, "paresthesia-free" spinal cord stimulation has spurred interests in its application for abdominal pain.[47] Traditionally based on the "gate control" theory of pain where nonpainful sensory inputs effectively "gate" off ascending pain signals, conventional paresthesia-based spinal cord stimulation delivers electrical impulses to the dorsal column of the spinal cord at a frequency of 2–1200 Hz with above-sensory threshold amplitudes. Comparatively, high-frequency stimulation utilizes subsensory threshold amplitudes with frequencies up to 10 kHz. As a result, high-frequency waveforms eliminate the often uncomfortable sensations of abdominal paresthesias and the need for intraoperative mapping during implant and revision surgeries. The analgesic mechanism of high-frequency stimulation remains unclear. However, it is postulated that afferent nerve signaling may be reduced from the activation of inhibitor interneurons with 10-kHz stimulation.[47]

Spinal cord stimulators, as expected with any implantable devices, carry complications including lead migration and associated loss of analgesic therapy, lead fracture, seroma, infection, dural puncture, epidural hematoma, or cord trauma. In addition, these devices also carry the risk of tolerance and a resulting loss of analgesia.[48–50] The need for repeat MRIs for surveillance of disease progression should be considered before spinal cord stimulation as devices may have limited MRI compatibility.

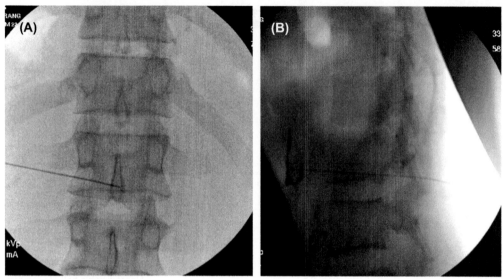

FIG. 12.2 Antecrural celiac plexus neurolysis under fluoroscopic guidance. Final needle position is shown in the **(A)** anteroposterior and **(B)** lateral views. Contrast medium outlining the plexus is seen in the lateral view **(B)**.

Intrathecal Drug Delivery Systems

Intrathecal drug delivery systems (IDDS) should be considered in patients with focal pain that is refractory to traditional systemic opioids or those who are unable to tolerate the side effects of opioids.[46,51] These are implantable devices with a tunneled intrathecal catheter connected to a reservoir system typically placed in a subcutaneous pocket in the abdomen. Medications (most often an opioid) are then delivered directly into the intrathecal space and programmed at a continuous rate with the option of providing additional scheduled and patient-controlled boluses. Before proceeding with the full implant, a trial of intrathecal opioids is often done to assess the patient's candidacy for permanent therapy. This may be achieved with either a single shot spinal injection or infusion via intrathecal or epidural catheter. Recent guidelines by the Polyanalgesic Consensus Conference indicate that patient with advanced disease and limited life expectancy may forego an intrathecal trial and proceed directly to the implant procedure.[52]

Cather placement is typically done with fluoroscopic guidance and introduced at the lumbar spinal level. Final tip placement should be in accordance with the dermatomal distribution of the patient's pain, with optimal placement for epigastric pain roughly being between the T6 and T8 vertebral bodies.[51,53]

There are three medications approved for IDDS by the US Food and Drug Administration: morphine, ziconotide, and baclofen. Ziconotide is an N-type calcium channel blocker that acts at the level of the dorsal horn to provide analgesia. Many other agents are used off-label in practice for IDDS, including hydromorphone, fentanyl, sufentanil, clonidine, and bupivacaine. Drug combinations, typically a combination of an opioid with either bupivacaine or clonidine, are utilized for mixed nociceptive and neuropathic pain disorders. A review of implant cases shows morphine to be an attractive first agent given its hydrophilic properties; however, in cases of escalating intrathecal narcotic requirement, bupivacaine has been added with success to reduce the concurrent opioid infusion dosage.[54–56]

Ziconotide is another nonnarcotic agent that can be infused in patients with pain refractory to opioids or with opioid-related side effects. A substantial portion of patients receiving intrathecal ziconotide experienced VAS score reductions of >50%. Risks include psychosis and other CNS-related side effects. Ziconotide may also be combined with narcotics to achieve analgesic synergy.[55,57,58]

IDDS carry risks of granuloma formation at the catheter tip, opioid tolerance, orthostatic hypotension, meningitis, and spinal cord injury. Fortunately, most of these serious adverse events are uncommon.[57,58] Table 12.2 shows commonly infused intrathecal agents and some comments about their usage.

TABLE 12.2
Commonly Used Intrathecal Infusion Agents.[52]

Intrathecal Agent	Maximum Intrathecal Dose Per Day[a]	Notes
Morphine	15 mg/day	Long term infusion associated with catheter tip granuloma. Hydrophilic, can cause respiratory depression, sedation, itching
Hydromorphone	10 mg/day	Can cause respiratory depression, sedation, itching
Fentanyl	1000 mcg/day	Hydrophobic, less risk for respiratory depression
Bupivacaine	15–20 mg/day	Can cause urinary retention, lower extremity weakness, hypotension
Ziconotide	19.2 mcg/day	Can cause fever, hypotension, nausea, confusion, somnolence, urinary retention N-type calcium channel blocker
Clonidine	600 mcg/day	Can cause hypotension, sedation, peripheral edema

[a] Dose may be increased for end of life care.

Tunneled Intraspinal Catheter Systems

Other options for chronic gastric cancer pain include tunneled epidural catheters and intrathecal infusions of analgesics. This is typically reserved for patients who have a life expectancy of less than 3 months as implantable intrathecal drug delivery systems may not be an option. Epidural catheters can be placed and tunneled after appropriate placement with typical loss-of-resistance methods, with or without fluoroscopic assistance. These catheters are connected to external portable infusion pumps. Patients with both chronic somatic and visceral abdominal pain experience relief after epidural implantation, with some data citing rates of up to 77% of patients achieving improvement in baseline pain scores.[29,51,59]

Alternative Therapies

Cognitive behavioral therapy (CBT) can help with achieving a sense of control over one's illness. CBT can also assist in developing coping skills, providing benefits for patients' sense of perceived pain and disability.[60,61]

Transcutaneous electrical nerve stimulation units may also provide benefits for severe cancer-related pain. Although not validated explicitly for gastric cancer, there has been some demonstrated benefit in managing other visceral cancer pain with minimal side effects.[62]

Transcranial magnetic stimulation is a nascent treatment modality with limited research in the management of chronic cancer pain. Treatment is carried out through targeted neural stimulation using a changing magnetic field, which is used to induce an electric current at a focal area of the brain. During the procedure, a magnetic coil is noninvasively placed on the patient's skull, and a magnetic field is induced. Effects can vary based on the frequency and intensity of the magnetic field.[63] Prior applications have included the management of Parkinsonian tremors and schizophrenia. The utility in transcranial magnetic stimulation in gastric cancer pain remains promising, but unproven. Limited studies have shown moderate benefit in pain scores for palliative care patients with cancer diagnoses who did not tolerate opioid analgesics.[64,65]

REFERENCES

1. Rawla P, Barsouk A. Epidemiology of gastric cancer: global trends, risk factors and prevention. *Przeglad Gastroenterol.* 2019;14:26–38. https://doi.org/10.5114/pg.2018.80001.
2. Bowles MJ, Benjamin IS. ABC of the upper gastrointestinal tract: cancer of the stomach and pancreas. *BMJ.* 2001;323(7326):1413–1416. https://doi.org/10.1136/bmj.323.7326.1413.
3. Karimi P, Islami F, Anandasabapathy S, Freedman ND, Kamangar F. Gastric cancer: descriptive epidemiology, risk factors, screening, and prevention, cancer epidemiol. *Prev. Biomarkers.* 2014;23:700–713. https://doi.org/10.1158/1055-9965.EPI-13-1057.
4. Siegel RL, Miller KD, Jemal A. Cancer statistics, 2019. *Ca - Cancer J Clin.* 2019;69(1):7–34. https://doi.org/10.3322/caac.21551.
5. WHO. WHO | WHO's cancer pain ladder for adults. *World Heal. Organ.* 2016. https://doi.org/2019.
6. Furness JB. The enteric nervous system and neurogastroenterology. *Nat Rev Gastroenterol Hepatol.* 2012;9(5):286–294. https://doi.org/10.1038/nrgastro.2012.32.
7. Wesselmann U. Chronic nonmalignant visceral pain syndromes of the abdomen, pelvis, and bladder and chronic urogenital and rectal pain. In: *Pain Curr. Understanding, Emerg. Ther. Nov. Approaches to Drug Discov.* 2003. https://doi.org/10.1201/9780203911259.ch20.

8. Nyberg P, Ylipalosaari M, Sorsa T, Salo T. Trypsins and their role in carcinoma growth. *Exp Cell Res.* 2006;312(8): 1219−1228. https://doi.org/10.1016/j.yexcr.2005.12.024.

9. Grant AD, Cottrell GS, Amadesi S, et al. Protease-activated receptor 2 sensitizes the transient receptor potential vanilloid 4 ion channel to cause mechanical hyperalgesia in mice. *J Physiol.* 2007;578(3):715−733. https://doi.org/10.1113/jphysiol.2006.121111.

10. Amadesi S, Cottrell GS, Divino L, et al. Protease-activated receptor 2 sensitizes TRPV1 by protein kinase Cε- and A-dependent mechanisms in rats and mice. *J Physiol.* 2006;575(2): 555−571. https://doi.org/10.1113/jphysiol.2006.111534.

11. Gebhart GF. Visceral pain - peripheral sensitisation. In: *Gut.* 2000. https://doi.org/10.1136/gut.47.suppl_4.iv54.

12. Deng J, You Q, Gao Y, et al. Prognostic value of perineural invasion in gastric cancer: a systematic review and meta-analysis. *PLoS ONE.* 2014;9(2):e88907. https://doi.org/10.1371/journal.pone.0088907.

13. Chen S-S, Zhang J-M. Progress in sympathetically mediated pathological pain. *J. Anesth. Perioper. Med.* 2015;2(4): 216−225. https://doi.org/10.24015/japm.2015.0029.

14. Mercadante S, Adile C, Giarratano A, Casuccio A. Breakthrough pain in patients with abdominal cancer pain. *Clin J Pain.* 2014;30(6):510−514. https://doi.org/10.1097/AJP.0000000000000004.

15. Mercadante S, Klepstad P, Kurita GP, Sjøgren P, Giarratano A. Sympathetic blocks for visceral cancer pain management: a systematic review and EAPC recommendations. *Crit Rev Oncol Hematol.* 2015;96(3): 577−583. https://doi.org/10.1016/j.critrevonc.2015.07.014.

16. Loprinzi CL, Reeves BN, Dakhil SR, et al. Natural history of paclitaxel-associated acute pain syndrome: prospective cohort study NCCTG N08C1. *J Clin Oncol.* 2011;29(11): 1472−1478. https://doi.org/10.1200/JCO.2010.33.0308.

17. Gastric Cancer. *Hopkins Med;* 2013. https://www.hopkinsmedicine.org/gastroenterology_hepatology/_pdfs/esophagus_stomach/gastric_cancer.pdf.

18. Wanebo HJ, Kennedy BJ, Chmiel J, Steele G, Winchester D, Osteen R. Cancer of the stomach: a patient care study by the American College of Surgeons. *Ann Surg.* 1993; 218(5):583−592. https://doi.org/10.1097/00000658-199321850-00002.

19. Xue H, yu Ge H, ying Miao L, et al. Differential diagnosis of gastric cancer and gastritis: the role of contrast-enhanced ultrasound (CEUS). *Abdom. Radiol.* 2017;42(3):802−809. https://doi.org/10.1007/s00261-016-0952-z.

20. Morgenstern L. The Virchow-Troisier node: a historical note. *Am J Surg.* 1979;138(5):703. https://doi.org/10.1016/0002-9610(79)90353-2.

21. Nersesyan H, Slavin KV. Current aproach to cancer pain management: availability and implications of different treatment options. *Therapeut Clin Risk Manag.* 2007;7(2): 113−120.

22. Magni G, Arsie D, De Leo D. Antidepressants in the treatment of cancer pain. *A survey in Italy, Pain.* 1987;29(3): 347−353. https://doi.org/10.1016/0304-3959(87)90049-2.

23. Walsh TD, MacDonald N, Bruera E, Shepard KV, Michaud M, Zanes R. A controlled study of sustained-release morphine sulfate tablets in chronic pain from advanced cancer. *Am. J. Clin. Oncol. Cancer Clin. Trials.* 1992;15(3):268−272. https://doi.org/10.1097/00000421-199206000-00018.

24. Ruoff G, Lema M. Strategies in pain management: new and potential indications for COX-2 specific inhibitors. *J Pain Symptom Manag.* 2003;24(1):18−27. https://doi.org/10.1016/S0885-3924(02)00628-0.

25. Onghena P, Van Houdenhove B. Antidepressant-induced analgesia in chronic non-malignant pain: a meta-analysis of 39 placebo-controlled studies. *Pain.* 1992;49(2): 205−219. https://doi.org/10.1016/0304-3959(92)90144-Z.

26. Ventafridda V, Bonezzi C, Caraceni A, et al. Antidepressants for cancer pain and other painful syndromes with deafferentation component: comparison of Amitriptyline and Trazodone. *Ital J Neurol Sci.* 1987;8(6):579−587. https://doi.org/10.1007/BF02333665.

27. Sindrup SH, Bach FW, Madsen C, Gram LF, Jensen TS. Venlafaxine versus imipramine in painful polyneuropathy: a randomized, controlled, trial. *Neurology.* 2003;60(8): 1284−1289. https://doi.org/10.1212/01.WNL.0000058749.49264.BD.

28. Tasmuth T, Härtel B, Kalso E. Venlafaxine in neuropathic pain following treatment of breast cancer. *Eur J Pain.* 2002; 6(1):17−24. https://doi.org/10.1053/eujp.2001.0266.

29. Lussier D, Portenoy RK. Adjuvant analgesics in management of cancer-related neuropathic pain. Encycl. Pain. 5th ed. 9. Wiley; 2006:571−591.

30. Mercadante S, Arcuri E, Tirelli W, Casuccio A. Analgesic effect of intravenous ketamine in cancer patients on morphine therapy: a randomized, controlled, double-blind, crossover, double-dose study. *J Pain Symptom Manag.* 2000; 20(4):246−252. https://doi.org/10.1016/S0885-3924(00)00194-9.

31. Tarumi Y, Watanabe S, Bruera E, Ishitani K. High-dose ketamine in the management of cancer-related neuropathic pain [1]. *J Pain Symptom Manag.* 2000;19(6):405−407. https://doi.org/10.1016/S0885-3924(00)00157-3.

32. Jackson K, Ashby M, Martin P, Pisasale M, Brumley D, Hayes B. "Burst" ketamine for refractory cancer pain. *J Pain Symptom Manag.* 2001;22(4):834−842. https://doi.org/10.1016/s0885-3924(01)00340-2.

33. Chung WJ, Pharo GH. Successful use of ketamine infusion in the treatment of intractable cancer pain in an outpatient. *J Pain Symptom Manag.* 2007;33(1):2−5. https://doi.org/10.1016/j.jpainsymman.2006.09.004.

34. Singh V, Gillespie TW, Harvey RD. Intranasal ketamine and its potential role in cancer-related pain. *Pharmacotherapy.* 2018;38(3):390−401. https://doi.org/10.1002/phar.2090.

35. Schug SA, Zech D, Dörr U. Cancer pain management according to WHO analgesic guidelines. *J Pain Symptom Manag.* 1990;5(1):27−32. https://doi.org/10.1016/S0885-3924(05)80006-5.

36. Corli O, Floriani I, Roberto A, et al. Are strong opioids equally effective and safe in the treatment of chronic cancer pain? A multicenter randomized phase IV "real life" trial on the variability of response to opioids. *Ann Oncol.* 2016;27(6):1107−1115. https://doi.org/10.1093/annonc/mdw097.

37. Raffa RB. Pharmacology of oral combination analgesics: rational therapy for pain. *J Clin Pharm Therapeut.* 2001;26(4): 257–264. https://doi.org/10.1046/j.1365-2710.2001.00355.x.

38. Ballantyne JC. Chronic opioid therapy and its utility in different populations. *Pain.* 2012;153(12):2303–2304. https://doi.org/10.1016/j.pain.2012.07.015.

39. Finch PM, Roberts LJ, Price L, Hadlow NC, Pullan PT. Hypogonadism in patients treated with intrathecal morphine. *Clin J Pain.* 2000;16(3):251–254. https://doi.org/10.1097/00002508-200009000-00011.

40. Practice guidelines for chronic pain management. *Anesthesiology.* 2010;112(4):810–833. https://doi.org/10.1097/aln.0b013e3181c43103.

41. Mohamed RE, Amin MA, Omar HM. Computed tomography-guided celiac plexus neurolysis for intractable pain of unresectable pancreatic cancer, Egypt. *J. Radiol. Nucl. Med.* 2017;48(3): 627–637. https://doi.org/10.1016/j.ejnm.2017.03.027.

42. Thompson GE, Moore DC, Bridenbaugh LD, Artin RY. Abdominal pain and alcohol celiac plexus nerve block. *Anesth Analg.* 1977;56(1):1–5. https://doi.org/10.1016/0304-3959(77)90117-8.

43. Nagels W, Pease N, Bekkering G, Cools F, Dobbels P. *Celiac Plexus Neurolysis for Abdominal Cancer Pain: A Systematic Review, Pain Med.* 8th ed. 14. United States); 2013: 1140–1163. In press.

44. John R, B D, R S. *Celiac Plexus Block.* StatPearls; 2020. https://www.ncbi.nlm.nih.gov/books/NBK531469/.

45. Eisenberg E, Carr DB, Chalmers TC. Neurolytic celiac plexus block for treatment of cancer pain: a meta-analysis. *Anesth Analg.* 1995;80(2):290–295. https://doi.org/10.1097/00000539-199502000-00015.

46. Kapural L, Bensitel T, Kapural A, et al. Technical aspects of spinal cord stimulation for managing chronic visceral abdominal pain: the results from the national survey. *Pain Med.* 2010;11(5):685–691. https://doi.org/10.1111/j.1526-4637.2010.00806.x.

47. Kapural L, Yu C, Doust MW, et al. Novel 10-kHz high-frequency therapy (HF10 therapy) is superior to traditional low-frequency spinal cord stimulation for the treatment of chronic back and leg pain. *Anesthesiology.* 2015;123(4): 851–860. https://doi.org/10.1097/ALN.0000000000000774.

48. Abram S. Effect of spinal cord stimulation for chronic complex regional pain syndrome Type I: five-year final follow-up of patients in a randomized controlled trial. *Yearb. Anesthesiol. Pain Manag.* 2009;108(2):292–298. https://doi.org/10.1016/s1073-5437(08)79081-8.

49. Bedder MD, Bedder HF. Spinal cord stimulation surgical technique for the nonsurgically trained. *Neuromodulation.* 2009; 12(1):1–19. https://doi.org/10.1111/j.1525-1403.2009.00194.x.

50. Kumar K, Hunter G, Demeria D. Spinal cord stimulation in treatment of chronic benign pain: challenges in treatment planning and present status, a 22-year experience. *Neurosurgery.* 2006;58(3):481–496. https://doi.org/10.1227/01.NEU.0000192162.99567.96.

51. Knight KH, Brand FM, Mchaourab AS, Veneziano G. Implantable intrathecal pumps for chronic pain: highlights and updates. *Croat Med J.* 2007;48(1):22–34.

52. Deer TR, Pope JE, Hayek SM, et al. The polyanalgesic Consensus conference (PACC): recommendations on intrathecal drug infusion systems best practices and guidelines. *Neuromodulation.* 2017;20:96–132. https://doi.org/10.1111/ner.12538.

53. Coombs DW, Fine N. Spinal anesthesia using subcutaneously implanted pumps for intrathecal drug infusion. *Anesth Analg.* 1991;73(2):226–231. https://doi.org/10.1213/00000539-199108000-00019.

54. Brogan SE, Winter NB, Okifuji A. Prospective observational study of patient-controlled intrathecal analgesia: impact on cancer-associated symptoms, breakthrough pain control, and patient satisfaction. In: *Reg. Anesth. Pain Med.* 4th ed. 40. 2015:375–396.

55. Staats PS, Yearwood T, Charapata SG, et al. Intrathecal ziconotide in the treatment of refractory pain in patients with cancer or AIDS: a randomized controlled trial. *J Am Med Assoc.* 2004;291(1):63–70. https://doi.org/10.1001/jama.291.1.63.

56. Onofrio BM, Yaksh TL, Arnold PG. Continuous low-dose intrathecal morphine administration in the treatment of chronic pain of malignant origin. *Obstet Gynecol Surv.* 1982; 37(4):270–271. https://doi.org/10.1097/00006254-198204000-00023.

57. Sjoberg M, Nitescu P, Appelgren L, Curelaru I. Long-term intrathecal morphine and bupivacaine in patients with refractory cancer pain: results from a morphine:bupivacaine dose regimen of 0.5:4.75 mg/ml. *Anesthesiology.* 1994; 80(2):284–297. https://doi.org/10.1097/00000542-199402000-00008.

58. Hassenbusch SJ, Pillay PK, Magdinec M, et al. Constant infusion of morphine for intractable cancer pain using an implanted pump. *J Neurosurg.* 1990;73(3):405–409. https://doi.org/10.3171/jns.1990.73.3.0405.

59. Mercadante S. Outcome and complications of epidural analgesia in patients with chronic cancer pain. *Cancer.* 1999;85:2492–2494. https://doi.org/10.1002/(sici)1097-0142(19990601)85:11<2493::aid-cncr29>3.0.co;2-u.

60. Tatrow K, Montgomery GH. Cognitive behavioral therapy techniques for distress and pain in breast cancer patients: a meta-analysis. *J Behav Med.* 2006;29(1):17–27. https://doi.org/10.1007/s10865-005-9036-1.

61. Gorin SS, Krebs P, Badr H, et al. Meta-analysis of psychosocial interventions to reduce pain in patients with cancer. *J Clin Oncol.* 2012;30(5):539–547. https://doi.org/10.1200/JCO.2011.37.0437.

62. Loh J, Gulati A. *The Use of Transcutaneous Electrical Nerve Stimulation (TENS) in a Major Cancer Center for the Treatment of Severe Cancer-Related Pain and Associated Disability, Pain Med.* 6th ed. 16. United States; 2015: 1204–1210.

63. Goudra B, Shah D, Balu G, et al. Repetitive transcranial magnetic stimulation in chronic pain: a meta-analysis. *Anesth Essays Res.* 2017;11(3):751–757. https://doi.org/10.4103/aer.aer_10_17.

64. Nizard J, Levesque A, Denis N, et al. Interest of repetitive transcranial magnetic stimulation of the motor cortex in the management of refractory cancer pain in palliative

care: two case reports. *Palliat Med.* 2015;29(6):564—568. https://doi.org/10.1177/0269216315574260.

65. Zeydi AE, Esmaeili R, Kiabi FH, Sharifi H. Repetitive transcranial magnetic stimulation as a promising potential therapeutic modality for the management of cancer-related pain: An Issue that merits further research. *Indian J Palliat Care.* 2017;23(1):109—110. https://doi.org/10.4103/0973-1075.197950.

CHAPTER 13

Colorectal Cancer

DANIEL J. PAK, MD • KRISHNA B. SHAH, MD

INTRODUCTION

Colorectal cancer (CRC) is the third most commonly diagnosed cancer globally and in the United States.[1] Although the incidence and mortality rates have been steadily declining over the last several decades likely due to earlier detection from standardized screening and mitigation of risk factors, there are still roughly 130,000 newly diagnosed cases and 50,000 deaths every year in the United States. The incidence is higher in people over the age of 65 and among males compared to females. Other risk factors for nonhereditary disease include smoking, obesity, sedentary lifestyle, inflammatory bowel disease, and race, with African Americans having the highest incidence rate among all ethnic groups in the United States.[1,2] Although the vast majority of new CRC cases are sporadic, there are a number of hereditary conditions that confer additional risk, including variants of familial adenomatous polyposis, MUTYH-associated polyposis, and Lynch syndrome.[3]

Compared to their global counterparts, the United States has a higher survival rate for CRC at 60%–65%.[4] These patients not only face challenges with pain management when they are being treated for their active disease, but a growing population of survivors faces the unexpected burden of treatment-related chronic pain syndromes as well. Almost one-third of cancer survivors experience chronic pain following curative treatment,[5] and there are very few guidelines for the treatment of chronic pain syndromes following cancer survivorship.

ETIOLOGY AND PATHOGENESIS

As previously stated, the majority of CRC cases occur sporadically with no known genetic predisposition. Sporadic carcinogenesis is secondary to progressive accumulation of genetic instabilities of the tumor suppressor genes and oncogenes.[3] Tumors develop from polyps, which are generally benign in nature. Although most hyperplastic polyps are nonneoplastic lesions, adenomas and a subset of hyperplastic polyps called serrated adenomas are considered precursors for CRC. The majority of all CRCs are adenocarcinomas, although lesions can infrequently be mucinous adenocarcinomas, sarcomas, lymphomas, and carcinoid tumors. Most cases occur in the proximal colon (41%) and rectum (28%).[1]

Tumor invasion into the bowel wall is seen with local disease. Direct invasion of neighboring organs occurs with more aggressive disease. Extension to the blood and lymphatic vessels leads to metastatic lesions, including involvement of the liver, lungs, bone, and brain. Patients with local disease expectedly have a better prognosis with a 5-year survival rate of roughly 90% compared to patients with metastases to distant organs, with a survival rate of 12.5%.[6]

The prevalence of pain among patients with CRC is high, with reported rates of 64%–79%.[7,8] Tumor infiltration causes luminal distention of the intestinal wall and nearby viscera, releasing inflammatory markers and activating nociceptors. Compression or invasion of the peripheral and central nervous system may also lead to neuropathic pain syndromes. The small intestine and colon up to the splenic flexure receives parasympathetic innervation from the vagus nerve and sympathetic innervation from the greater (T5–T9) and lesser (T10–T11) thoracic splanchnic nerves.[9] These nerves then synapse via the celiac and superior mesenteric plexuses. The gastrointestinal tract distal to the splenic flexure has sympathetic innervation from the lumbar splanchnic nerves (L1–L2) via the inferior mesenteric plexus.

CLINICAL FEATURES

Patients with early-stage CRC are frequently asymptomatic and identified through screening.

Signs and symptoms of CRC are often due to tumor growth into the intestinal lumen or neighboring viscera, thereby indicating relatively advanced disease. The most common symptom is change in bowel habits.[10] Large masses lead to narrow-caliber stools or even complete

Interventional Management of Chronic Visceral Pain Syndromes. https://doi.org/10.1016/B978-0-323-75775-1.00011-8

bowel obstruction, particularly if the tumor is located near the transition zone of the small and large bowels. Patients with rectal cancers often present with loose stools with sensations of inadequate evacuation. Colicky abdominal pain is common, which may be due to partial bowel obstruction or peritoneal disease. Patients can also have hematochezia or melena depending on the location of the tumor. Darker red stools (melena) suggest a more proximal source whereas bright-red rectal bleeding (hematochezia) indicates a distal source. Alternatively, many patients present with iron deficiency anemia from occult bleeding. Other general warning signs include fatigue, unintended weight loss, anorexia, nausea, and vomiting.

Patients with hepatic involvement can have right upper quadrant abdominal pain consistent with hepatic distention syndrome. Those with bone metastases may have deep, aching bony pain that is worse with movement and even pathologic fractures. Tumor infiltration into the posterior abdominal wall or peritoneum is experienced as epigastric or midback pain that is worse when lying down and improved when sitting up.

As previously mentioned, many patients who are successfully treated with their disease experience chronic pain syndromes as a sequelae. Chemotherapy-induced peripheral neuropathy (CIPN) secondary to demyelination or axonal injury from exposure to platinum (i.e., oxaliplatin) and taxane (docetaxel) based compounds are known to cause numbness and dysesthesias in the lower extremities in a "stocking-glove" distribution.[11] Other potential neurologic deficits include weakness and ataxias.

Radiation therapy also causes axonal nerve injury and tissue ischemia. Although recent advancements in conformal radiation therapy have been able to reduce the amount of exposure to normal tissue, injury to the lumbosacral plexus during abdominal radiation can present as neuropathic pain and weakness of the lower extremities. Radiation-induced enteropathy also presents as chronic abdominal pain, bowel obstruction, and malabsorption. These symptoms may not appear for years after the last radiation treatment.

Postsurgical pain is common and often a result of cutaneous nerve entrapment at the lateral border of the rectus abdominis muscle. Patients classically present with very localized anterior abdominal wall pain that is exacerbated with Valsalva maneuvers (Carnett's sign).[12] Iatrogenic injury to other peripheral nerves may also occur during surgery and repeated procedures lead to the formation of intraabdominal adhesions and bowel obstruction.

DIAGNOSIS

When CRC is suspected, colonoscopy is a versatile diagnostic tool and the gold standard for identifying lesions through direct visualization. Biopsies may also be taken and polyps can be removed during the same procedure.

Computed tomography (CT) colonography, also known as virtual colonoscopy, utilizes cross-sectional CT images to produce three-dimensional views of the interior of the colon to simulate the views that might be obtained with traditional colonoscopy.[13] Ingestible capsule endoscopy also allows direct visualization of the colon. Equipped with a miniature video camera and the ability to take images as the capsule passes through the gastrointestinal tract, capsule endoscopy has been approved in the United States by the Food and Drug Administration (FDA) for patients who have had an incomplete colonoscopy.[14]

When a diagnosis of CRC has been confirmed, additional imaging modalities are used for clinical staging. CT imaging of the chest, abdomen, and pelvis is obtained for surgical planning before resection surgery. Magnetic resonance imaging may also be used to identify hepatic lesions if liver metastases are suspected given its superior sensitivity compared to CT. Positron emission tomography-CT is another imaging modality that assesses distant and occult disease; this is utilized when assessing for recurrent disease and is rarely used at the time of initial diagnosis.

Laboratory testing of serum markers, such as carcinoembryonic antigen (CEA), assesses tumor burden and monitors for recurrence after curative treatment.[15] However, given that CEA levels are not always elevated at the time of diagnosis, it is not recommended as a screening or staging tool.

The newest screening guidelines by the American Cancer Society recommends that individuals with an average risk of CRC should undergo regular screening starting at the age of 45 with either a stool-based test (i.e., guaiac-based fecal occult blood test or fecal immunochemical test) or visual exam (colonoscopy, flexible sigmoidoscopy).[16]

DIFFERENTIAL DIAGNOSIS

Several nonmalignant syndromes present with similar symptoms as CRC. Patients with irritable bowel syndrome have recurrent abdominal discomfort with changes in stool frequency and consistency. Inflammatory bowel disease is also associated with weight loss, hematochezia/melena, abdominal discomfort, and changes in bowel consistency. It is important to note that the average age of onset for inflammatory bowel disease at 20–40 years is younger than with CRC. Other sources of rectal bleeding, such as hemorrhoids and diverticulosis, should also be ruled out.

Metastatic disease from other primary cancers also presents almost identically to CRC. Therefore, the primary source must be identified when there is suspicion for disseminated disease.

PHYSICAL EXAM

A comprehensive physical exam should be completed with a focus on the abdominal and rectal exams. Although early-stage disease may not reveal exam findings, the advanced disease presents with the general appearance of pallor, jaundice, and lethargy. A physical exam can demonstrate abdominal tenderness, palpable abdominal or rectal masses, lymphadenopathy, hepatomegaly, ascites, and macroscopic rectal bleeding.

TREATMENT

Opioids

Opioid-based therapy is still considered the mainstay treatment for patients with moderate to severe CRC-related pain. The World Health Organization (WHO) analgesic ladder (Fig. 13.1) is the conventionally accepted approach for opioid treatment.[17,18]

Opioids are administered to patients with moderate-to-severe pain, with oral opioids being the most common route of delivery. Although morphine-based medications have traditionally been the most accepted agents, the recognition that individuals have varying responses to different μ-agonists has led practitioners to adopt opioid rotation to identify the most effective agent that minimizes side effects.[18,19] Therefore, while the WHO analgesic ladder generally recommends the use of weak opioids such as tramadol and codeine for moderate pain, stronger opioids such as oxycodone or morphine at lower doses should be considered as an alternative.[17] There is no significant difference in the analgesic effect or tolerability of oxycodone compared to morphine for moderate-to-severe cancer pain.[20]

For opioid-naive patients, immediate-release (IR) oral opioids are recommended for break-through pain[21]. The dose should be carefully titrated if the patient endorses inadequate relief. The frequency of administration may also be adjusted if the patient complains of a short duration of relief. The general duration of action for immediate-release formulations is 4 h with some variation depending on renal and hepatic function. Fixed scheduled dosing of extended-release opioids should then be considered for patients with inadequate control with as needed (PRN) usage of IR formulations. This provides maintenance relief while allowing for PRN doses for breakthrough pain. If a patient is unable to tolerate oral medications and a long-acting opioid is desired, then transdermal fentanyl should be considered. Other routes of rapid fentanyl delivery for breakthrough pain include transmucosal lozenge, sublingual tablet, and nasal spray.

If patients experience intolerable side effects or inadequate relief, the opioid rotation should be considered. In these cases, the equianalgesic dose of the new opioid should be reduced by 20%–30% to account for incomplete cross-tolerance. Attention to a patient's neuropsychological function and tolerance to side effects is essential to provide individualized therapy.

Chronic opioid use in cancer survivors remains controversial. Survivors often experience psychosocial hardship, including depression and anxiety, which increases their risk for dependency and misuse. All attempts should be made to reduce opioid use while utilizing adjuvant medications and interventions when appropriate. When these alternative modalities have failed, the benefits and risks of continuing chronic opioids must be weighed. Should opioid use be deemed appropriate, use of a low dose regimen (<90 mg/day morphine equivalence) is recommended with close follow-up.[22] If worsening pain is encountered, tumor relapse should be ruled out.

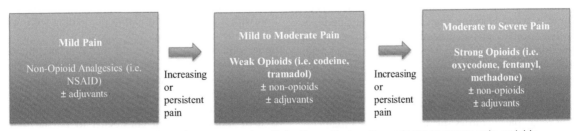

FIG. 13.1 **WHO guidelines for cancer pain relief.** For patients with moderate-to-severe pain, opioids should be considered from the start of therapy.

Nonopioid Analgesics

Nonopioid analgesics should be utilized when possible. Acetaminophen and nonsteroidal antiinflammatory drugs (NSAIDs) may be used alone or in conjunction with opioids. NSAIDs, which have antiinflammatory and antipyretic properties, are more efficacious for bone and inflammatory pains.[19] The efficacy of NSAIDs with opioids is unclear, with some studies demonstrating benefit and others showing no additional efficacy compared to the use of NSAID or opioid alone.[18,21] The use of these medications may be limited due to their renal, gastrointestinal, hematological, and cardiac toxicity profiles.

Corticosteroids are commonly used in late-stage disease for anorexia, analgesia, and nausea. Bisphosphonates are also often given in conjunction with glucocorticoids, such as dexamethasone and prednisone, for malignant bone pain.

CIPN remains a debilitating problem for patients who receive chemotherapy. The overall incidence rate is estimated to be 38% in survivors, and the mainstay pharmacologic options include antidepressants and anticonvulsants.[23] Duloxetine and venlafaxine, both serotonin and norepinephrine reuptake inhibitors, have been shown to be superior to placebo in treating CIPN. Tricyclic antidepressants (TCAs), such as amitriptyline and nortriptyline, are also used for treating neuropathic pain, though their efficacy for CIPN remains inconclusive. Gabapentinoids, such as gabapentin and pregabalin, are anticonvulsants used for treating nonmalignant neuropathic pain and should be considered as well. In fact, pregabalin has been shown to provide greater analgesia with significantly improved opioid-sparing effects compared to gabapentin and TCAs.[24]

Intranasal ketamine may be considered to reduce oral opioid requirements or if patients do not tolerate opioids. The nares and sinus cavities have an abundant vascular supply, which allows for efficient systemic absorption. Additionally, intranasal delivery has greater bioavailability compared to oral delivery due to the absence of the first-pass metabolism. The data is limited to intranasal ketamine for cancer pain. Intranasal ketamine is typically made from a compound pharmacy with a specially prepared nasal spray to deliver a mist of atomized medication. Dosing can be used with 100 mg ketamine per ml, with 10 mg or 0.1 mL administered per puff, given 3–4 times per day.[25]

Celiac Plexus Block, Neurolysis

The celiac plexus carries the afferent, parasympathetic, and sympathetic innervation of the upper abdominal viscera, including the ascending and transverse colon. It lies in the retroperitoneum on the anterolateral surface of the aorta at the level of the T12 and L1 vertebrae. Image-guided block and neurolysis of the celiac plexus is used to treat intractable abdominal pain from CRC of the ascending or transverse colon as well as metastatic disease to other abdominal viscera (i.e., liver).

Celiac plexus neurolysis may be performed with an anterior or posterior approach with fluoroscopic or CT-guided imaging. Posterior approaches are performed with the patient lying prone, most commonly utilizing the antecrural or retrocrural techniques, which refers to the site of injection. The antecrural and retrocrural sites are the spaces anterior and posterior, respectively, to the crura of the diaphragm. The antecrural approach is effective for targeting the celiac plexus while the retrocrural approach targets the splanchnic nerves.[9]

When performing the posterior retrocrural technique under fluoroscopy, the needle is inserted at the level of the L1 transverse process and advanced until the tip is just past the anterior surface of the T12–L1 vertebral bodies. For the antecrural technique, a single needle is inserted using a left posterior paramedian approach and advanced through the posterior and anterior walls of the aorta to get access to the plexus (Fig. 13.2). The use of CT has become increasingly popular as well because of the ability to visualize the retroperitoneal anatomy and spread of the neurolytic agent. The bilateral posterior antecrural approach (Fig. 13.3) is the most commonly performed technique for CT-guided neurolysis.[9]

An anterior approach with the patient positioned supine may also be taken. Under the guidance of ultrasound or CT, a single needle is advanced to the level of the celiac artery. Puncture of other visceral organs may occur with this technique; therefore anatomic considerations must be taken into account for each patient. Endoscopic ultrasound-guided celiac plexus blocks have also recently come into favor because of the ability to directly inject into the individual celiac ganglia.[26]

Diagnostic blocks may be performed with a local anesthetic such as lidocaine or bupivacaine in combination with a corticosteroid before proceeding with permanent neurolysis. Neurolytic injections are typically done with 50%–100% ethanol or 4%–10% phenol, which causes necrotic damage to neural structures. Unlike phenol, ethanol has no initial local anesthetic effect. Therefore, it is recommended to inject local anesthetic 5 min before administering ethanol. Ethanol is used most often and considered to be the more destructive agent.

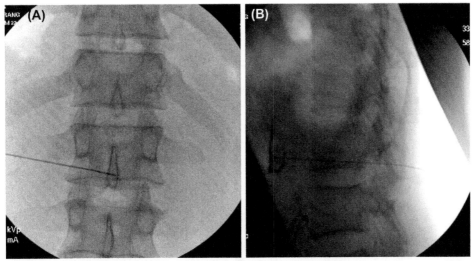

FIG. 13.2 **Antecrural celiac plexus neurolysis under fluoroscopic guidance.**   Final needle position is shown in the (**A**) anteroposterior and (**B**) lateral views. Contrast medium outlining the plexus is seen in the lateral view (**B**).

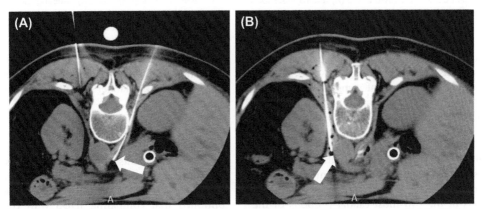

FIG. 13.3 **Bilateral antecrural celiac plexus neurolysis under CT guidance.** Axial CT images demonstrate needle tips (*arrow*) at the (**A**) right celiac ganglion and (**B**) left celiac ganglion.

The most common complication from celiac plexus neurolysis is orthostatic hypotension and diarrhea from the blockade of the sympathetic fibers. Other less common but serious complications include retroperitoneal hemorrhage, abdominal aortic dissection (more frequently associated with the antecrural approach), paraplegia from injury to lumbar segmental arteries, surrounding organ injury, and pneumothorax.[27]

Superior Hypogastric Block, Neurolysis

The superior hypogastric plexus carries the afferent, parasympathetic, and sympathetic innervation for the pelvic viscera and bowel distal to the left colonic flexure.

Like the celiac plexus, it is located in the retroperitoneum and situated bilaterally along the anterior surface of the L5 vertebral body.[27] CT or fluoroscopically guided neurolysis of the superior hypogastric plexus is appropriate for patients with CRC of the sigmoid colon and intractable abdominal or pelvic pain.

This procedure is most commonly performed with a posterior approach with the patient prone. Two needles are inserted with a paramedian approach and directed anterolaterally until the tips sit at the anterior border of the L5–S1 interspace (Fig. 13.4). Aspiration of the needle should always be done to avoid intravascular injection of the iliac vessels. As with celiac plexus blocks,

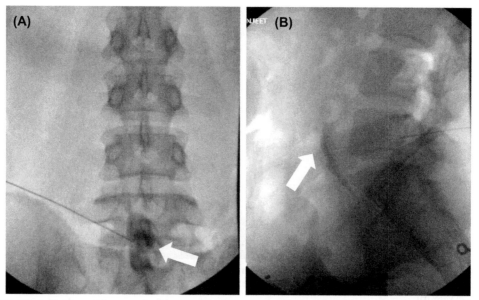

FIG. 13.4 **Single needle superior hypogastric plexus neurolysis under fluoroscopic guidance.** Final needle position is shown in the **(A)** anteroposterior and **(B)** lateral views. Contrast medium outlining the plexus is shown by the *arrow*.

neurolysis is typically reserved for patients with advanced disease.

Common complications of superior hypogastric blocks include intravascular injection, retroperitoneal hematoma, bowel or bladder incontinence, and discitis.

Ganglion Impar Block, Neurolysis

The ganglion impar, also known as the ganglion of Walther, is situated in the retroperitoneum just anterior to the coccyx at the level of the sacrococcygeal junction and consists of the two most caudal portions of the sympathetic ganglia.[28] It provides afferent and sympathetic innervation for organs in the pelvis, including the distal rectum. A blockade of this structure is performed with image guidance for CRC patients with rectal or perineal pain.

The transcoccygeal approach under fluoroscopy is perhaps most popular since it allows the shortest needle trajectory while avoiding surrounding structures. The patient is positioned prone and the needle is advanced through the sacrococcygeal ligament until the tip is just posterior to the rectum (Fig. 13.5). The block can also be done in the lateral position with the needle advanced through the anococcygeal ligament until the tip is directed to the sacrococcygeal junction.[28] Neurolysis, cryoablation, and radiofrequency ablation of the plexus may then be performed.

Complications from this procedure are rare, though perforation of the rectum and bladder is possible. Sexual, bowel, and bladder dysfunction may also be observed.

Intrathecal Drug Delivery Systems

The use of intrathecal drug delivery systems (IDDS) is considered in patients with focal pain that is refractory to traditional systemic opioids or those who are unable to tolerate the side effects of opioids. A randomized controlled trial comparing IDDS with conventional medical management in patients with refractory cancer pain demonstrated a reduction in visual analog scale (VAS) pain scores, reduced drug toxicity, and improved survival compared to comprehensive medical management.[29]

Several factors should be considered when choosing candidates for this therapy, including the patient's life expectancy, support systems, ability to continue regular clinic follow-ups (for refills, dose adjustments), expectations of the therapy, and psychological status. Medications are delivered directly into the intrathecal space through an indwelling catheter that is connected to a reservoir system implanted in a subcutaneous pocket typically in the abdomen. The catheter tip is placed according to the corresponding dermatomal distribution of the patient's pain; for abdominal coverage, we

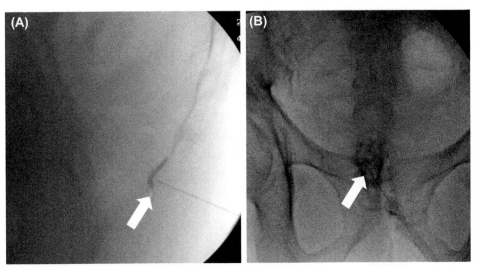

FIG. 13.5 Transcoccygeal approach for ganglion impar block under fluoroscopic guidance. Final needle position is shown in the (**A**) lateral and (**B**) anteroposterior views. Contrast medium outlining the structure is shown by the *arrows*.

suggest that the tip be placed at the level of the T9 or T10 vertebral body. The pump is programmed to deliver a set dosage of medication at a continuous rate with the option of also providing scheduled and patient-controlled boluses.

Before proceeding with the implant, a trial of intrathecal opioids either by single-shot spinal injection or infusion via intrathecal catheter is often done to assess the potential benefit of the therapy and any side effects. Although epidural infusion can also be used as a trial modality, it has been demonstrated to overestimate the effective intrathecal dosages once the permanent system is implanted.[30] More recently, recommendations from the Polyanalgesic Consensus Conference (PACC) indicate that a trial may not be required for cancer patients with advanced disease and limited survival time.[31]

There are currently three medications approved for IDDS by the US FDA: morphine, ziconotide, and baclofen. Ziconotide is an N-type calcium channel blocker that acts at the level of the dorsal horn to provide analgesia. Several other agents are commonly used off-label in practice for IDDS, including hydromorphone, fentanyl, sufentanil, clonidine, and bupivacaine. Drug combinations, generally a combination of an opioid with either bupivacaine or clonidine, are also utilized for mixed nociceptive and neuropathic pain disorders. Recent PACC algorithms (Table 13.1) provide recommendations on drug choice to guide clinicians based on the hierarchy of studies by the US Preventative Services Task Force.[32,33] It should be noted that the use

of off-label agents is not recommended by the PACC unless FDA-approved agents are contraindicated or have been deemed ineffective.

Tunneled Intraspinal Catheter Systems

In cases where the patient has a terminal prognosis with less than 3 months of life expectancy and fails to achieve adequate pain relief with systemic opioids, one may consider an epidural or intrathecal catheter that is tunneled subcutaneously and attached to an external infusion pump. This is a less invasive and more cost-effective approach compared to an internalized IDDS with a subcutaneous pump. Infection is perhaps the most common concern with any chronic indwelling catheter. However, a systematic review of tunneled intrathecal catheters found an overall infection risk rate of 1.4% for deep infections and 2.3% for superficial infections, which are relatively low and comparable to infection rates with other implanted subcutaneous ports.[34] For patients who are discharged home or to another care facility, it is essential that they have the necessary education and support to manage the external pump device.

Spinal Cord Stimulation

Spinal cord stimulation (SCS) is considered in patients with chronic abdominal pain resistant to traditional medical and interventional therapies. SCS devices deliver electrical stimulation to the dorsal column of the spinal cord to modulate ascending and descending pain signals. The mechanisms and details of SCS are

TABLE 13.1
PACC Recommendations for Intrathecal Medications for Cancer Pain Syndromes With Localized Nociceptive or Neuropathic Pain.[31]

Evidence Level[a]					
I	Ziconotide		Morphine		
II-1	Fentanyl		Morphine or fentanyl + bupivacaine		
II-3	Hydromorphone	Hydromorphone + bupivacaine		Morphine or hydromorphone or fentanyl + ziconotide	
III	Hydromorphone or morphine or fentanyl + clonidine	Ziconotide + bupivacaine	Ziconotide + clonidine	Hydromorphone or morphine or fentanyl + bupivacaine + ziconotide	Sufentanil
III	Sufentanil + ziconotide	Sufentanil + bupivacaine	Baclofen	Sufentanil + clonidine	Bupivacaine + clonidine + ziconotide
III	Sufentanil + bupivacaine + clonidine			Bupivacaine + clonidine	
III	Opioid[b] + bupivacaine + clonidine + adjuvants[c]				

a Based on the hierarchy of studies by the US Preventative Services Task Force.[32]
b All known intrathecal opioids.
c Includes midazolam, ketamine, octreotide.

discussed in more detail in other chapters of this textbook. Traditionally used for chronic back pain, radicular pain, and complex regional pain syndrome, there is now limited literature demonstrating analgesic benefit with reduced VAS pain scores and opioid use for patients with chronic visceral abdominal pain.[35] No studies have specifically examined its efficacy for visceral cancer pain syndromes. If SCS is considered for a patient with colorectal cancer pain, physicians need to consider the need for further magnetic resonance imaging that may be limited with an SCS device.

REFERENCES

1. Siegel RL, Miller KD, Fedewa SA, et al. Colorectal cancer statistics, 2017. *CA Cancer J Clin.* 2017;67(3):177–193.
2. Jemal A, Siegel R, Xu J, Ward E. Cancer statistics, 2010. *CA Cancer J Clin.* 2010;60(5):277–300.
3. Yamagishi H, Kuroda H, Imai Y, Hiraishi H. Molecular pathogenesis of sporadic colorectal cancers. *Chin J Cancer.* 2016;35(1):4.
4. Burgers K, Moore C, Bednash L. Care of the colorectal cancer survivor. *Am Fam Physician.* 2018;97(5):331–336.
5. Drury A, Payne S, Brady A-M. The cost of survival: an exploration of colorectal cancer survivors' experiences of pain. *Acta Oncol.* 2017;56(2):205–211.
6. DeSantis CE, Lin CC, Mariotto AB, et al. Cancer treatment and survivorship statistics, 2014: cancer treatment and survivorship statistics, 2014. *CA Cancer J Clin.* 2014;64(4): 252–271.
7. Chiu TY, Hu WY, Chen CY. Prevalence and severity of symptoms in terminal cancer patients: a study in Taiwan. *Support Care Cancer.* July 2000;8(4):311–313.
8. Vainio A, Auvinen A. Prevalence of symptoms among patients with advanced cancer: an international collaborative study. Symptom Prevalence Group. *J Pain Symptom Manage.* 1996;12(1):3–10.
9. Kambadakone A, Thabet A, Gervais DA, Mueller PR, Arellano RS. CT-guided celiac plexus neurolysis: a review of anatomy, indications, technique, and tips for successful treatment. *Radiographics.* 2011;31(6):1599–1621.
10. Thompson MR, O'Leary DP, Flashman K, Asiimwe A, Ellis BG, Senapati A. Clinical assessment to determine the risk of bowel cancer using symptoms, age, mass and iron deficiency anaemia (Sami). *Br J Surg.* 2017;104(10): 1393–1404.
11. Brown TJ, Sedhom R, Gupta A. Chemotherapy-induced peripheral neuropathy. *JAMA Oncol.* 2019;5(5):750.
12. Akhnikh S, de Korte N, de Winter P. Anterior cutaneous nerve entrapment syndrome (ACNES): the forgotten diagnosis. *Eur J Pediatr.* 2014;173(4):445–449.
13. Levine MS, Yee J. History, evolution, and current status of radiologic imaging tests for colorectal cancer screening. *Radiology.* 2014;273(2 Suppl):S160–S180.
14. Pasha SF. Applications of colon capsule endoscopy. *Curr Gastroenterol Rep.* 2018;20(5):22.
15. Duffy MJ. Carcinoembryonic antigen as a marker for colorectal cancer: is it clinically useful? *Clin Chem.* 2001;47(4): 624–630.
16. Wolf AMD, Fontham ETH, Church TR, et al. Colorectal cancer screening for average-risk adults: 2018 guideline update from the American cancer Society: ACS colorectal cancer screening guideline. *CA Cancer J Clin.* 2018;68(4): 250–281.
17. World Health Organization. *WHO guidelines for the pharmacological and radiotherapeutic management of cancer pain in adults and adolescents;* 2018. http://www.ncbi.nlm.nih.gov/books/NBK537492/.
18. Portenoy RK. Treatment of cancer pain. *Lancet Lond Engl.* 2011;377(9784):2236–2247.
19. Portenoy RK, Lesage P. Management of cancer pain. *Lancet Lond Engl.* 1999;353(9165):1695–1700.
20. Guo K-K, Deng C-Q, Lu G-J, Zhao G-L. Comparison of analgesic effect of oxycodone and morphine on patients with moderate and advanced cancer pain: a meta-analysis. *BMC Anesthesiol.* 2018;18(1):132.
21. Scarborough BM, Smith CB. Optimal pain management for patients with cancer in the modern era: pain Management for Patients with Cancer. *CA Cancer J Clin.* 2018; 68(3):182–196.
22. Carmona-Bayonas A, Jiménez-Fonseca P, Castañón E, et al. Chronic opioid therapy in long-term cancer survivors. *Clin Transl Oncol.* 2017;19(2):236–250.
23. Hershman DL, Lacchetti C, Dworkin RH, et al. Prevention and management of chemotherapy-induced peripheral neuropathy in survivors of adult cancers: American society of clinical oncology clinical practice guideline. *J Clin Oncol.* 2014;32(18):1941–1967.
24. Mishra S, Bhatnagar S, Goyal GN, Rana SPS, Upadhya SP. A comparative efficacy of amitriptyline, gabapentin, and pregabalin in neuropathic cancer pain: a prospective randomized double-blind placebo-controlled study. *Am J Hosp Palliat Med.* 2012;29(3): 177–182.
25. Singh V, Gillespie TW, Harvey RD. Intranasal ketamine and its potential role in cancer-related pain. *Pharmacotherapy.* 2018;38(3):390–401.
26. Yasuda I, Wang H-P. Endoscopic ultrasound-guided celiac plexus block and neurolysis. *Dig Endosc.* 2017;29(4): 455–462.
27. De Leon-Casasola OA. Critical evaluation of chemical neurolysis of the sympathetic Axis for cancer pain. *Cancer Control.* March 2000;7(2):142–148.
28. Gunduz OH, Kenis Coskun O. Ganglion blocks as a treatment of pain: current perspectives. *J Pain Res.* 2017;10: 2815–2826.
29. Smith TJ, Staats PS, Deer T, et al. Randomized clinical trial of an implantable drug delivery system compared with comprehensive medical management for refractory cancer pain: impact on pain, drug-related toxicity, and survival. *J Clin Oncol.* 1, 2002;20(19):4040–4049.
30. Maniker AH, Krieger AJ, Adler RJ, Hupert C. Epidural trial in implantation of intrathecal morphine infusion pumps. *N J Med.* 1991;88(11):797–801.

31. Deer TR, Provenzano DA, Hanes M, et al. The Neurostimu-lation Appropriateness Consensus Committee (NACC) recommendations for infection Prevention and management. *Neuromodulation*. 2017;20(1):31−50.

32. Deer TR, Pope JE, Hayek SM, et al. The polyanalgesic consensus conference (PACC): recommendations on intrathecal drug infusion systems best practices and guidelines: intrathecal therapy best practices and guidelines. *Neuromodulation*. February 2017;20(2): 96−132.

33. Harris RP, Helfand M, Woolf SH, et al. Current methods of the US preventive services Task Force: a review of the process. *Am J Prev Med*. 2001;20(3 Suppl):21−35.

34. Aprili D, Bandschapp O, Rochlitz C, Urwyler A, Ruppen W. Serious complications associated with external intrathecal catheters used in cancer pain patients: a systematic review and meta-analysis. *Anesthesiology*. 2009;111(6):1346−1355.

35. Kapural L, Nagem H, Tlucek H, Sessler DI. Spinal cord stimulation for chronic visceral abdominal pain. *Pain Med Malden Mass*. 2010;11(3):347−355.

CHAPTER 14

Chronic Pancreatitis

ANOKHI D. MEHTA, MD • R. JASON YONG, MD

INTRODUCTION

Chronic pancreatitis describes a syndrome of chronic inflammation of the pancreas. Treatment of chronic pancreatitis involves supplementation for malnutrition and pancreatic enzyme deficiencies, and treatment for chronic pain that develops.[1] Chronic pancreatitis is estimated to cost the healthcare system approximately 150 million dollars in the United States.[1] Managing the pain of pancreatitis adequately could help reduce morbidity and reduce this cost burden. In this chapter, we will review chronic pancreatitis followed by the various pain treatments available for this chronic condition.

ETIOLOGY, PATHOGENESIS, AND CLINICAL FEATURES

There are several different known etiologies including alcohol, smoking, genetic causes, anatomic abnormalities, and ductal obstruction. Smoking, in particular, is associated with chronic pancreatitis even when adjusting for alcohol intake.[2] It is a progressive, ongoing inflammatory syndrome involving mononuclear cell infiltration and activation of pancreatic stellate cells. This leads to fibrosis and loss of acinar and islet cells.[3,4] An initial insult with alcohol or tobacco occurs and this incites the first episode of acute pancreatitis. At this time, inflammatory cells are recruited. Repeated insults incite further episodes of acute pancreatitis that activates stellate cells and begins the process of fibrogenesis.[4] Pancreatitis can also have idiopathic or autoimmune causes. In these cases, it is unknown what provokes the initial episode of pancreatitis. Complications of pancreatitis include but are not limited to biliary obstruction, duodenal obstruction, portal vein thrombosis, vascular aneurysms, pseudocysts, and bleeding.[4]

DIAGNOSIS

The standard for diagnosis had been the triad of diabetes mellitus, steatorrhea, and pancreatic calcifications visible on abdominal radiographs. It is now known that this will only be seen in end-stage disease. Measuring of pancreatic enzymes and endoscopic ultrasound, magnetic resonance imaging (MRI), or computed tomography (CT) can help diagnose pancreatitis earlier in the course of disease.[4] On MRI and CT, one could see pancreatic atrophy and/or calcifications with irregularities in the pancreatic duct.[5] Clinically, epigastric pain is typically seen and can be debilitating; this pain is thought to be due to "increased pressure in the ductal system and/or neuroplastic changes."[4] Managing pain can become the single most prominent component of disease management in chronic pancreatitis.

PHYSICAL EXAM FINDINGS

Chronic pancreatitis pain typically presents as epigastric pain radiating toward the back. A thorough history should be taken to assess the intensity of pain, if the pain is constant or intermittent, exacerbating factors, mitigating factors, and impact of pain on activities of daily living and quality of life.[6] Physical exam should include a full, thorough abdominal exam but should also include a general physical examination of other systems (cardiovascular, pulmonary, etc.). A full neurological exam should be performed as well. On exam, one could find tenderness to palpation in the epigastric region. It is important to remember that earlier in the course of the disease, an abdominal exam could potentially be normal with no tenderness to palpation elicited. This highlights the importance of ordering

Interventional Management of Chronic Visceral Pain Syndromes. https://doi.org/10.1016/B978-0-323-75775-1.00010-6

pancreatic enzyme labs and imaging if one has a high clinical suspicion for pancreatitis. As mentioned previously, imaging options include endoscopic ultrasound, CT, or MRI for the diagnosis of pancreatitis.[6]

TREATMENT

Lifestyle modifications and conservative therapies: Treating pain often becomes the focal point of chronic pancreatitis management. Lifestyle modifications are imperative to discuss. Tobacco and alcohol cessation are an important component of reducing the likelihood of disease progression, which, in turn, has an impact on pain[6]. Pancreatic enzyme replacement therapy has been shown in being effective in pain reduction as well and patients should be referred to a gastroenterologist for evaluation.[5]

To manage the pain, conservative management with oral medications should be attempted first. Initially, over the counter analgesics can be attempted if there are no contraindications. This includes acetaminophen and antiinflammatories. If pain is not adequately managed by over the counter analgesics, then prescription-strength medications are to be attempted. All nonopioid options should be exhausted before trialing opioids. This includes gabapentinoids and tricyclic antidepressants. In a randomized, double-blinded, placebo-controlled trial, it was found that pregabalin is associated with reduced central sensitization in pain related to chronic pancreatitis.[7] Tricyclic antidepressants (TCAs) such as nortriptyline or amitriptyline can be trialed as well.

If gabapentinoids or TCAs prove ineffective, then tramadol, a weak opioid, can be trialed next. A discussion including risks of tolerance, dependence, and addiction should be done with the patient regarding chronic opioid therapy. If tramadol proves ineffective, oral opioids, such as hydrocodone or oxycodone, can be considered with caution paying careful attention to dose.[7] The lowest possible dose to achieve pain relief is recommended.

Referral to a pain psychologist for coping strategies is another conservative management option that should be utilized. Cognitive behavioral therapy has been utilized for managing chronic pain. It teaches coping mechanisms and alters thoughts and perception for patients to approach their pain. Understanding how to cope and manage pain flares is crucial in positive long-term outcomes.

Interventional procedures: In addition to oral medications for pain management, there are several interventional therapies available.

Celiac plexus block may be considered in patients with chronic upper abdominal pain secondary to chronic pancreatitis. Typically, this procedure is done for patients with pancreatic cancer or upper abdominal malignancies, but it is reasonable to consider this procedure in patients with chronic pancreatitis who are refractory to oral medications.

Please refer to Chapter 13 for technique and different approaches to the celiac plexus block. For chronic pancreatitis, local anesthetic (8–10 mL of 2% lidocaine or 0.25% bupivacaine) with corticosteroid can be administered. A study found that patients with chronic pancreatitis who experienced pain relief had 2 months of relief with a subset of patients receiving minimal to no pain relief.[8] Expectations should be discussed with patients before proceeding with celiac plexus block for chronic pancreatitis. If patients do have adequate relief but short term, then neurolysis with alcohol or phenol can be considered.

Neuromodulation: If the above interventions are not effective, surgical pain management techniques can be considered. Spinal cord stimulation (SCS) for abdominal visceral pain has been performed with significant pain relief, although research into this specific area is limited (see Figs. 14.1 and 14.2). Khan et al. reported five cases of chronic nonalcoholic pancreatitis that were treated with SCS. Leads were placed midline along the dorsal column, with the electrode tips at the T5–T6 vertebral bodies. In one instance, the leads were placed at the T5–T8 levels. All five patients experienced at least 50% pain relief and significantly reduced their opioid usage.[9]

In a separate retrospective study of 35 patients with chronic visceral abdominal pain, 26 reported pancreatitis-related pain. Overall, patients with permanent implants demonstrated reduced opioid usage.[10] Furthermore, in a systematic review regarding the use of SCS for chronic pancreatitis, reviewers found that there was a greater than 50% reduction in pain during the reported follow-up periods.[11]

Targeted drug delivery: Intrathecal pumps are another surgical pain management technique that can be considered for refractory cases. Kongkam and colleagues published a case series of 13 patients with a history of intractable pancreatitis who underwent intrathecal pump placement.[12] Catheter tip placement varied from T1 to T9. Multiple intrathecal agents were utilized, including morphine, hydromorphone, and adjuvants such as clonidine and bupivacaine. Global pain scores showed improvement at 1 year follow-up, and the vast majority of the patients were weaned significantly in their oral opioids.

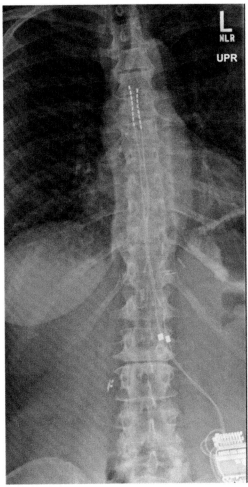

FIG. 14.1 Anteroposterior fluoroscopic view of spinal cord stimulation system implanted for chronic pancreatitis.

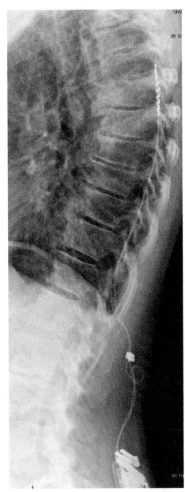

FIG. 14.2 Lateral fluoroscopic view of spinal cord stimulation system implanted for chronic pancreatitis.

REFERENCES

1. Lew D, Afghani E, Pandol S. Chronic pancreatitis: current status and challenges for prevention and treatment. *Dig Dis Sci.* 2017;62(7):1702−1712.
2. Law R, Parsi M, Lopez R, Zuccaro G, Stevens T. Cigarette smoking is independently associated with chronic pancreatitis. *Pancreatology.* 2010;10(1):54−59.
3. Gupte AR, Forsmark CE. Chronic pancreatitis. *Curr Opin Gastroenterol.* 2014;30(5):500−505.
4. Kleeff J, Whitcomb DC, Shimosegawa T, et al. Chronic pancreatitis. *Nat Rev Dis Primer.* 2017;3(1).
5. Pham A, Forsmark CE. Chronic pancreatitis: review and update of etiology, risk factors, and management. In: *F1000Research.* 2018.
6. Dominguez-Munoz JE, Drewes AM, Lindkvist B, et al. Recommendations from the United European Gastroenterology evidence-based guidelines for the diagnosis and therapy of chronic pancreatitis. *Pancreatology.* 2018; 18(8):847−854.
7. Bouwense SAW, Olesen SS, Drewes AM, Poley J-W, van Goor H, Wilder-Smith OHG. Effects of pregabalin on central sensitization in patients with chronic pancreatitis in a randomized, controlled trial. Eldabe S, editor. *PLoS One.* 2012;7(8):e42096.
8. Leung JW, Bowen-Wright M, Aveling W, Shorvon PJ, Cotton PB. Coeliac plexus block for pain in pancreatic cancer and chronic pancreatitis. *Br J Surg.* 1983;70(12): 730−732.
9. Khan YN, Raza SS, Khan EA. Spinal cord stimulation in visceral pathologies: table 1. *Pain Med.* 2006;7(Suppl 1): S121−S125.
10. Kapural L, Nagem H, Tlucek H, Sessler DI. Spinal cord stimulation for chronic visceral abdominal pain. *Pain Med.* 2010;11(3):347−355.

11. Ratnayake CB, Bunn A, Pandanaboyana S, Windsor JA. Spinal cord stimulation for management of pain in chronic pancreatitis: a systematic review of efficacy and complications. *Neuromodulation Technol Neural Interface.* 2019:1–7.

12. Kongkam P, Wagner DL, Sherman S, et al. Intrathecal narcotic infusion pumps for intractable pain of chronic pancreatitis: a pilot series. *Am J Gastroenterol.* 2009; 104(5):1249–1255.

CHAPTER 15

Chronic Postsurgical Pain

CATHY HE, MD • R. JASON YONG, MD

INTRODUCTION

The development of chronic pain after surgery is an important and often overlooked problem.[1] Chronic postsurgical pain (CPSP) can dramatically impair quality of life, limit postoperative rehabilitation, and strain patient–physician relationships.

The incidence of CPSP varies widely by study and surgical procedure, but can range from low estimates of 5% to as high as 85%.[2] CPSP after abdominal surgeries specifically have been reported to range from 19% for emergent laparotomy,[3] 5%–32% after hysterectomy,[4] 10%–52% after inguinal hernia repair,[5] and 5%–42% after cholecystectomy.

The exact pathophysiology of CPSP is poorly understood but is theorized to be the result of maladaptive and persistent pain sensitization. Preexisting pain syndromes, surgical site complications, and recurrence of the primary disease process should be ruled out and a spatiotemporal relationship to surgery is required to diagnose CPSP.

Management primarily focuses on prevention through effective perioperative analgesia and minimization of surgical trauma. Once established, CPSP management should target inciting pain mechanisms, which can be diverse. For instance, abdominal surgery may result in chronic visceral pain from injury to the organs themselves or from the development of scarring and adhesions postoperatively. Conversely, abdominal wall pain may represent referred pain from intraabdominal sources or may be the result of an abdominal wall neuroma or nerve compression.

A comprehensive approach is crucial and includes physical and psychological therapies in addition to multimodal pharmacotherapy. A range of interventions and surgical procedures have been reported for patients who do not improve with conservative therapies.

ETIOLOGY AND PATHOGENESIS

The mechanistic underpinnings of CPSP are poorly understood. Development of CPSP is presumed to be multifactorial, representing the complex interplay from surgical, genetic, psychological, and perioperative factors.[6,7] Chronic pain may arise from a background of acute postsurgical pain or may develop later after an asymptomatic period.

Intraoperative nerve injury is associated with the development of CPSP. Surgeries with nerve damage, deliberate or inadvertent, demonstrate the highest prevalence of CPSP.[2,6] Accordingly, many patients exhibit signs and symptoms consistent with neuropathic pain, such as hyperalgesia and sensory disturbances.[8] However, not all CPSP is neuropathic and not all patients with known nerve damage go on to develop chronic pain.

As with all chronic pain syndromes, CPSP is thought to be due to aberrant peripheral and central sensitization.[7,9] Surgery inherently imparts tissue damage upon surrounding tissues. As part of the adaptive response to this injury, peripheral and central sensitization can develop. These neuroplastic changes induce a state of hypersensitivity intended to protect during times when the risk for injury is greatest. As the surgical site heals, inflammation resolves and the noxious stimuli are removed, the upregulation of peripheral and central neurons usually returns to baseline. However, in a subset of patients, pain sensitization persists.[6,7] In some cases, this may be due to ongoing nociceptive activation.[6] For instance, implanted mesh or excessive scarring can compress or stretch nerves, eliciting ongoing pain signals. In other cases, however, there may not be an obvious source of ongoing inflammation. In these instances, inadequate inhibitory pain pathways may prevent the appropriate downregulation of pain sensitization.

Although the exact mechanisms that lead to CPSP are not yet known, there are well-described risk factors that shed insight into the pathogenesis (Table 15.1). The most consistent risk factor to develop chronic postoperative pain is pain itself. The presence of preoperative pain and the duration and intensity of postoperative acute pain are strong risk factors for CPSP. Pain is also strongly affected by psychological

Interventional Management of Chronic Visceral Pain Syndromes. https://doi.org/10.1016/B978-0-323-75775-1.00023-4

TABLE 15.1
Risk Factors for Developing Chronic Postsurgical Pain[7].

PREOPERATIVE FACTORS

Pain >1 month duration

Female gender

Advanced age

Psychological comorbidities (i.e., anxiety, depression)

Genetics (i.e., COMT mutations)

INTRAOPERATIVE FACTORS

Operative duration >3 h

Surgeon experience

Nerve injury

POSTOPERATIVE FACTORS

Poorly controlled postoperative pain

Pain upon discharge

Radiation or chemotherapy (neurotoxicity)

conditions. Anxiety, depression, and pain catastrophizing are predictive of CPSP, and chronic pain in general.

CLINICAL FEATURES

The clinical presentation of CPSP can be highly variable. Chronic pain most commonly arises from uncontrolled or high intensity acute postoperative pain.[7] However, patients can present months later after an intervening asymptomatic period, sometimes termed the honeymoon period.[10] Neuropathic pain findings are common in CPSP, such as allodynia, hyper- or hypoalgesia, or dysesthesia in both somatic and visceral structures.[7,8]

CPSP may present with visceral pain features including diffuse, poorly localized pain that is often crampy, colicky, and achy in nature.[4] The diffuse distribution is the result of visceral convergence in which relatively few afferent fibers innervate each visceral organ and then converge on overlapping spinal dorsal horn neurons.[11] Visceral pain tends to be highly associated with autonomic features including nausea, vomiting, sweating, pallor as well as functional bowel and bladder disorders.[12]

Pain is generally described at the surgical site but can also be referred or remote somatic areas. Abdominal wall pain may be the result of referred visceral pain

due to somato-visceral convergence or may be the result of pain originating in the abdominal wall structures as a result of surgical injury, such as the ilioinguinal nerve during hernia repair. Carnett's test may differentiate abdominal wall pain from visceral pain. It is performed by palpating the area with the patient supine and abdomen relaxed. The patient is then asked to tighten the abdominal muscles (by lifting their head and shoulder off the bed), and the area is palpated again. Abdominal wall pain will be increased when the abdominal muscles are contracted, whereas intraabdominal sources of pain will decrease from guarding by rigid overlying musculature.

As always, clinicians should maintain a high suspicion accompanying comorbidities and mood disorders, particularly anxiety and depression, which are commonly reported in CPSP patients.

DIAGNOSIS

The diagnostic criteria for CPSP have evolved since the first description in 1999 by Crombie et al.[1] Table 15.2 displays the established diagnostic criteria as well as recently proposed modifications.

A temporal relationship between surgery and the onset of pain is imperative to the diagnosis. This may be straightforward if there is a new onset of pain postoperatively. However, many operative conditions commonly present with presurgery pain (i.e., incarcerated inguinal hernia, cholecystitis) that can confuse the diagnostic picture. In these cases, there must be a significant increase in pain intensity to be classified as CPSP. Additionally, pain that differs in characteristics or distribution would be suggestive of CPSP.

Although previously thought to always be an extension of acute postsurgical pain, recent evidence notes that CPSP can arise sometimes many months postoperatively after an asymptomatic period.[13,14] A delayed onset of pain should raise suspicion for a neuropathic mechanism, as painful neuromas and compression neuropathies can develop over a protracted period.

In addition to a temporal relationship, there must also be an identifiable spatial relationship between surgery and pain. Pain is frequently located directly at the surgical site. This can be at the cutaneous level or in the deeper visceral tissues. Hypoesthesia is indicative of a nerve injury and is suggestive of a neuropathic pain component.[8] Conversely, hypersensitivity to stimuli may be present, which is associated with an inflammatory pain component or neuropathic etiology.[6,8]

TABLE 15.2
Diagnostic Criteria for Chronic Postsurgical Pain.

TRADITIONAL CRITERIA[19]

1.	Pain develops after a surgical procedure
2.	Pain persists for at least 2 months
3.	Other causes are excluded (i.e., ongoing infection or cancer recurrence)
4.	Pain from a preexisting pain problem is excluded

UPDATED CRITERIA[10]

1.	Pain begins, increases, or changes in characteristic postoperatively
2.	Pain persists for at least 3 months and significantly affects quality of life
3.	Pain is either a continuation of acute postoperative pain into a chronic condition, or develops after an asymptomatic period
4.	Pain is localized to the surgical site or is referred to an anatomically appropriate sensory distribution
5.	Other causes of pain are excluded (i.e., ongoing infection or cancer recurrence)

Adapted from Werner, M. Defining persistent postsurgical pain. *Br J Anaesth.* 2014.

Pain does not always exist at or near the surgical site. Chronic visceral pain can be referred to as corresponding cutaneous dermatomes due to robust viscerosomatic convergence. Importantly, neuropathic pain from direct or indirect nerve injuries can be projected to a remote sensory distribution that corresponds to the implicated nerve. Clinicians should attempt to anatomically identify suspected lesions based on history and physical exam findings to determine if remote pain may be a manifestation of CPSP.

PHYSICAL EXAM FINDINGS

Given the diverse presentation of CPSP, the approach to the physical exam should be systematic to identify the underlying pain mechanisms. The surgical site should be examined thoroughly, beginning first with the incision and surrounding skin. Infection and wound healing issues should be ruled out. The site should be evaluated for thermal and tactile hypoesthesia, allodynia, and hyperalgesia.

If a specific nerve injury is suspected, a Tinel's test should be performed in which the examiner percusses over the course of the nerve in question. It is positive when a focal area of pain is palpated, and when percussed, generates pain and/or paranesthesia's in the distribution of that nerve.[15] This would be suggestive of a painful neuroma or compression neuropathy. Diagnostic blocks may be performed to confirm findings.

Examination of deeper structures within the surgical field should also be performed. Common postoperative complications, such as ileus, delayed gastric emptying, or ongoing disease processes should be evaluated.

Diagnostic imaging including ultrasonography, computed tomography scans, and magnetic resonance imaging can be considered as part of the diagnostic workup to identify and rule out any other causes.

TREATMENT

Emphasis is placed on preventing the development of CPSP. When possible, preexisting pain and other modifiable risk factors should be well controlled before surgical interventions. Preemptive and preventative analgesia aimed at limiting sensitization is crucial, particularly in high-risk patients. It is important to provide adequate analgesia throughout the entire period of inflammation, again with the goal of preventing pain sensitization. Regional, local, and multimodal analgesia appear to reduce the risk of CPSP and have been well described elsewhere; the details are beyond the scope of this chapter.

A. Pharmacologic: Nonsteroidal antiinflammatory drugs (NSAIDs) can be well suited to reduce the risk of CPSP as well as to treat ongoing pain that may be the result of occult inflammation. Topical NSAIDs may also be of value by reducing cutaneous hypersensitivity.[6,7] Similarly, anticonvulsants like pregabalin have demonstrated the ability to reduce CPSP development and may greatly aid in the reduction of neuropathic pain symptoms once developed.[7] Opioids may have limited utility for short-term treatment, but do not generally demonstrate efficacy in the long-term management of CPSP and may in fact worsen outcomes.[7] Antidepressants, particularly serotonin-norepinephrine reuptake inhibitors, have demonstrated strong efficacy for the treatment of neuropathic pain in multiple randomized trials.[2,7] Side effects are usually well tolerated, but effects may not be seen for many weeks.

B. Injections: Injections of local anesthetics and corticosteroids play an important role in both diagnosing and treating CPSP.[2] Local anesthetics can help localize lesions. A successful or positive block requires the presence of transient hypoesthesia in the distribution of the targeted nerve in addition to a reduction in pain scores for at least the duration of the block. The addition of corticosteroids aims to break the cycle of inflammation and sensitization and may lead to long-term pain reduction.[2] Intraabdominal sources of pain may be targeted with a variety of sympathetic blocks, although one must remember that the sympathetic innervation of organs has wide overlap, and thus, a single nerve block may not suffice. The splanchnic nerves and celiac plexus blocks (refer to Pancreatic Cancer chapter) target stomach, small bowel, pancreas, renal, and proximal large bowel sources of pain. The superior hypogastric plexus block (refer to Chronic Prostatitis chapter) has been described to treat distal colon, bladder, and pelvic pain sources. The ganglion impar (refer to Coccydynia chapter) has demonstrated efficacy in the treatment of rectal, pelvic, scrotal, and perineal pain. Abdominal wall may be relieved with anterior abdominal cutaneous nerve, iliohypogastric, ilioinguinal blocks (refer to postsurgical pelvic pain), or transverse abdominis plane blocks (refer to Chronic Abdominal Wall Pain chapter).

C. Advanced Procedures: Nerve injuries that demonstrate transient responses to nerve blocks may benefit from chemical or radiofrequency neurolysis to achieve more long-lasting pain relief. Conventional tonic spinal cord stimulation (SCS) is an established treatment for neuropathic pain. It has demonstrated efficacy in the treatment of chronic abdominal pain in several trials. Typically, electrodes stimulate the dorsal column of the spinal cord at 40−70 Hz, producing paresthesia. Although the mechanism is unclear, it is thought that the stimulation of the dorsal column activates supraspinal pain modulatory pathways, releases inhibitory neurotransmitters, and downregulates sympathetic output results in pain relief.[16] Recent studies suggest high frequency, low amplitude SCS may be more efficacious. A study of 10 kHz SCS reduced pain scores by 50% or more in 78% of implanted patients at 12 months.[17] Lead tips are generally positioned between T5−T8 for abdominal pain and T11−T12 for lower abdominal or pelvic pain.

Intrathecal drug delivery system (IDDS) can be considered for refractory pain. IDDS delivers medications directly into the intrathecal space via an indwelling catheter that is attached to a reservoir typically placed in the abdomen. The catheter tip is placed according to the patient's dermatomal distribution of pain. Before proceeding with a permanent pump implant, an epidural trial or intrathecal trial is done to determine the efficacy of this treatment. FDA has approved morphine, baclofen, and ziconotide for intrathecal use and multiple off-label medications have been used as well (please refer to Pancreatic Cancer chapter).

D. Surgical Interventions: Removal of hardware, mesh, or other implants can remove the persistent inflammatory source in some cases. When painful neuromas are the primary source of pain, as confirmed by diagnostic nerve blocks, surgical resection is an appropriate intervention. Traditional measures involved resecting the neuroma and burying the proximal end of the nerve in muscle. However, recent evidence demonstrates improved outcomes when the nerve end is reconstructed or directed to reinnervate muscle.[18] Generalized intraabdominal pain with no clear source will likely not respond to further surgical intervention.

E. Other: A range of psychological therapies including cognitive-behavioral therapy have demonstrated efficacy. Physical therapies including desensitization, acupuncture, and functional restoration therapy may be beneficial. Lifestyle modifications and trigger avoidance can also help improve the quality of life.

REFERENCES

1. Crombie IK, Davies HT, Macrae MA. Cut and thrust: antecedent surgery and trauma among patients attending a chronic pain clinic. *Pain*. 1998;76(1−2):167−171.
2. Thapa T, Euasobhon P. Chronic postsurgical pain: current evidence for prevention and management. *Korean J Pain*. 2018;31(3):155−173.
3. Tolstrup MB, Thorup T, Gogenur I. Chronic pain, quality of life and functional impairment after emergency laparotomy. *World J Surg*. 2019;43(1):161−168.
4. Brandsborg B. Pain following hysterectomy: epidemiological and clinical aspects. *Dan Med J*. 2012;59(1):4374.
5. Nikkolo C, Lepner U. Chronic pain after open inguinal hernia repair. *Postgrad Med*. 2016;128(1):69−75.
6. Fregoso G, Want A, Tseng K, et al. Transition from acute to chronic pain: evaluating risk for chronic postsurgical pain. *Pain Physician*. 2019;22(5):479−488.
7. Richebé P, Capdevila X, Rivat C. Persistent postsurgical pain: pathophysiology and preventative pharmacologic considerations. *Anesthesiology*. 2018;129(3):590−607.
8. Kehlet H, Jensen TS, Woolf CJ. Persistent postsurgical pain: risk factors and prevention. *Lancet*. 2006;367(9522): 1618−1625.
9. Reddi D, Curran N. Chronic pain after surgery: pathophysiology, risk factors and prevention. *Postgrad Med*. 2014; 90(1062):222−227.
10. Werner MU, Kongsgaard UEI. Defining persistent postsurgical pain: is an update required? *Br J Anaesth*. 2014; 113(1):1−4.

11. Hoffman D. Understanding multisymptom presentations in chronic pelvic pain: the inter-relationships between the viscera and myofascial pelvic floor dysfunction. *Curr Pain Headache Rep.* 2011;15(5):343–346.

12. Gebhart GF, Bielefeldt K. Physiology of visceral pain. *Comp Physiol.* 2016;6(4):1609–1633.

13. Reinpold WM, Nehls J, Eggert A. Nerve management and chronic pain after open inguinal hernia repair: a prospective two phase study. *Ann Surg.* 2011;254(1):163–168.

14. Gartner R, Jensen MB, Nielsen J, et al. Prevalence of and factors associated with persistent pain following breast cancer surgery. *JAMA.* 2009;302(18):1985–1992.

15. Davis EN, Chung KC. The Tinel sign: a historical perspective. *Plast Reconstr Surg.* 2004;114(2):494–499.

16. Kapural L. *Chronic Abdominal Pain: An Evidence-Based, Comprehensive Guide to Clinical Management.* 1st ed. Springer; 2015.

17. Kapural L, Narouze SN, Janicki TI, et al. Spinal cord stimulation is an effective treatment for the chronic intractable visceral pelvic pain. *Pain Med.* 2006;7(5):440–443.

18. Dumanian GA, Potter BK, Mioton LM, et al. Targeted muscle reinnervation treats neuroma and phantom pain in major limb amputees: a randomized clinical trial. *Ann Surg.* 2019;270(2):238–246.

19. Macrae WA. Chronic pain after surgery. *Br J Anaesth.* 2001; 87(1):88–98.

CHAPTER 16

Chronic Abdominal Wall Pain

JOSIANNA HENSON, MD • NARAYANA VARHABHATLA, MD

INTRODUCTION

Between 10% and 30% of patients presenting to gastroenterologists with chronic abdominal pain have chronic abdominal wall pain (CAWP).[1] These patients often undergo unnecessary procedures and tests while their diagnosis is delayed by 2 years on average, adding more than $6700 in direct healthcare costs.[2] An appropriate diagnosis and correct treatment of abdominal wall pain can often be curative. The abdominal wall is supplied by the T7–T12 nerve roots, and the nerves can be affected at the level of the nerve roots or at the distal branches where they make a right-angle turn at the lateral edge of the rectus abdominis muscle.[3] The distal branches are particularly prone to causing pain, either from surgical changes or scar tissue. Applegate coined the term abdominal anterior cutaneous nerve entrapment syndrome (ACNES) for this pathology.[4] It is usually felt as a sharp, localized pain, worse with activity, and is independent of eating or bowel habits.[4,5] Diagnosis is notoriously difficult and relies almost exclusively on history and physical findings. CAWP can be seen at any age, but predominantly affects women. Carnett's test is often the most consistent physical exam finding to aid diagnosis. Interventions for CAWP include transversus abdominis plane (TAP) block, ACNES block, neuromodulation, and surgical neurectomy, which are preferable to long-term medical management.[5,6]

ETIOLOGY AND PATHOGENESIS

The abdominal wall consists of several muscle layers. The paired rectus muscles are found in the midline. Laterally, from superficial to deep, lie the external abdominal oblique, the internal abdominal oblique, and the transversus abdominis muscles. The abdominal wall is innervated by the anterior branches of the intercostal nerves of T7–T12.[7] These nerves travel in a plane between the internal oblique and the transversus abdominis, where they are a target for the TAP block.

They then pierce the posterior rectus sheath and make a 90-degrees turn through a fibrous sheath to become the anterior cutaneous nerves, and subsequently make another 90 degrees° turn beneath the skin.[3]

The differential diagnosis of CAWP is extensive and includes peripheral nerve entrapment or traumatic injury, referred pain from the abdominal or thoracic viscera, T7–T12 radicular lesions, herpes zoster, painful rib, myofascial trigger points, and rectus sheath hematoma.[5] The most commonly discussed cause of CAWP is anterior cutaneous nerve entrapment syndrome (ACNES), which is caused by the entrapment of a cutaneous branch of the lower intercostal nerve (T7–T12). Many patients previously diagnosed with functional abdominal pain syndromes have a component of abdominal wall pain.[8]

Peripheral nerve entrapment of the anterior cutaneous branches of the lower intercostal nerves can be caused by surgical trauma or anatomical variations of the anterior intercostal neurovascular bundle and surrounding structures in the abdominal wall. This can occur when a surgical incision directly damages the cutaneous nerve, or when scar tissue formation (or suture) impinges on a cutaneous nerve causing iatrogenic ACNES.[8] In patients who have not had abdominal surgery, the nerve is most commonly entrapped at the lateral border of the rectus muscle. Here, the neurovascular bundle travels through a fibrous ring in the rectus sheath that can compress the structures and produce the symptoms of ACNES.[3]

CLINICAL PRESENTATION

Pain is the dominant finding in CAWP, and the specific presentation is variable. Patients typically report 1–3 months of well-localized pain. The pain may range from mild to debilitating, and the pain itself may be aching, burning, or dull.[6] Patients will often be able to point to the exact area of pain (as opposed to patients with visceral abdominal pain, which is poorly localized),

Interventional Management of Chronic Visceral Pain Syndromes. https://doi.org/10.1016/B978-0-323-75775-1.00018-0

and may report a history of pain improving with manual application of pressure to the painful area.[1] The pain can also radiate posteriorly over a thoracic dermatome.[2] Increased abdominal pressure or conditions such as obesity exacerbate the pain. A history of prior abdominal surgery may also point to a diagnosis of CAWP, as cutaneous nerve entrapment may occur due to the formation of scar tissue or suture placement.[9,10]

DIAGNOSIS

In one survey, only 26% of internists were able to diagnose and choose the appropriate diagnostic step when given a classic vignette of chronic abdominal wall pain.[6] Patients who present to their primary care provider or gastroenterologist for abdominal pain may have diagnostic workup completed to rule out any structural abnormalities or malignancies. Labs can include comprehensive metabolic panel, complete blood count, and liver enzymes and diagnostic imaging may include abdominal X-ray and computed tomography of abdomen and pelvis.

The diagnosis of CAWP is based on history and physical exam. The first step in diagnosis in CAWP is differentiating it from visceral abdominal pain. Although this differentiation can be difficult, in general, visceral abdominal pain is diffuse and poorly localized, while abdominal wall pain is well localized by the patient.[11] If there is confusion, diagnostic injections may clarify the diagnosis.[3,4] This includes infiltration of a local anesthetic directly into the point of tenderness, as well as abdominal wall blocks such as TAP blocks, rectus sheath blocks, erector spinae plane blocks, and paravertebral nerve blocks. Improvement of alleviation of the pain with a diagnostic block points to the abdominal wall as the cause of the pain.

A differential epidural block has also been described to help differentiate between visceral, central, and abdominal wall pain.[12] This involves the placement of a thoracic epidural that is initially injected with saline (as a placebo) and then incremental doses of local anesthetics. The physiologic basis for this exam relies on the theory that sympathetic and visceral afferent nerves are more sensitive to local anesthetic than large cutaneous sensory fibers. Therefore, the time point at which the patient's pain is relieved by the local anesthetic (or returns after the local anesthetic boluses are discontinued) can help elucidate the source of the pain. Furthermore, if the patient's abdominal pain is not relieved with any dose of local anesthetic, this may indicate a centrally mediated pain syndrome. However, the interpretation of this block is very subjective, and the interaction between local anesthetic and nerve fibers is unpredictable and

nonstandard between patients. Therefore, this test is not recommended as an initial step in the diagnostic workup.

PHYSICAL EXAM FINDINGS

Several physical exam findings are pathognomonic for abdominal wall pain. Carnett's test is the most well-described physical exam finding.[13,14] To perform this test, the patient is placed in the supine position with the knees flexed to relax the abdominal wall. In the relaxed position, the painful area is initially palpated. Then, the patient is asked to tighten the musculature of the abdominal wall by lifting the head and shoulders off the bed. The test is positive if there is increased tenderness with increased abdominal wall tension (indicating that the pain arises from the abdominal wall). If the pain is intraabdominal in origin, it is more likely that pain will decrease with increased abdominal wall tension, as the tensed abdominal muscles guard the abdominal viscera.[3]

Additional physical exam findings include a fixed location of tenderness, superficial tenderness, or point tenderness over the abdominal wall with less than 2.5 cm of diameter. An allodynic response may occur when pinching the skin overlying the painful area, which is known as the "pinch test."[5]

TREATMENT

There are no evidence-based guidelines regarding the treatment of CAWP, and there are few high-quality studies. Therefore, most of the treatments described are based on expert opinion or chronic pain interventions studied for other etiologies of chronic pain. The treatment of CAWP can include pharmacologic interventions, injections, advanced procedures, surgical interventions, as well as physical therapy.

Pharmacologic

Systemic pharmacotherapy is usually first-line for most pain syndromes, but in ACNES this is not the case. NSAIDs, acetaminophen, weak opioids, anticonvulsants, and antidepressants provide partial benefit. Therefore, it would be reasonable to try conservative therapy with standard neuropathic medications. This would include anticonvulsant (i.e., gabapentin, pregabalin) and antidepressant (serotonin and norepinephrine reuptake inhibitors, tricyclic antidepressants) medications.

Injections

Injection of local anesthetic with steroids directly into the localized area of pain may provide significant long-term relief for CAWP. One study demonstrated that 91% of patients suspected to have CAWP experienced greater than 50% pain relief after a local anesthetic-steroid injection.[3] More recent reports of ultrasound-guided cutaneous nerve injections describe the technique of the procedure, lasting up to 10 months after two injections.[15] The target of an ultrasound-guided cutaneous nerve injection is between the rectus abdominis and the linea semilunaris, approximately 1 cm medial to the linea semilunaris. If the area of pain is more difficult to localize, abdominal wall blocks such as transversus abdominis plane blocks (TAP), rectus sheath blocks, and paravertebral nerve blocks may also have diagnostic as well as a therapeutic benefit in the treatment of CAWP.

A TAP block anesthetizes the nerves more proximally, between the internal oblique and transversus abdominal muscles. It reliably provides analgesia below the umbilicus, though it may not adequately cover above the umbilicus.[16] It can be performed laterally, posteriorly, or subcostally (see Figs. 16.1 and 16.2). This block may be used for diagnostic or therapeutic purposes in the setting of CAWP if more focal injections are not helpful.

A rectus sheath block may also be used for diagnostic or therapeutic purposes in chronic abdominal wall pain. The block is performed below the costal margin in the plane between the posterior rectus sheath and the transversalis fascia, and it provides sensory block along the midline of the abdomen.[17] It has been advocated for use in pediatrics, where pain localization is more difficult to achieve.

A less common approach is to use a paravertebral nerve block both for diagnosis and treatment of CAWP. The block is performed under ultrasound by the placement of local anesthetic along with the paravertebral space, which contains sympathetic as well as intercostal nerves. It provides a large unilateral somatic and sympathetic blockade.[18]

Advanced Procedures

Refractory abdominal wall pain may also benefit from advanced procedures that have been studied for chronic visceral abdominal pain or other types of peripheral neuropathies. There is some evidence that peripheral neuropathic pain can be treated with local injection of botulinum toxin, though to our knowledge no studies have been done on this intervention specifically for CAWP.[19] An older report from McGrady describes 44 patients who underwent a stimulation-guided 6% phenol injection.[20] A 23-g insulated needle was inserted into the anterior rectus sheath. Final needle placement was obtained when the pain was elicited at 0.5 V. Moreover, 1 mL of 6% phenol was injected and patients were followed up at varying time intervals. Complete or partial relief for up to 6 months was seen in 26 out of 28 (94%) of patients.

Spinal cord stimulator implantation has demonstrated some efficacy in chronic abdominal pain. However, the studies performed up to this point have evaluated spinal cord stimulation for chronic visceral abdominal pain, rather than abdominal wall pain.[21] Peripheral nerve stimulation is successful in the treatment of neuropathic pain from nerve entrapment, and could also be considered in the treatment of ACNES but this specific indication is not described in the literature.

Surgical Interventions

An anterior neurectomy is an option for patients not responding to or having short relief from conservative measures. A recent randomized double-blinded trial of 44 patients diagnosed with ACNES compared

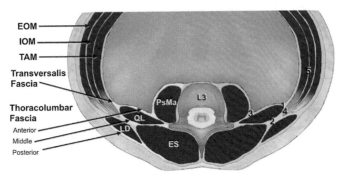

FIG. 16.1 Cross-section of posterolateral abdominal wall at L3 level showing the transversalis fascia and the anterior, middle, and posterior layers of the thoracolumbar fascia. Numbers relate to the needle endpoints: (1) lateral QL (QL1) block, (2) posterior QL (QL2) block, (3) transmuscular QL (QL3 or anterior) block, (4) posterior TAP block, and (5) lateral TAP block. (Reproduced from Onwochei, D. N., J. Børglum, A. Pawa. Abdominal wall blocks for intra-abdominal surgery. *BJA Educ* 2018;18(10):317–322.)

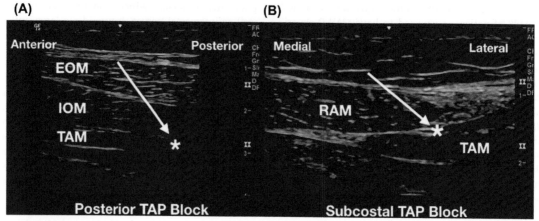

FIG. 16.2 Ultrasound images of a **(A)** posterior transversus abdominal plane block and **(B)** subcostal transversus abdominal plane block. The arrow represents the trajectory of the needle, while the asterisk indicates the location for deposition of local anesthetic. (Reproduced from Onwochei, D. N., J. Børglum, A. Pawa. Abdominal wall blocks for intra-abdominal surgery. *BJA Educ* 2018;18(10):317–322.)

surgical neurectomy to sham surgery.[22] 73% of the treated patients versus. 18% of the sham surgery patients reported at least 50% pain response. The benefit is noted to last up to 32 months.[23] Lindestmo et al. advocate for patient referral to a surgeon if conservative treatment in combination with three local injections does not relieve the abdominal pain.[9] The surgeon can then perform a fascial release at the lateral border of the rectus fascia or a surgical neurectomy.

CONCLUSION

Chronic abdominal wall pain is often mistaken for visceral pain, which can result in unnecessary diagnostic testing as well as delay in diagnosis and treatment. The diagnosis can be made with an appropriate history and physical exam. In patients with focal pain, positive Carnett's test, and a history of abdominal surgery, CAWP should be suspected. Confirmatory blocks include the infiltration of local anesthetic and steroid into the location of maximal pain. Other options include a plane block such as the rectus sheath or the TAP block. In refractory cases, referral to a surgeon for fascial release of nerve entrapment is indicated, and peripheral or spinal cord stimulation devices may also be considered.

REFERENCES

1. Friedenberg FK, Gissen Brown JR, Bernstein GR, Erlich AC. Chronic abdominal wall pain. *J Clin Gastroenterol.* 2016; 50(10):828–835.
2. Thompson C, Goodman R, Rowe WA. Abdominal wall syndrome: a costly diagnosis of exclusion. *Gastroenterology.* 2001;120:A637.
3. Scheltinga MR, Roumen RM. Anterior cutaneous nerve entrapment syndrome (ACNES). *Hernia.* 2018;22:507–516.
4. Applegate WV. Abdominal cutaneous nerve entrapment syndrome (ACNES): a commonly overlooked cause of abdominal pain. *Perm J.* 2002;6(3):20.
5. Sweetser S. Abdominal wall pain: a common clinical problem. *Mayo Clinic Proc.* 2019;94(2). Elsevier.
6. Koop H, Koprdova S, Schürmann C. Chronic abdominal wall pain: a poorly recognized clinical problem. *Dtsch Ärzteblatt Int.* 2016;113(4):51.
7. Tsai H-C, Yoshida T, Chuang TY, et al. Transversus abdominis plane block: an updated review of anatomy and techniques. *BioMed Res Int.* 2017;2017.
8. van Assen T, de Jager-Kievit JW, Scheltinga MR, et al. Chronic abdominal wall pain misdiagnosed as functional abdominal pain. *J Am Board Fam Med.* 2013;26:738–744.
9. Lindsetmo R-O, Stulberg J. Chronic abdominal wall pain—a diagnostic challenge for the surgeon. *Am J Surg.* 2009;198:129–134.
10. De Andres J, Perotti L, Palmisani S, Perez VLV, Asensio-Samper JM, Fabregat G. Chronic pain due to postsurgical intra-abdominal adhesions: therapeutic options. In: *Chronic Abdominal Pain.* Springer; 2015:77–87.
11. Costanza C. Chronic abdominal wall pain: clinical features, health care costs, and long term outcome. *Clin Gastroenterol Hepatol.* 2004;2:395–399.
12. McCollum D, Stephen CR. The use of graduated spinal anesthesia in the differential diagnosis of pain of the back and lower extremities. *South Med J.* 1964;57:410–416.
13. Srinivasan R, Greenbaum DS. Chronic abdominal wall pain: a frequently overlooked problem. *Am J Gastroenterol.* 2002;97:824.

14. Carnett JB. Intercostal neuralgia as a cause of abdominal pain and tenderness. *Surg Gynecol Obstet.* 1926;42:625−632.

15. Hong MJ, Kim YD, Seo DH. Successful treatment of abdominal cutaneous entrapment syndrome using ultrasound guided injection. *Korean J Pain.* 2013;26:291−294.

16. Støving K, Rothe C, Rosenstock CV, Aasvang EK, Lundstrøm LH, Lange KH. Cutaneous sensory block area, muscle-relaxing effect, and block duration of the transversus abdominis plane block: a randomized, blinded, and placebo-controlled study in healthy volunteers. *Reg Anesth Pain Med.* 2015;40:355−362.

17. Skinner AV, Lauder GR. Rectus sheath block: successful use in the chronic pain management of pediatric abdominal wall pain. *Pediatr Anesth.* 2007;17:1203−1211.

18. Richardson J, Lönnqvist PA, Naja Z. Bilateral thoracic paravertebral block: potential and practice. *Br J Anaesth.* 2011; 106:164−171.

19. Jeynes LC, Gauci CA. Evidence for the use of botulinum toxin in the chronic pain setting—a review of the literature. *Pain Pract.* 2008;8:269−276.

20. McGrady EM, Marks RL. Treatment of abdominal nerve entrapment syndrome using a nerve stimulator. *Ann R Coll Surg Engl.* 1988;70:120−122.

21. Kapural L. Spinal cord stimulation for chronic abdominal pain. In: *Neuromodulation.* Elsevier; 2018:1379−1386.

22. Boelens OB, van Assen T, Houterman S, et al. A double-blind, randomized, controlled trial on surgery for chronic abdominal pain due to anterior cutaneous nerve entrapment syndrome. *Ann Surg.* 2013;257:845−849.

23. van Assen T, Boelens OB, van Eerten PV, et al. Long-term success rates after an anterior neurectomy in patients with an abdominal cutaneous nerve entrapment syndrome. *Surgery.* 2015;157:137−143.

FURTHER READING

1. McGarrity TJ, Peters DJ, Thompson C, McGarrity SJ. Outcome of patients with chronic abdominal pain referred to chronic pain clinic. *Am J Gastroenterol.* 2000;95:1812.

2. Chrona E, Kostopanagiotou G, Damigos D, Batistaki C. Anterior cutaneous nerve entrapment syndrome: management challenges. *J Pain Res.* 2017;10:145−156.

CHAPTER 17

Chronic Mesenteric Ischemia

SALIM ZERRINY, MD • R. JASON YONG, MD

INTRODUCTION

Chronic mesenteric ischemia develops due to insufficient blood flow within the splanchnic vasculature, most typically in the presence of a gradually occlusive disease state like atherosclerosis. An estimated one-fifth of the elderly population lives with some degree of significant stenosis within their mesenteric vasculature, but they often remain asymptomatic due to sufficient collateralization. However, when the blood supply fails to meet the demand, symptoms referred to as "splanchnic syndrome" develop, highlighted by postprandial pain, which in turn leads to food fear and weight loss.

Once diagnosed, lifestyle modifications are recommended, though a majority of patients ultimately require invasive treatment via percutaneous endovascular revascularization or open surgical revascularization. Before corrective surgical treatment, pain can be temporized with interventions such as celiac plexus and epidural blocks. For nonsurgical candidates, the placement of a spinal cord stimulator (SCS) can be considered.

ETIOLOGY AND PATHOGENESIS

A majority of cases of chronic mesenteric ischemia are due to atherosclerotic narrowing, although rare causes include median arcuate ligament syndrome, fibromuscular dysplasia, aortic or mesenteric dissection, vasculitis (polyarteritis nodosum, Takayasu's disease), and retroperitoneal fibrosis.

The three major vessels that supply the abdomen are the celiac trunk (esophagus, stomach, proximal duodenum, liver, gallbladder, pancreas, and spleen), superior mesenteric artery (distal duodenum, jejunum, ileum, and colon to the splenic flexure), and the inferior mesenteric artery (descending colon, sigmoid colon, and rectum). Approximately 18% of the elderly (>65) are thought to have significant stenosis in one of their splanchnic vessels without any known prior symptoms, and only 1.3% are thought to have two or more significantly stenotic vessels.[1] Despite this, many patients remain asymptomatic in the setting of sufficient perfusion supplied by collateral vessels. One area at high risk is the splenic flexure, as it is a vulnerable area between territories of SMA (Superior Mesenteric Artery) and IMA (Inferior Mesenteric Artery) vasculature distribution. The majority of cases of mesenteric ischemia involve narrowing of the origins of the celiac or SMA, although the single-vessel disease was found to occur much more commonly in the celiac artery than SMA (81% vs. 19%, respectively).[2]

CLINICAL FEATURES

As previously mentioned, a vast majority of patients who have atherosclerotic mesenteric vasculature are asymptomatic due to the extensive splanchnic collaterals. Most patients who are symptomatic are over age 60 and are three times more likely to be female.[3] An estimated 60% of patients have a smoking history and 50% have been shown to have known vascular disease.[4]

The result of poor perfusion to the gut causes symptoms referred to as splanchnic syndrome: postprandial pain (i.e., intestinal angina), food fear, weight loss, and 50% of patients have an epigastric bruit.[5] The pain after eating is typically described as colicky, dull, and crampy. This pain often occurs within the first hour and subsides over the following 2 h, although this time may be longer in meals with high-fat content. It is typically localized in the epigastrium with occasional radiation to the back. The pain is thought to occur secondary to arterial steal. Blood is diverted from the intestinal to the gastric circulation and this develops when food is in the stomach, thus explaining its temporal nature.[6] Patients with a constellation of symptoms including weight loss, postprandial pain, adapted eating patterns, and diarrhea were 60% likely to have chronic mesenteric ischemia, whereas they were only 13% likely if none of these symptoms were present.[7] A third of patients have been shown to have symptoms that were less typical such as nausea, vomiting, early satiety, and lower gastrointestinal tract (GI) bleeding

Interventional Management of Chronic Visceral Pain Syndromes. https://doi.org/10.1016/B978-0-323-75775-1.00008-8

(secondary to foregut ischemia due to celiac artery insufficiency).[6] If a thrombus forms, symptoms can progress and cause what is known as acute on chronic mesenteric ischemia, in which morbidity and mortality are much higher.

DIAGNOSIS

Diagnosis of chronic mesenteric ischemia is initially clinical, requiring symptoms of splanchnic syndrome, diarrhea/malabsorption, or vomiting. Initial diagnosis can be difficult, as many of the symptoms overlap with other etiologies, such as malignancy. An inability to pinpoint an alternate etiology in those experiencing the aforementioned symptoms should highly increase suspicion for chronic mesenteric ischemia. Some studies have demonstrated that the time from symptoms to diagnosis is approximately 1.5 years on average.[8] For an official diagnosis, one must have significant stenosis in two or more of the mesenteric vessels (>70% narrowing of the celiac artery, SMA or IMA). However, due to the vascular supplies' vast collateral network, all but approximately 5% of patients were found to be asymptomatic even with complete occlusion of a single mesenteric artery.

Per guidelines set by the American College of Radiology, computed tomography angiography of the abdomen and pelvis with intravenous contrast is the initial imaging of choice (Fig. 17.1). It has high sensitivity in identifying or excluding atherosclerotic disease in the mesenteric vessels and is also helpful in ruling out other intraabdominal pathologies as the cause of symptoms. Magnetic resonance angiography (MRA) with contrast-enhancement is an alternative noninvasive imaging option, as it has high sensitivity in detecting proximal stenotic region within the mesenteric vasculature, though this is unreliable at detecting more distal lesions. In patients who cannot tolerate contrast loads, noncontrast MR angiography has proven to be an accurate method for detecting stenosis in the celiac trunk and superior mesenteric artery.[9] In the event that the noninvasive imaging techniques are deemed equivocal, the next step would be to perform arteriography with possible intervention when necessary.

In an outpatient setting, it is often reasonable to first perform a duplex ultrasound of the mesenteric vasculature as a screening tool. It has a high negative predictive value of 99% for high-grade stenosis, which helps justify the pursuit of alternative causes of abdominal pain in the setting of a negative study.[10] It is important to note that although duplex ultrasound is sensitive in diagnosing stenosis, it cannot diagnose intestinal ischemia.

Functional studies are being investigated for their possible role in the diagnosis of chronic mesenteric ischemia. Such modalities as tonometry may be utilized to assess intraluminal pH of the intestines to identify tissue ischemia.[11] Currently, there are additional

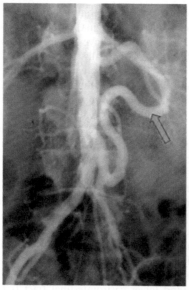
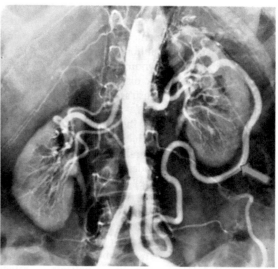

FIG. 17.1 Viscero-visceral collateral pathways in chronic mesenteric ischemia: arc of Riolan (arrows) is a collateral pathway between the superior mesenteric artery (SMA) and inferior mesenteric artery (IMA).

functional studies being assessed for their clinical utility including visible light spectroscopy oximeters and MR venography to assess mucosal saturations and blood flow, respectively.

PHYSICAL EXAM FINDINGS

On physical examination, there are typically no specific findings. Pain may be present but is nonlocalized. When present, its onset often occurs within 30 min following a meal and worsens over the course of an hour, classically resolving within 1–3 h. Approximately 80% of patients exhibit some degree of weight loss, some of whom will be cachectic with signs of severe malnutrition. Additionally, patients may show evidence of diffuse atherosclerotic disease, including coronary artery disease and peripheral vascular disease. Upon auscultation, approximately 50% will be found to have an epigastric abdominal bruit.

TREATMENT

Pharmacologic

Antiplatelet agents are often used as secondary prevention in those with atherosclerotic disease. If there is evidence of acute thrombus formation, systemic anticoagulation is then indicated. Proton pump inhibitors have shown some value given evidence of decreased oxygen demand of the gastric mucosa. Antispasmodic agents (i.e., papaverine hydrochloride) and nitrates have been shown to be helpful in attenuating symptoms of intestinal angina.

Revascularization

Revascularization is typically only warranted if symptoms are present with evidence of severe stenosis of the splanchnic vessels. When the need for vascularization arises, the two options are open surgical reconstruction (aortomesenteric and celiac bypass grafting, endarterectomy, and mesenteric reimplantation) and percutaneous transluminal angioplasty (PTA). PTA is becoming the more favored option given improvements in the technique. However, open surgical techniques may be preferred in patient populations where intravenous contrast loads are contraindicated. Systematic reviews of both techniques have shown no significant difference in perioperative mortality and 3-year cumulative survival between the two groups.[12]

Injection Therapy

For patients with chronic abdominal pain, interventional pain techniques have been demonstrated to be effective adjunctive treatments. Patients may gain temporary relief

with procedures like epidural blocks, which in turn may suggest benefit from the placement of more permanent devices like intrathecal pumps for refractory patients. To date, studies assessing the effectiveness of visceral blockade has been highly variable and included a limited number of patients. In a retrospective study by Rizk et al., patients with chronic visceral abdominal pain were evaluated and treated with the differential thoracic epidural regional blockade, also known as differential neural blocks.[13] Incremental doses of local anesthetic are infused through the epidural catheter with subsequent blockade of the nerve supply to visceral organs, such as the celiac, hypogastric and splanchnic nerves. In Rizk et al. study, 81 patients underwent differential thoracic epidural regional block. Among this group, 70.4% of the patients reported a successful block, described as >50% reduction in their visual analog scale pain score. The findings of this study also suggested that more intense initial pain scores led to a greater degree of pain alleviation from the block.

Intrathecal Drug Delivery Systems

Intrathecal drug delivery systems (IDDS) deliver medications directly into the intrathecal space through an indwelling catheter that is connected to a reservoir system implanted in a subcutaneous pocket typically in the abdomen (Fig. 17.2). Currently, FDA approved medications for IDDS are morphine, baclofen, and ziconotide. Additive and off-label medications include fentanyl,

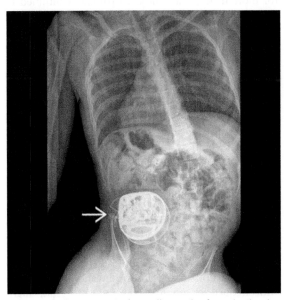

FIG. 17.2 Anteroposterior radiograph of cerebral palsy patient displays an intrathecal baclofen infusion pump (arrow).

bupivacaine, clonidine, and hydromorphone among others. Opioids are most commonly used, and often as monotherapy, with subsequent additional of agents often guided by the Polyanalgesic Consensus Conference recommendations.[14] Before placement of IDDS, an epidural or intrathecal trial is performed to determine the potential benefit of treatment. Alternatively, a single shot spinal may also be done. The catheter tip is placed according to the corresponding dermatomal distribution of the patient's pain.

Neuromodulation

SCS is a longer-term interventional pain technique that has been conventionally used to treat a variety of chronic pain conditions such as complex regional pain syndrome and failed back surgery syndrome. In recent years, their use has been expanded to treat a variety of conditions causing chronic visceral pain, with case series demonstrating long-term improvement in pain scores and decreased opioid use. In a study by Kapural et al., 35 patients received SCS for their chronic visceral abdominal pain.[15] The majority of patients had SCS leads placed at the level of the T5 or T6 vertebral bodies for generalized, epigastric, or periumbilical pain, and a subset of patients with lower abdominal pain had leads placed at the T11 and T12 levels. Two of these patients specifically were suffering from mesenteric ischemia. Twenty-eight patients received permanent implants following a positive trial, and 19 patients were followed for more than 1 year. These 19 patients continued to have sustained pain relief and a decrease in opioid use at 6 months and 1-year follow-up.

The mechanism of action is traditionally thought to be through the generation of paresthesias in the receptive field of the spinal segment, which is thought to occur through antidromic activation of primary efferent fibers. An additional proposed mechanism is based on the spinal gating theory, which suggests that the stimulation of large afferent nerve fibers causes a reduction in sympathetic outflow and small diameter visceral fibers transmission.[16]

Recent development of high frequency, "paresthesia-free" spinal cord stimulation has spurred renewed interests in its application for abdominal pain. Although conventional paresthesia-based spinal cord stimulation delivers electrical impulses to the dorsal column of the spinal cord at a frequency of 2–1200 Hz with above-sensory threshold amplitudes, high-frequency stimulation utilizes subsensory threshold amplitudes with frequencies up to 10 kHz. As a result, high-frequency waveforms eliminate the often uncomfortable sensations of abdominal paresthesias and the

need for intraoperative mapping during implant and revision surgeries. The analgesic mechanism of high-frequency stimulation remains unclear. However, it is postulated that afferent nerve signaling may be reduced from the activation of inhibitor interneurons with 10-kHz stimulation.[17]

SCS has become further refined with the advent of burst stimulation, a modality where periods of high-frequency impulses are delivered (five pulses at 500 Hz, 40 times per second). This is thought to be effective due to mimicry of the central nervous system firing of neurons and its effect on medial pain pathways, thereby influencing the emotional components of pain perception.[18] Similar to other neuromodulation modalities, burst stimulation's efficacy in treating chronic abdominal pain has yet to be thoroughly investigated. In a retrospective review by Richter et al., three patients with various forms of chronic abdominal pain underwent BurstDR SCS paddle lead and pulse generator placement following a successful trial stimulation period.[19] SCS lead tips were positioned between the levels of the T6 and T8 vertebral bodies with paresthesia mapping done intraoperatively. In a 24-month-long follow-up period, two out of the three patients reported complete resolution of pain, and the third patient reported a 60% decrease in pain. Additionally, patients were found to have satisfaction in the quality of life, decrease in monthly pain episodes, and decrease in opioid use. Although the evidence-to-date has been promising, higher-powered studies are required to adequately assess the efficacy of SCS modalities in patients with chronic abdominal pain such as mesenteric ischemia.

Dorsal root ganglion (DRG) stimulation is an alternate stimulation-based therapy that has recently increased in popularity, particularly for the treatment of areas that have been difficult to treat with traditional dorsal column stimulation, including the abdomen. The DRG is a collection of sensory nerve cell bodies that are located bilaterally at each spinal level and can be accessed percutaneously for focused stimulation of particular dermatomes.[20] In a case presentation by Justiz and Smith assessing chronic abdominal pain due to pancreatitis, they had successful treatment results with bilateral T8 and T10 DRG lead placements in a 16-year-old patient with hereditary pancreatitis.[21] Although this patient did not have mesenteric ischemia, it is important to note that DRG stimulation can be considered in patients with refractory abdominal pain.

To date, research regarding interventional techniques has been quite limited, as stimulation of the receptive field of the spinal segment cannot be mimicked transcutaneously, making it difficult to blind and conduct proper randomized control trials. In the setting of ischemic pain, the mechanism of SCS analgesia is felt to be partially attributed to the restoration of the oxygen supply and demand mismatch through the redistribution of blood flow. Vasodilation with neuromodulation may occur directly through action on the sympathetic nervous system or through the release of vasodilatory substances by sensory fibers.[22]

Conservative Management

In patients who are diagnosed incidentally and are without the clinical manifestations of ischemia, management is often conservative. Lifestyle changes include smoking cessation, treatment of risk factors for atherosclerosis, changes in diet (small, more frequent meals), low protein and fat diet, inhibition of gastric acid secretion, and improved gastric mucosal blood flow via proton pump inhibitors (helps decrease GI metabolic demand). Nutritional assessments are particularly useful given the degree of significant weight loss associated with the condition.

REFERENCES

1. Biolato M, Miele L, Gasbarrini G, Grieco A. Abdominal angina. *Am J Med Sci.* 2009;338:389–395.
2. Hansen KJ, Wilson DB, Craven TE, et al. Mesenteric artery disease in the elderly. *J Vasc Surg.* 2004;40:45–52. https://doi.org/10.1016/j.jvs.2004.03.022.
3. Keese M, Schmitz-Rixen T, Schmandra T. Chronic mesenteric ischemia: time to remember open revascularization. *World J Gastroenterol.* 2013;19(9):1333–1337. https://doi.org/10.3748/wjg.v19.i9.1333.
4. Veenstra RP, ter Steege RW, Geelkerken RH, et al. The cardiovascular risk profile of atherosclerotic gastrointestinal ischemia is different from other vascular beds. *Am J Med.* 2012;125:394.
5. Kolkman JJ, Bargeman M, Huisman AB, et al. Diagnosis and management of splanchnic ischemia. *World J Gastroenterol.* 2008;14:7309–7320.
6. Poole JW, Sammartano RJ, Boley SJ. Hemodynamic basis of the pain of chronic mesenteric ischemia. *Am J Surg.* 1987;153:171.
7. ter Steege RW, Sloterdijk HS, Geelkerken RH, et al. Splanchnic artery stenosis and abdominal complaints: clinical history is of limited value in detection of gastrointestinal ischemia. *World J Surg.* 2012;36:793.
8. Oderich GS. Current concepts in the management of chronic mesenteric ischemia. *Curr Treat Options Cardiovasc Med.* 2010;12:117.
9. Cardia PP, Penachim TJ, Prando A, et al. Non-contrast MR angiography using three-dimensional balanced steady-state free-precession imaging for evaluation of stenosis in the celiac trunk and superior mesenteric artery: a preliminary comparative study with computed tomography angiography. *Br J Radiol.* 2017;90:20170011.
10. Nicoloff AD, Williamson WK, Moneta GL, et al. Duplex ultrasonography in evaluation of splanchnic artery stenosis. *Surg Clin North Am.* 1997;77:339.
11. Walley KR, Friesen BP, Humer MF, Phang PT. Small bowel tonometry is more accurate than gastric tonometry in detecting gut ischemia. *J Appl Physiol.* 1998;85:1770.
12. Cai W, Li X, Shu C, et al. Comparison of clinical outcomes of endovascular versus open revascularization for chronic mesenteric ischemia: a meta-analysis. *Ann Vasc Surg.* 2015;29:934.
13. Rizk MK, Tolba R, Kapural L, et al. Differential epidural block predicts the success of visceral block in patients with chronic visceral abdominal pain. *Pain Pract.* 2012;12(8):595–601. https://doi.org/10.1111/j.1533-2500.2012.00548.x.
14. Deer TR, Pope J, Hayek SM. The Polyanalgesic Consensus Conference (PACC) recommendations on intrathecal drug infusion systems best practices and guidelines. *Neuromodulation.* 2017;20:96–132.
15. Kapural L, Hassan N, Tlucek H, Sessler DI. Spinal cord stimulation for chronic visceral abdominal pain. *Pain Med.* 2010; 11(3):347–355. https://doi.org/10.1111/j.1526-4637.2009.00785.x.
16. Qin C, Lehew R, Khan K, Wienecke G, Foreman R. Spinal cord stimulation modulates intraspinal colorectal visceroreceptive transmission in rats. *Neurosci Res.* 2007;58(1):58–66. https://doi.org/10.1016/j.neures.2007.01.014.
17. Kapural L, Gupta M, Paicius M, et al. Treatment of chronic abdominal pain with 10-KHz spinal cord stimulation. *Clin Transl Gastroenterol.* 2020;11(2):e00133. https://doi.org/10.14309/ctg.0000000000000133.
18. De Ridder D, Plazier M, Kamerling N, Menovsky T, Vanneste S. Burst spinal cord stimulation for limb and back pain. *World Neurosurg.* 2013;80:642–649.
19. Richter B, Novik Y, Bergman JJ, Tomycz ND. The efficacy of BurstDR spinal cord stimulation for chronic abdominal pain: a clinical series. *World Neurosurgery.* 2020;138: 77–82. https://doi.org/10.1016/j.wneu.2020.02.075.
20. Deer T, Levy R, Kramer J, et al. Dorsal root ganglion stimulation yielded higher treatment success rate for complex regional pain syndrome and causalgia at 3 and 12 months: a randomized comparative trial. *Pain.* 2017;158:669–681.
21. Justiz R, Smith N. *Thoracic DRG Stimulation for Chronic Abdominal Pain Due to Hereditary Pancreatitis.* Las Vegas: North American Neuromodulation Society; 2017.
22. Foreman RD. *Neural Mechanisms of Spinal Cord Stimulation.* Vol. 107. 2012.

CHAPTER 18

Inflammatory Bowel Disease

MARK ABUMOUSSA, MD • MERON SELASSIE, MD • M. GABRIEL HILLEGASS, MD

INTRODUCTION

Inflammatory bowel disease (IBD) is a chronic inflammatory condition that comprises two different clinical diseases of the gastrointestinal tract: Crohn's disease (CD) and ulcerative colitis (UC).[1] The Centers for Disease Control and Prevention approximates that IBD affects over 3 million US adults, approximately 1.3% of the population, with the prevalence increasing yearly. It is more common than previously believed. IBD has a bimodal distribution, with peaks at 15–30 years of age and another at 50–80 years of age. Americans of Jewish descent are among those found to have an increased prevalence.[2] It is also important to note that the incidence of IBD is rising in children, with about 25% of all diagnosed cases occurring in patients under the age of 18.[4] The two entities of IBD, CD and UC, have many shared characteristics; however, they are distinguished by certain pathologic and clinical findings.

ETIOLOGY AND PATHOGENESIS

There are many factors that are known to contribute to the pathogenesis of IBD. These include environmental, genetic, immune, and bacterial.[3] The combined effects of these factors result in dysregulated immune responses that cause the gastrointestinal inflammation that characterizes IBD. Crohn's disease is classically described as transmural inflammation characterized by skip lesions that can involve the entire GI tract, from mouth to anus. The transmural inflammation may lead to fibrosis and strictures, as well as obstruction of the colon. Ulcerative colitis on the other hand solely involves the mucosa of the colon, invariably affecting the rectum and extends proximally to other regions of the colon. Both CD and UC tend to have a relapsing and remitting course. With improving technology and research, the pathogenesis of IBD has been found to include other components of the inflammatory process, including immunopathogenic components of epithelial cells, endothelial cells, cellular components, and inflammatory mediators.[1] Interestingly, smoking has been found to be one of the most important modifiable risk factors for Crohn's disease, whereas it may confer a protective benefit for ulcerative colitis.[5]

CLINICAL FEATURES

Although there are shared signs and symptoms in UC and CD, there are features of IBD that are uniquely specific to each. Over 50% of IBD patients have a chief complaint of abdominal/pelvic pain on presentation. Chronic pelvic pain has been reported in about 14% of IBD.[6] Pain can be from acute inflammation during relapses, partial or full bowel obstructions due to strictures or adhesions, fistulas, abscesses, or chronic pain from visceral hypersensitivity. Fever, weakness, and diarrhea are also common complaints. About 90% of patients affected with Crohn's disease report bloody diarrhea, whereas patients with UC have a main complaint of cramping that subsides with defecation. Both forms of IBD can lead to reduced appetite and, in turn, unintended weight loss.

Given that IBD causes a chronic systemic inflammatory state, a new emphasis has been put on symptoms that occur outside of the GI tract, called extraintestinal manifestations (EIM). It has been estimated that 6%–47% of adult patients and approximately 25% of pediatric patients are affected by EIMs.[7] The most common form of EIMs occurs in the musculoskeletal system in the form of peripheral and axial joint disease. Some examples of these commonly include metacarpophalangeal joint arthropathies that are usually self-limiting, to the more severe form of ankylosing spondylitis and sacroiliitis.[8] Cutaneous manifestations of IBD occur in the form of erythema nodosum and pyoderma gangrenosum; however, most dermatological manifestations are usually associated as a complication of IBD therapies.[9] Ocular manifestations of IBD are well known, however, rare with only 2%–5% of IBD patients developing them. These manifestations include uveitis and scleritis.[7] Hepatobiliary conditions are also

Interventional Management of Chronic Visceral Pain Syndromes. https://doi.org/10.1016/B978-0-323-75775-1.00012-X

associated with IBD, with up to 50% of IBD patients developing a hepatobiliary manifestation at some point in their disease process.[10] Primary sclerosing cholangitis is the most common. It is seen mostly in patients with CD, affecting up to 7.5% of these patients with a predisposition toward middle-aged men.[7]

DIAGNOSIS

IBD is diagnosed via endoscopic evidence of inflammatory changes to the digestive tract as well as chronic changes seen on histology from tissue biopsy. Upper endoscopy and colonoscopy are the two modalities most commonly used, while flexible sigmoidoscopy or capsule endoscopies are alternative options. It is important to rule out other causes of GI discomfort and/or bleeding with an extensive medical history, lab tests for infectious causes, and other imaging modalities for anatomical causes of obstruction including cancer and other masses.

PHYSICAL EXAM FINDINGS

Physical exam findings are typically nonspecific in IBD. Visceral abdominal pain is a common finding, with or without abdominal palpation. Cachexia may be seen in severe cases in which anorexia is related to unrelenting abdominal pain and related GI symptoms. Cutaneous findings of erythema nodosum and pyoderma gangrenosum may be seen. Given the common involvement of joints, signs of arthropathy such as metacarpal and phalangeal warmth and swelling may be observed. Further, stiffness and loss of range of motion along the spinal column due to ankylosing spondylitis is another possible EIM finding. Due to the recurring and often debilitating nature of the disease, many patients often suffer from a psychiatric standpoint. It is prudent to evaluate for anxiety, depression, and any maladaptive behavior or thought patterns (e.g., catastrophizing) as these mental health conditions are often comorbid with the disease.[12]

TREATMENT

Pain management in IBD is complicated and often requires an interdisciplinary approach with coordination of care among primary care, gastroenterologists and other medical specialists, pain management, and mental health providers. Chronic abdominal pain with visceral hypersensitivity complicated by significant mental health disease and/or maladaptive coping skills and thought patterns may require patient-centered care plans to educate both the patient and their network of

support for successful treatment outcomes. It is always important to make the distinction between pain of an acute exacerbation (i.e., relapse) of IBD versus chronic visceral pain when determining the treatment plan. Evaluations for active clinical disease and relapses should be managed by the gastroenterologist. Patients with IBD are always at risk for surgical interventions should an obstruction, fistula, perforation, abscess, or other severe complications develop.

Lifestyle Modification and Conservative Therapies

Regular aerobic exercise, mindfulness-based stress reduction, meditation, and yoga are all self-management interventions that can be learned and implemented to help patients reduce stress and promote a healthy lifestyle and resiliency. These should be discussed as part of the interdisciplinary treatment plan

Pharmacologic

Most of the disease-specific medical treatments will be managed by a gastroenterologist. These may include antiinflammatory medications such as corticosteroids or aminosalicylates, immunosuppressive agents (e.g., azathioprine), or newer biologic drugs that block tumor necrosis factor, integrins, cytokines, or transcription factors.

NSAIDs

These are typically effective when used for pain related to arthropathies from EIMs; however, in general, they should be avoided as a specific treatment for IBD-related visceral pain. The inhibition of cyclooxygenase and subsequent reduction of prostaglandin can adversely affect the intestinal mucosa, which is already pathologically altered in IBD.

Adjuvant analgesics—SNRIs, TCAs, SSRIs, AEDs

There are no randomized controlled trials demonstrating the effectiveness of these classes of medications on IBD-related symptoms or disease progression. The SNRIs and SSRIs would be indicated for the treatment of comorbid anxiety and depression when appropriate. The SNRIs, TCAs, and AEDs may also be beneficial for the treatment of central sensitization and visceral hypersensitivity.

Opioids

Use with caution and close monitoring for chronic visceral pain. Well-defined short opioid courses for acute pain related to IBD relapses or surgery may be appropriate until remission and surgical healing occur, respectively. A bowel regimen must be implemented as toxic megacolon is a risk with opioid use in IBD. Narcotic bowel syndrome is another concern with chronic opioid use because frequently recurring abdominal pain makes it difficult to distinguish active IBD pain from this opioid-related adverse effect.

Novel therapies

New molecular targets are being studied, but translational research is still being developed. One such marker that is gaining interest is the bioactive peptide nociceptin.[12] It has been shown that this peptide is involved in pain signaling and reversal of stress-induced analgesia. Further, it has also been implicated in the pathophysiology of IBD suggesting that targeting this peptide may not only alleviate pain but also help affect the chronic course of the disease.[12,13] Other molecular pathways of interest involve transient receptor potential (TRP) channels (e.g., TRPV1/TRPA1 mixed antagonists and TRPV4 antagonists) and cytokine signaling utilizing Janus kinase inhibitors.[12]

Psychological Interventions

There has been an increased interest in determining the efficacy and role of psychotherapy (including psychodynamic therapy, cognitive behavioral therapy, systemic therapy, brief therapy, supportive therapy, patient education, and coping skills) and other psychological interventions in IBD treatment. In 1989, Drossman commented on the impairment that IBD can have on many aspects of the patient's life but emphasized that emotional behavior might be the most negatively affected of all.[14] As this approach has gained traction, multiple authors have reported that IBD activity may be closely related to corresponding increases and decreases in anxiety/depression and the degree of psychological disturbance appears to correlate with disease severity.[15,16] This has led to the hypothesis that the improvement of psychosocial factors may have consequences on both the patient's psychosocial well-being, as well as the course of IBD itself. This has been controversial in the literature with conflicting results.

A large Cochrane systematic review in 2011 aimed to address this question. Twenty-one studies were selected, including both randomized controlled trials as well as observational studies. Their objective was to assess the effects of psychological interventions in IBD and resulting disease activity. The review concluded that there was no evidence for the efficacy of psychological therapy in adult patients with IBD. However, it was suggested that

in adolescents psychologic interventions may be beneficial and more research is needed in this specific population.[17]

Dietary Restrictions

Patients with IBD often have a strong interest in implementing dietary modifications into their treatment plan for controlling and managing their IBD. There is evidence that dietary factors may influence the risk of developing and/or further worsening intestinal mucosal inflammation. There is a known link between the environment, especially diet, and the composition of the gut microbiome. However, there is currently a paucity of rigorous data from controlled trials and translational research to allow for patient guidelines.[18] Reported diets with success include carbohydrate-free, gluten-free, specific carbohydrate diet, the fermentable oligosaccharides, disaccharides, and monosaccharides diet and the Paleolithic diet.[18] Each of these diets manipulates the types of substances the gut is exposed to in a way that is supposed to reduce inflammation. However, essentially all food groups have been self-reported by patients to exacerbate their symptoms with a high degree of individual variability. Therefore, patients are often instructed to be aware of their diet, make note of which foods exacerbate their symptoms, and tailor their eating habits to their specific requirements.

Interventional Pain Management

There have not been any interventional pain modalities that have been reported to aid in the treatment of pain specifically from IBD.[19] However, in patients with visceral sensitization, there may be a role for neuromodulation of the dorsal columns or dorsal horns in the regions of the spinal cord that correspond to innervation of the gut. Kapural and colleagues (2010) published a case series on 35 consecutive spinal cord stimulation (SCS) trials for chronic visceral abdominal pain. Epidural access can be obtained from the lumbar region (Fig. 18.1). They placed the electrode in the midline with the tips at T5–T6 (Fig. 18.2) for epigastric/periumbilical pain or T11–L1 for lower abdominal/pelvic pain. Most of the patients had a primary diagnosis of pancreatitis or adhesive disease. There was no diagnosis of IBD. Moreover, 86% had a successful trial (>50% reduction in pain). Nineteen patients were followed for a year and their average visual analog scale pain scores were 50% of baseline at 1 year.[20] Further, a national survey published the same year analyzed 70 cases of SCS utilized for chronic visceral pain of which only 4 failed the SCS trial. Sixty-six patients were implanted with

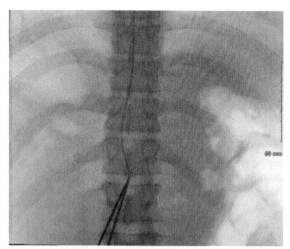

FIG. 18.1 Epidural access obtained at T12/L1 interspace with a paramedian approach for an SCS trial.

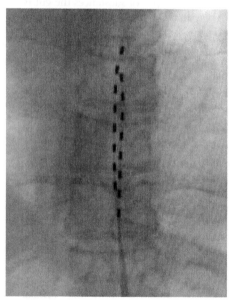

FIG. 18.2 Spinal cord stimulator lead tips at the top of the T5 vertebral body.

midline electrode tips at T5—6 and significant sustained pain relief (>50% reduction in pain) and a significant reduction in opioid consumption was found at an average follow-up of 84 weeks.[21]

A recent development in neuromodulation has been the ability to modulate the activity of the glial cells in the spinal cord. This may hold promise for certain chronic pain states in which central sensitization has occurred as emerging research has implicated activated glia in perpetuating CNS inflammation and sensitization. It will take years for this translational research to be conducted in various chronic pain populations, but the application to the IBD population seems plausible.

Surgical Management

Ultimately, surgical interventions such as colectomies and ostomies are options for treatment in severe cases of IBD.[11] As mentioned earlier, acute surgical interventions may be required for complications related to IBD as well.

REFERENCES

1. De Souza H, Fiocchi C. Immunopathogenesis of IBD: current state of the art. *Nat Rev Gastroenterol Hepatol*. 2015; 13(1):13—27.
2. Inflammatory bowel disease is more common than earlier studies showed. *J Am Med Assoc*. 2016;316(24):2590.
3. Roberts H, Rai S, Pan J. Extraintestinal manifestations of inflammatory bowel disease and the influence of smoking. *Digestion*. 2014;90(2):122—129.
4. Yu YR, Rodriguez JR. Clinical presentation of Crohn's, ulcerative colitis, and indeterminate colitis: symptoms, extraintestinal manifestations, and disease phenotypes. *Semin Pediatr Surg*. 2017;26:349—355.
5. Biedermann L, Fournier N, Misselwitz B, et al. High rates of smoking especially in female Crohn's disease patients and low use of supportive measures to achieve smoking cessation–data from the Swiss IBD Cohort Study [published correction appears in J Crohns Colitis. 2016 Jun;10(6): 754]. *J Crohns Colitis*. 2015;9(10):819-829.
6. Rapkin AJ, Mayer EA. Gastroenterological causes of chronic pelvic pain. *Obstet Gynecol Clin N Am*. 1993;20: 663—683.
7. Vavricka SR, Schoepfer A, Scharl M. Extraintestinal manifestations of inflammatory bowel disease. *Inflamm Bowel Dis*. 2015;21(8):1982—1992.
8. Brakenhoff L, Van der Heijde DM, Hommes DW. IBD and arthropathies: a practical approach to its diagnosis and management. *Gut*. 2011;60(10):1426—1435.
9. Levine JS, Burakoff R. Extraintestinal manifestations of inflammatory bowel disease. *Gastroenterol Hepatol*. 2011; 7(4):235—241.
10. Ott C, Scholmerich J. Extraintestinal manifestations and complications in IBD. *Nat Rev Gastroenterol Hepatol*. 2013;10(10):585—595.
11. Sobczak M, Fabisiak A, Murawska N, et al. Current overview of extrinsic and intrinsic factors in etiology and progression of inflammatory bowel diseases. *Pharmacol Rep*. 2014;66(5):766—775.
12. Zielinska A, Salalga M, Wlodarczyk M. Focus on current and future management possibilities in inflammatory bowel disease-related chronic pain. *Int J Colorectal Dis*. 2019;34(2):217—227.
13. Sobczak M, Mokrowiecka A, Cygankiewicz AI, et al. Anti-inflammatory and antinociceptive action of an orally

available nociceptin receptor agonist SCH 221510 in a mouse model of inflammatory bowel diseases. *J Pharmacol Exp Therapeut.* 2014;348(3):401–409.

14. Drossman DA, Patrick DL, Mitchell CM, Zagami EA, Appelbaum MI. Health-related quality of life in inflammatory bowel disease: functional status and patient worries and concerns. *Dig Dis Sci.* 1989;34(9):1379–1386.
15. Porcelli P, Leoci C, Guerra V. A prospective study of the relationship between disease activity and psychologic distress in patients with inflammatory bowel disease. *Scand J Gastroenterol.* 1996;31(8):792–796.
16. Mawdsley JE, Rampton DS. Psychological stress in IBD: new insights into pathogenic and therapeutic implications. *Gut.* 2005;54(10):1481–1491.
17. Timmer A, Preiss JC, Motschall E, Rücker G, Jantschek G, Moser G. Psychological interventions for treatment of

inflammatory bowel disease. *Cochrane Database Syst Rev.* 2011;16(2):CD006913.
18. Hou JK, Lee D, Lewis J. Diet and inflammatory bowel disease: review of patient-targeted recommendations. *Clin Gastroenterol Hepatol.* 2014;12(10):1592–1600.
19. Docherty MJ, Jones RC, Wallace MS. Managing pain in inflammatory bowel disease. *Gastroenterol Hepatol.* 2011;7(9):592–601.
20. Kapural L, Nagem H, Tlucek H, Sessler DI. Spinal cord stimulation for chronic visceral abdominal pain. *Pain Med.* 2010;11(3):347–355.
21. Kapural L, Deer T, Yakovlev A, et al. Technical aspects of spinal cord stimulation for managing chronic visceral abdominal pain: the results from the national survey. *Pain Med.* 2010;11(5):685–691.

CHAPTER 19

Irritable Bowel Syndrome

JESSICA BEATTY, MD • NARAYANA VARHABHATLA, MD

INTRODUCTION

IBS has a worldwide prevalence rate of 5%–20%[1,2] and makes up ~25% of "functional gastrointestinal disorders" diagnoses. Functional abdominal pain is difficult to define, diffuse (not localized), and not associated with structural or biochemical changes.[3] IBS, specifically, is characterized by chronic abdominal pain, altered bowel habits (diarrhea or constipation), and the absence of any alarm findings. The pain and symptoms of IBS often last a lifetime and have a significant impact on quality of life (QOL). A meta-analysis of 18 studies from the United States and the United Kingdom calculated the annual *direct* cost of *each* IBS patient (drugs, procedures, and doctors visits) to be $348–$8750 and the annual *indirect* cost (loss of work days and decreased productivity) to be $355–$3444.[4,5] Within the United States, IBS has an annual direct cost of $228 million in doctors' visits and $80 million in drugs.[5] IBS patients are significant utilizers of the healthcare system. It is estimated that IBS cases make up 25%–50% of the annual referrals seen by a gastroenterologist.[6,7] In short, IBS has a significant impact on healthcare utilization, the global economy, and on patients' QOL. It is worth understanding how to diagnose and manage this syndrome's hallmark feature — abdominal pain.

ETIOLOGY AND PATHOGENESIS

The chronic abdominal pain of IBS, like most chronic pain, is multidimensional (peripheral sensory, affective emotional, and cognitive central nervous system) and multifactorial, including changes in physiology at the peripheral and central level. Signals from the colon are conveyed to the spinal cord through first and second-order neurons and then travel to the brain via the spinothalamic, spinoreticular, and spinomesencephalic pathways. These tracts then project to the somatosensory cortex, which functions to discriminate the location of painful signals, whether they are somatic or visceral in origin. These tracts also project to the perigenual anterior cingulate cortex and midcingulate cortex within the

limbic system.[2,8] These areas of the limbic system function in the regulation and handling of pain affect as well as behavioral response modification.[9]

It is believed that the central feature of functional gastrointestinal disorders (FGID), like IBS, is a change within the central nervous system's modulation and processing of painful peripheral signals. There may also be an abnormal or increased peripheral signal originating from the gut. Changes at the peripheral level may be due to food, stress, visceral inflammation, menses, previous surgery, or acute gastrointestinal infection.[7,10] This enhanced peripheral signal can be further accentuated by spinal or central level hyperexcitability — leading to a state of visceral hyperalgesia (exaggerated sense of pain) or allodynia (pain that results from a nonnoxious stimulus) in IBS patients.[11,12] Heightened peripheral sensitivity has a role at the beginning of the IBS pain process. It is the CNS, however, not the periphery that leads to chronic pain in IBS patients. Central regulation, not peripheral sensitivity, is the primary factor in chronic pain related to IBS. Patients with psychiatric disease, significant life stress, sexual or physical trauma, poor relational support, and poor coping skills demonstrate more severe and more chronic pain, as well as poorer health outcomes.[13–16]

CLINICAL FEATURES

IBS is characterized by chronic abdominal pain and altered bowel habits. The chronic abdominal pain of IBS is usually "crampy" in nature with varying intensity and intermittent exacerbations. Severity can range from mild and episodic pain to severe and unrelenting.[1,17,18] The pain is typically related to defecation; sometimes relieved with defecation, sometimes exacerbated by it.[19] Stress and food commonly worsen the pain. A bloated sensation and frequent flatulence or belching are other common associated symptoms.

A patient's description of their pain can be a valuable insight into the origin or components of a multifactorial etiology.[8] A "nauseating," "sharp," or "stabbing" description is consistent with a strong emotional

Interventional Management of Chronic Visceral Pain Syndromes. https://doi.org/10.1016/B978-0-323-75775-1.00003-9

component and therefore limbic origin. "Constant" and not affected by eating or defecation is unlikely to be associated with an abnormality in GI motility. When a patient describes their abdominal pain, and it is couched amidst several other pain complaints, there is likely a component of central sensitization. When the patient's abdominal pain is part of a series of pains over their lifetime, the clinician has to be concerned for impaired limbic modulation as a preeminent factor.

IBS is as much behavioral as it is symptomatic, but IBS cannot be diagnosed by behavioral changes alone. It is important to evaluate the patient's cognitive and emotional patterns from a biopsychosocial model — recognizing that a patient's behavior reflects how they are evaluating, reacting to, and handling their symptoms. Many behaviors are maladaptive and present an opportunity for the clinician to intervene and counsel healthier, more effective habits. It is not uncommon to discover concurrent psychiatric comorbidities, "unresolved loss, a history of abuse, poor social support, and maladaptive coping skills."[8] Referral to a mental health professional can be of great value, and help in the amelioration of a patient's symptoms. Additionally, a trusting and therapeutic relationship can be an avenue by which more healthful habits are fostered.

DIAGNOSIS

There are no diagnostic biomarkers specific for IBS; it is a clinical diagnosis of exclusion. It is this workup process that contributes to the heavy health care utilization and economic burden previously described. While many physicians may not feel comfortable without first completing a thorough workup,[20] other etiologies should be investigated only as directed by history and physical exam findings.[17,21] The Rome Foundation Criteria is the current standard for diagnosing FGIDs and IBS. It builds and expands on the original Manning criteria[22] and incorporates a *combination* of symptoms to increase the sensitivity and specificity to diagnose IBS. The latest version, the Rome IV criteria, was published in May 2016 (Table 19.1).[13,17,23,24]

For the diagnosis of IBS, Rome IV requires:
- the presence of recurrent abdominal pain
- on average at least 1 day/week in the last 3 months
- with symptom onset at least 6 months before diagnosis

Additionally, the pain must be associated with at least two of the three following symptoms:
(1) Related to defecation (either increasing or decreasing the pain)
(2) Associated with a change in stool frequency
(3) Associated with a change in stool appearance

"Alarm" or "red flag symptoms" must be absent. These include unintended weight loss, blood in the stool, nocturnal symptoms, fever, family history of serious gastrointestinal disease (e.g., colorectal cancer, inflammatory bowel disease, or celiac disease), new onset of IBS symptoms after age 50, or an abnormal finding on physical exam. A complete blood count, c-reactive protein, and celiac panel are high yield, relatively low cost, and commonly recommended as part of the routine, initial evaluation.[2,21] A thyroid panel, fecal calprotectin, and stool analysis can also be considered based on history and physical exam. Again, patients with a clinical presentation consistent with the Rome criteria, who lack any red flags on H&P, warrant only a basic evaluation — after which the clinician can feel comfortable making a diagnosis of IBS.[25,26]

PHYSICAL EXAM FINDINGS

The purpose of the physical exam should be to allay patient anxiety, to meet patient expectations, and to rule out organic disease.

Abdominal Exam

- The clinician should palpate for internal changes such as an enlarged liver, abdominal mass, or signs of bowel obstruction.

TABLE 19.1
Rome IV Criteria for Diagnosis of IBS

Presence of recurrent abdominal pain, on average at least 1 day/week in the last 3 months, with symptom onset at least 6 months before diagnosis, with 2 of the 3 below criteria:

- Abdominal pain related to defecation (either increasing or decreasing the pain)
- Associated with a change in stool frequency
- Associated with a change in stool appearance

- Observe for the "closed eyes sign" whereby someone with a functional origin to their abdominal pain is more likely to keep their eyes closed during abdominal palpation, whereas the patient with an organic etiology is more likely to hold their eyes open.[27] The thought is that the patient with organic disease wants to watch the doctor and avoid severe pain when able.

Pelvic Exam

- Warranted when there are lower abdomen and/or pelvic symptoms on history or a change in menses or vaginal discharge.

Digital Rectal Examination

- Particularly important when there are symptoms of incontinence or dyschezia in the history. Also valuable to identify a dysfunctional sphincter, paradoxical pelvic floor contraction, dyssynergic defecation, fecal impaction, or rectal cancer.

  Note: Pelvic, digital, and perianal examinations are typically performed by gastroenterologists or primary care physicians before a pain consultation, and repeating this exam is not necessary.

TREATMENT

Cultivating a trusting doctor–patient relationship is paramount.[28,29] Patients who have a good rapport with their physicians have fewer IBS-related follow-up visits.[30] Psychiatric and functional comorbidities are common among IBS patients. An educational discussion about the unifying concept that explains many of their symptoms (central sensitization) can be relieving and therapeutic in and of itself.[2] The treatment of IBS includes both pharmacologic and nonpharmacologic interventions, and there is no data to support any one agent or modality as first-line therapy for IBS.

Pharmacologic Agents

Of the pharmacologic interventions, there are central and peripherally acting modalities. The peripherally acting agents work at the gut level — treating the bloating, cramping, and abnormal bowel movements of IBS. Many of these agents take advantage of the deranged serotonin (5HT) levels found at the peripheral gut level in IBS. These agents include the antispasmodics (e.g., pinaverium, mebeverine, colpermin, hyoscyamine, and dicyclomine) that mechanistically are anticholinergic, smooth muscle relaxants (Table 19.2). Serotonergic agents (e.g., alosetron and tegaserode) also work at the peripheral level as 5HT3 receptor antagonists and 5HT4 receptor agonists. Peripherally acting medications are not designed to treat the pain of IBS; however, they are an important complement and in some mild cases may provide sufficient symptom management.

TABLE 19.2 Pharmacologic Agents for IBS

Type	Agents	Therapeutic Mechanism of Action
Antispasmodics	• Pinaverium • Mebeverin • Colpermin • Hyoscamine • Dicyclomine	• Smooth muscle relaxants to decrease GI spasms
Serotonergic agents	• Alosetron • Tegaserode	• Alosetron: $5\text{-}HT_3$ antagonist to slow gut motility • Tegaserode: $5\text{-}HT_4$ agonist, $5\text{-}HT_{2B}$ antagonist to simulate gut motility

Serotonin reuptake inhibitors	• Serotonin reuptake inhibitors (SSRIs)
	  • Fluoxetine, paroxetine
	• Selective serotonin-norepinephrine reuptake inhibitors (SNRIs)
	  • Venlafaxine, duloxetine
	• Tricyclic antidepressants (TCAs)
	  • Amitriptyline, imipramine
		• Increases serotonin by inhibiting serotonin reuptake

In moderate-to-severe cases, where pain is the primary and most distressing symptom, centrally acting agents are preferred. Serotonin reuptake inhibitors are the preeminent classes of medication that should be used in treating moderate to severe IBS. This class includes selective serotonin reuptake inhibitors (SSRIs), selective serotonin-norepinephrine reuptake inhibitors (SNRIs), and tricyclic antidepressants (TCAs). Additional agents to consider include atypical antipsychotics such as quetiapine and other antidepressants such as mirtazapine and buspirone. Although classically considered psychiatric medications, these agents are equally appropriate in the treatment of IBS. It may be helpful to educate patients that the antidepressants, particularly the TCAs, are given at lower doses than those used in the management of depression. As discussed previously, psychiatric comorbidities are not uncommon among the IBS population, therefore antidepressants may contribute to patients' overall mental health. Additionally, and independently, TCAs and SNRIs are recommended in the treatment of other chronic pain disorders. It is for these reasons that antidepressants play a central role in the medical management of IBS pain.

When initiating medication(s), consider the unique patient profile and choose the agent whose direct effects, and side effects, work to their advantage. For example, the TCAs tend to be constipating and less anxiolytic. Mirtazapine is an appetite stimulation, antiemetic, and anxiolytic. Quetiapine is anxiolytic, restores normal sleep patterns, and "has direct analgesic effects, particularly in severe IBS."[31] Buspirone is a strong anxiolytic agent and effectively treats symptoms of dyspepsia and early satiety by increasing "gastric compliance and relaxation."[2] There is an important phenomenon called "augmentation therapy" whereby medications are used in combination, at lower doses, to maximize therapeutic effect and minimize adverse side effects.[32] In keeping with this approach, clinicians are advised to start medications at a low dose, titrate to response, and not hesitate to initiate additional medications instead of increasing a single agent to the maximum dose.

Many IBS patients are reticent to start an antidepressant — either out of concern for how it will make them feel in their head or because it suggests the disease is "all in their head." It behooves the clinician to come to the conversation prepared to present *all* the treatment options in a delicate and balanced fashion. A disarming and effective approach might be this, "the same drugs can be used for different reasons; at higher doses antidepressants treat depression, at lower doses they are effective in pain relief."[2]

Behavioral Therapy

Lastly, there are nonpharmacologic psychologic-focused interventions, which serve an important role in the management of IBS pain. Recommended modalities include cognitive-behavioral therapy (CBT), interpersonal psychodynamic therapy, hypnosis, stress reduction, and mindfulness meditation.[33]

CBT has garnered the most attention and study, and the research seems to bear out consistently positive results — suggesting that CBT plays an important complementary part in the treatment of IBS symptoms.[34-36] In the largest randomized placebo-controlled study to date, it was found that 12 weekly CBT sessions were significantly more beneficial than placebo for female patients with moderate to severe FGIDs.[37] The goal of CBT in IBS is to help the patient identify and correct distorted, unhelpful beliefs regarding their symptoms and build helpful, personalized coping skills. Interpersonal therapy works from the assumption that symptoms are related to and exacerbated by interpersonal, relational difficulties and that symptoms can be alleviated by resolving relational conflict. There has been research to suggest that interpersonal psychodynamic therapy improves symptoms and reduces disability and IBS-related healthcare costs.[38-40] In children with functional abdominal pain and IBS, psychosomatic approaches to management decreased abdominal pain in 70%−89% of cases.[41] CBT psychodynamic therapy can be conducted on an individual or group basis.

Stress reduction and mindfulness meditation aim to counteract the physiologic effects of the stress created by IBS symptoms. These techniques are often taught in conjunction with CBT as effective coping mechanisms. They have been shown to improve symptoms and QOL and reduce stress levels in IBS patients.[42,43]

Lastly, gut-targeted hypnosis uses guided imagery to produce muscle relaxation and improvements in gut function and symptoms. Interestingly, hypnosis is not only effective at acutely improving IBS symptoms and QOL,[44,45] it's positive effects have been shown to persist long term.[44-47]

Patient buy-in, an internal locus of control, rapport with the therapist, and early response — these are all predictors of a favorable outcome with behavioral, psychologic intervention.[48] Patient preference should dictate the choice of intervention. Importantly, the clinician should not hesitate to initiate this type of therapy at the outset, alongside pharmacologic agents. Likewise, behavioral interventions are particularly appropriate for the patient who does not want to take medications or the patient whose symptoms have not responded to pharmacologic intervention.[49,50] Guided imagery over four weekly sessions has shown benefit in decreasing pain days and missed activities in a small study of 22 children.[41] The problem with a lot of these studies is that psychosomatic interventions are often intermixed making it difficult to tease out which are actually beneficial. These interventions carry low risk beyond the time required, and thus can all be attempted. However, CBT has the most evidence and should be tried first.

REFERENCES

1. Enck P, Aziz Q, Barbara G, et al. Irritable bowel syndrome. *Nat Rev Dis Prim.* 2016;2(16014). https://doi.org/10.1038/nrdp.2016.14.
2. Dekel R, Drossman DA, Sperber AD. Abdominal pain in irritable bowel syndrome (IBS). In: Kapural L, ed. *Chronic Abdominal Pain: An Evidence-Based, Comprehensive Guide to Clinical Management.* New York, NY: Springer; 2015: 59–67.
3. Noe JD, Li BU. Navigating recurrent abdominal pain through clinical clues, red flags, and initial testing. *Pediatr Ann.* 2009;38(5):259–266.
4. Maxion-Bergemann S, Thielecke F, Abel F, Bergemann R. Costs of irritable bowel syndrome in the UK and US. *Pharmacoeconomics.* 2006;24(1):21–37. https://doi.org/10.2165/00019053-200624010-00002.
5. Sandler RS, Everhart JE, Donowitz M, et al. The burden of selected digestive disease in the United States. *Gastroenterology.* 2002;122(5):1500–1511. https://doi.org/10.1053/gast.2002.32978.
6. Malone MA. Irritable bowel syndrome. *Prim Care Clin Off Pract.* 2011;38(3):433–447. https://doi.org/10.1016/j.pop.2011.05.003.
7. Drossman DA, Camilleri M, Mayer EA, Whitehead WE. *Gastroenterology.* 2002;123(6):2108–2131. https://doi.org/10.1053/gast.2002.37095.
8. Drossman DA. Functional abdominal pain syndrome. *Clin Gastroenterol Hepatol.* 2004;2(5):353–365. https://doi.org/10.1016/s1542-3565(04)00118-1.
9. Fuchs PN, Peng YB, Boyette-Davis JA, Uhelski ML. The anterior cingulate cortex and pain processing. *Front Integr Neurosci.* 2014;8(35). https://doi.org/10.3389/fnint.2014.00035.
10. Sperber AD, Drossman DA. Review article: the functional abdominal pain syndrome. *Aliment Pharmacol Therapeut.* 2011;33(5):514–524. https://doi.org/10.1111/j.1365-2036.2010.04561.x.
11. Coderre TJ, Katz J, Vaccarino AL, Melzack R. Contribution of central neuroplasticity to pathological pain: review of clinical and experimental evidence. *Pain.* 1993;52(3): 259–285. https://doi.org/10.1016/0304-3959(93)90161-h.
12. Mayer EA, Gebhart GF. Basic and clinical aspects of visceral hyperalgesia. *Gastroenterology.* 1994;107(1):271–293. https://doi.org/10.1016/0016-5085(94)90086-8.
13. Thompson WG, Longstreth GF, Drossman DA, Heaton KW, Irvine EJ, Muller-Lissner SA. Functional bowel disorders and functional abdominal pain. *Gut.* 1999; 45(2):43–47. https://doi.org/10.1136/gut.45.2008.ii43.
14. Drossman DA, Creed FH, Olden KW, Svedlund J, Toner BB, Whitehead WE. Psychological aspects of the functional gastrointestinal disorders. *Gut.* 1999;45(2): 25–30. https://doi.org/10.1136/gut.45.2008.ii25.
15. Drossman DA, Whitehead WE, Toner BB, et al. What determines severity among patients with painful functional bowel disorders? *Am J Gastroenterol.* 2000;95(4):974–980. https://doi.org/10.1111/j.1572-0241.2000.01936.x.
16. Drossman DA, Li Z, Leserman J, Toomey TC, Hu YJ. Health status by gastrointestinal diagnosis and abuse history. *Gastroenterology.* 1996;110(4):999–1007. https://doi.org/10.1053/gast.1996.v110.pm8613034.
17. Longstreth GF, Thompson WG, Chey WD, Houghton LA, Mearin F, Spiller RC. Functional bowel disorders. *Gastroenterology.* 2006;130(5):1480–1491. https://doi.org/10.1053/j.gastro.2005.11.061.
18. Swarbrick ET, Hegarty JE, Bat L, Williams CB, Dawson AM. Site of pain from the irritable bowel. *Lancet.* 1980;2(8192): 443–446. https://doi.org/10.1016/s0140-6736(80)91885-1.
19. Simren M, Palsson OS, Whitehead WE. Update on Rome IV criteria for colorectal disorders: implications for clinical practice. *Curr Gastroenterol Rep.* 2017;19(4):15. https://doi.org/10.1007/s11894-017-0554-0.
20. Spiegel BM, Farid M, Esrailian E, Talley J, Chang L. Is irritable bowel syndrome a diagnosis of exclusion?: a survey of primary care providers, gastroenterologists, and IBS experts. *Am J Gastroenterol.* 2010;105(4):848–858. https://doi.org/10.1038/ajg.2010.47.
21. Grayson M. Irritable bowel syndrome. *Nature.* 2016; 533(7603). https://doi.org/10.1038/533S101a.
22. Manning AP, Thompson WG, Heaton KW, Morris AF. Towards positive diagnosis of the irritable bowel. *Br Med J.* 1978;2(6138):653–654. https://doi.org/10.1136/bmj.2.6138.653.
23. Drossman DA, Thompson WG, Talley NJ. Identification of sub-groups of functional gastrointestinal disorders. *Int J Gastroenterol.* 1990;3:159–172.
24. Drossman DA, Hasler WL. Rome IV-functional GI disorders: disorders of gut-brain interaction. *Gastroenterology.* 2016;150(6):1257–1261. https://doi.org/10.1053/j.gastro.2016.03.035.
25. Vanner SJ, Depew WT, Paterson WG, et al. Predictive value of the Rome criteria for diagnosing the irritable bowel syndrome. *Am J Gastroenterol.* 1999;94(10):2912–2917. https://doi.org/10.1111/j.1572-0241.1999.01437.x.
26. Hammer J, Eslick GD, Howell SC, Altiparmak E, Talley NJ. Diagnostic yield of alarm features in irritable bowel syndrome and functional dyspepsia. *Gut.* 2004;53(5): 666–672. https://doi.org/10.1136/gut.2003.021857.
27. Gray DWR, Dixon JM, Collin J. The closed eyes sign: an aid to diagnosing non-specific abdominal pain. *Br Med J.* 1988; 297:837. https://doi.org/10.1136/bmj.297.6652.837.

28. Tanaka Y, Kanazawa M, Fukudo S, Drossman DA. Bio-psychosocial model of irritable bowel syndrome. *J Neurogastroenterol Motility.* 2011;17(2):131–139. https://doi.org/10.5056/jnm.2011.17.2.131.

29. Drossman DA. Psychosocial sound bites: exercises in the patient- doctor relationship. *Am J Gastroenterol.* 1997;92:1418–1423.

30. Owens DM, Nelson DK, Talley NJ. The irritable bowel syndrome: long-term prognosis and the physician-patient interaction. *Ann Intern Med.* 1995;122(2):102–112. https://doi.org/10.7326/0003-4819-122-2-199501150-00005.

31. Grover M, Dorn SD, Weinland SR, Dalton CB, Gaynes BN, Drossman DA. Atypical antipsychotic quetiapine in the management of severe refractory functional gastrointestinal disorders. *Dig Dis Sci.* 2009;54(6). https://doi.org/10.1007/s10620-009-0723-6.

32. Drossman DA. Beyond tricyclics: new ideas for treating patients with painful and refractory functional gastrointestinal symptoms. *Am J Gastroenterol.* 2009;104(12):2897–2902. https://doi.org/10.1038/ajg.2009.341.

33. National Institute of Health and Care Excellence. *CG61. Irritable Bowel Syndrome in Adults: Diagnosis and Management of Irritable Bowel Syndrome in Primary Care.* NICE; 2008.

34. Blanchard EB, Lackner JM, Sanders K, et al. A controlled evaluation of group cognitive therapy in the treatment of irritable bowel syndrome. *Behav Res Ther.* 2007;45(4):633–648. https://doi.org/10.1016/j.brat.2006.07.003.

35. Kennedy TM, Chalder T, McCrone P, et al. Cognitive behavioral therapy in addition to antispasmodic therapy for irritable bowel syndrome in primary care: randomized controlled trial. *Health Technol Assess.* 2006;10(19):1–67. https://doi.org/10.3310/hta10190.

36. Lackner JM, Jaccard J, Krasner SS, Katz LA, Gudleski GD, Holroyd K. Self-administered cognitive behavioral therapy for moderate to severe irritable bowel syndrome: clinical efficacy, tolerability, feasibility. *Clin Gastroenterol Hepatol.* 2008;6(8):899–906. https://doi.org/10.1016/j.cgh.2008.03.004.

37. Drossman DA, Toner BB, Whitehead WE, et al. Cognitive-behavioral therapy versus education and desipramine versus placebo for moderate to severe functional bowel disorders. *Gastroenterology.* 2003;125(1):19–31. https://doi.org/10.1016/s0016-5085(03)00669-3.

38. Creed F, Fernandes L, Guthrie E, et al. The cost-effectiveness of psychotherapy and paroxetine for severe irritable bowel syndrome. *Gastroenterology.* 2003;124(2):303–317. https://doi.org/10.1053/gast.2003.50055.

39. Guthrie E, Creed F, Dawson D, Tomenson B. A controlled trial of psychological treatment for the irritable bowel syndrome. *Gastroenterology.* 1991;100(2):450–457. https://doi.org/10.1016/0016-5085(91)90215-7.

40. Hyphantis T, Guthrie E, Tomenson B, Creed F. Psychodynamic interpersonal therapy and improvement in interpersonal difficulties in people with irritable bowel syndrome. *Pain.* 2009;145(1–2):196–203. https://doi.org/10.1016/j.pain.2009.07.005.

41. Chiou E, Nurko S. Functional abdominal pain and irritable bowel syndrome in children and adolescents. *Therapy.* 2011;8(3):315.

42. Blanchard EB, Schwarz SP, Suls JM, et al. Two controlled evaluations of multicomponent psychological treatment of irritable bowel syndrome. *Behav Res Ther.* 1992;30(2):175–189. https://doi.org/10.1016/0005-7967(92)90141-3.

43. Gaylord SA, Palsson OS, Garland EL, et al. Mindfulness training reduces the severity of irritable bowel syndrome in women: results of a randomized controlled trial. *Am J Gastroenterol.* 2011;106(9):1678–1688. https://doi.org/10.1038/ajg.2011.184.

44. Lindfors P, Unge P, Arvidsson P, et al. Effects of gut-directed hypnotherapy on IBS in different clinical settings-results from two randomized, controlled trials. *Am J Gastroenterol.* 2012a;107(2):276–285. https://doi.org/10.1038/ajg.2011.340.

45. Lindfors P, Unge P, Nyhlin H, et al. Long-term effects of hypnotherapy in patients with refractory irritable bowel syndrome. *Scand J Gastroenterol.* 2012b;47(4):414–420. https://doi.org/10.3109/00365521.2012.658858.

46. Gonsalkorale WM, Houghton LA, Whorwell PJ. Hypnotherapy in irritable bowel syndrome : a large-scale audit of a clinical service with examination of factors influencing responsiveness. *Am J Gastroenterol.* 2002;97(4):954–961. https://doi.org/10.1111/j.1572-0241.2002.05615.x.

47. Gonsalkorale WM, Miller V, Afzal A, Whorwell PJ. Long term benefits of hypnotherapy for irritable bowel syndrome. *Gut.* 2003;52(11):1623–1629. https://doi.org/10.1136/gut.52.11.1623.

48. Lackner JM, Gudleski GD, Keefer L, Krasner SS, Powell C, Katz LA. Rapid response to cognitive behavior therapy predicts treatment outcome in patients with irritable bowel syndrome. *Clin Gastroenterol Hepatol.* 2010;8(5):426–432. https://doi.org/10.1016/j.cgh.2010.02.007.

49. Spiller R, Aziz Q, Creed F, et al. Guidelines on the irritable bowel syndrome: mechanisms and practical management. *Gut.* 2007;56(12):1770–1798. https://doi.org/10.1136/gut.2007.119446.

50. Fukudo S, Kaneko H, Akiho H, et al. Evidence-based clinical practice guidelines for irritable bowel syndrome. *J Gastroenterol.* 2015;50(1):11–30. https://doi.org/10.1007/s00535-014-1017-0.

CHAPTER 20

Postherpetic Neuralgia

ALINA BOLTUNOVA, MD • NEEL D. MEHTA, MD

INTRODUCTION

Postherpetic neuralgia (PHN) is a neuropathic pain syndrome that occurs following an acute episode of herpes zoster, commonly known as *shingles*. As with other manifestations of neuropathic pain, the pain of PHN is caused by a lesion of the somatosensory pathway of the nervous system.[1] The management of neuropathic pain conditions such as PHN is often challenging as many patients have an inadequate response to treatment.[2] Although pharmacologic and other noninvasive therapies are typically tried first, interventional treatments may be considered for refractory cases.[3]

PHN is the most common complication of herpes zoster infection. Acute herpes zoster (AHZ) results from the reactivation of the latent varicella-zoster virus (VZV) and is characterized by a painful skin rash that involves the dermatome innervated by the affected sensory ganglion.[4] PHN manifests as pain that persists in the same area as the herpes zoster rash following resolution of the rash. The most common definition refers to PHN as pain that persists for more than 3 months; however, this is an arbitrary distinction and other definitions include neuralgia ranging from 1to 6 months after rash onset.[5] Pain associated with this condition can last for months to years after healing of the rash.[6]

There are approximately one million cases of AHZ annually in the United States, and one in three individuals will develop AHZ in their lifetime.[7] The frequency and severity of PHN increases with age.[8] The incidence of PHN in patients with AHZ increases from 5% in individuals younger than 60%−20% in those 80 years or older (Fig. 20.1).[9] Aside from advanced age, risk factors for the development of PHN following an episode of AHZ include prodromal sensory symptoms (pain or abnormal sensations before the onset of the rash), severe rash, immune compromise, and greater acute pain.[10,11]

ETIOLOGY AND PATHOGENESIS

VZV, a double-stranded herpes virus, is the causative agent of herpes zoster. Primary infection with VZV results in varicella (*chickenpox*), typically seen in childhood. The virus subsequently lies dormant in the sensory ganglion following the resolution of the infection. Impairment of cellular immunity, as occurs with increasing age or immunosuppression, allows for reactivation of the virus.[12] VZV reactivation results in viral particle migration from the sensory ganglion to the dorsal horn of the spinal cord and to the surface of the skin. This process is accompanied by an immune response and inflammation.[13]

The pathophysiology of PHN is complex and involves central and peripheral nerve injury. Viral reactivation and propagation lead to changes in the processing of central nervous system signals and peripheral nerve damage.[8,14,15] These damaged peripheral neurons generate spontaneous discharges and develop a lowered action potential threshold, resulting in exaggerated responses to stimuli.[8,14] Similarly, central nerve injury leads to an augmented response to nociceptor input.[14]

CLINICAL FEATURES

Herpes zoster develops as a unilateral, erythematous papular rash that in many instances affects a single dermatome, or occasionally two contiguous dermatomes. Frequently affected dermatomes include the cervical, mid-to-lower thoracic, and trigeminal regions.[12,16] Pain associated with AHZ precedes the onset of the rash and typically lasts 2−4 weeks.[17] The rash evolves into grouped vesicles, which subsequently form pustules that ulcerate and form scabs.[10] The rash typically lasts 7−10 days, though complete healing may take up to 4 weeks. Scarring and changes in pigmentation may be seen after the healing of the rash.[8] Although the pain

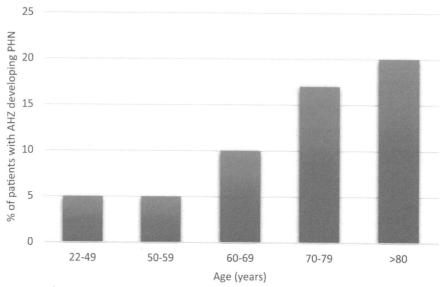

FIG. 20.1 Percentage of patients with herpes zoster developing PHN by age group. (Source: Yawn BP, Saddier P, Wollan PC, St Sauver JL, Kurland MJ, Sy LS. A population-based study of the incidence and complication rates of herpes zoster before zoster vaccine introduction. *Mayo Clin Proc.* 2007;82(11): 1341–1349.)

of AHZ resolves for most individuals, approximately 10% of patients develop PHN.[17,18]

Patients with PHN may report one or more of the following patterns of pain: constant burning or aching pain, intermittent lancinating or shock-like pain, and pain provoked by a normally nonpainful stimulus (allodynia) or disproportionate pain to a noxious stimulus (hyperalgesia).[8,19,20] Approximately 90% of patients have allodynia.[21,22] Patients frequently exhibit sensory deficits in the affected area, particularly loss of tactile, pinprick, and thermal sensation.[21,22]

The physical and psychosocial aspects of life may be disrupted in individuals suffering from PHN. Patients may exhibit impaired appetite, sleep disturbances, depression, diminished libido, and decreased energy levels.[23] Patients also report decreased quality of life and interference with their activities of daily living due to the pain.[23,24]

DIAGNOSIS

The diagnosis of PHN is based on clinical presentation, and thus a thorough medical history and physical examination is essential. Routine history taking should include the patient's symptoms and quality of the pain, vaccination history, and impact of pain on daily life.[8] The Zoster Brief Pain Inventory is a validated tool that can be used to assist in the assessment of pain and discomfort for patients with PHN.[25]

PHN diagnosis is usually straightforward as it is usually pain that persists for over 3 months in the same affected area as the episode of AHZ.[20] However, diagnosis may be more difficult if the rash resolves or if the patient does not remember the rash.[26] Consideration of PHN risk factors—including older age, severe rash, severe pain with AHZ, and localization to the trigeminal or brachial plexus dermatomes—may also aid in diagnosis.[26]

Laboratory tests are not typically needed for the diagnosis of PHN. Rarely, the neuropathic pain of AHZ can occur in the absence of a rash (*zoster sine herpete*). The diagnosis of this condition may require the detection of VZV DNA in cerebrospinal fluid.[27,28]

DIFFERENTIAL DIAGNOSIS

Patient history and clinical findings may help to differentiate herpes zoster from other skin conditions and PHN from other neuropathies and pain syndromes. Herpes zoster can be mistaken for impetigo, candidiasis, herpes simplex virus, contact dermatitis, drug-related eruptions, insect bites, autoimmune blistering disease, and dermatitis herpetiformis.[26,29] The differential diagnosis of PHN includes trigeminal neuralgia, migraine headache, cluster headache, peripheral neuropathy, paroxysmal hemicrania, nerve tumor, and traumatic nerve injury.[30]

PHYSICAL EXAM FINDINGS

A physical examination should include a comparison of the sensory findings on the affected side to that of the contralateral side.[19,31] The affected area may display hyperalgesia and allodynia upon application of mechanical or thermal stimuli.[26,32] In some patients, the involved dermatome(s) may also demonstrate decreased sensation to temperature, touch, and pinprick.[33] Scarring may be identified on exam due to the cutaneous changes related to the episode of AHZ.[20] Changes in autonomic function including increased sweating may also be present on physical exam.[26]

TREATMENT

There is no single therapy that reliably alleviates PHN.[34] PHN is most effectively treated with a multimodal analgesic approach that utilizes multiple therapies with different mechanisms of action.[26] Treatment can include a range of therapies including systemic medications, topical medications, interventional procedures, surgeries, and nontraditional treatments. Long-term therapies are often needed as the pain associated with the condition may last for years.[19]

Pharmacologic

The initial treatment should be tailored to patient preferences, comorbidities, concomitant medication use, and desired medication side effect profiles. Common pharmacologic agents used for the treatment of PHN include anticonvulsants, antidepressants, topical agents, and opioids (Table 20.1).

Anticonvulsant medications are first-line therapies that have been shown to be effective in relieving the pain of PHN. Gabapentin and pregabalin are two oral anticonvulsants that are FDA approved for the management of PHN. Gabapentin is initiated at 100 – 300 mg at bedtime and titrated to analgesic effect at a range of 1800 – 3600 mg in divided doses. A systemic review showed that gabapentin at daily doses of 1800 – 3600 mg provided a significant improvement in pain levels and quality of life measures including sleep, fatigue, and depression in individuals with moderate to severe pain due to PHN.[35] Pregabalin is structurally related to gabapentin. Pregabalin can be initiated at doses of 150 mg per day in once a day or in two divided doses and titrated up to 600 mg per day until adequate pain relief is achieved.[36] Pregabalin is associated with pain intensity reduction at daily doses of 150, 300, and 600 mg.[37] Common side effects of these medications include somnolence, dizziness, xerostomia, and weight gain.[38]

Tricyclic antidepressants (TCAs) including amitriptyline and nortriptyline are also considered to be first-line treatments for PHN and their efficacy is supported by clinical data.[17] Amitriptyline or nortriptyline can be started at 10 mg nightly and titrated up to effect with a maximum daily dose of 150 mg as tolerated.[33,39] Unfortunately, the use of TCAs is limited by their side effect profiles. TCAs are associated with anticholinergic effects such as xerostomia, sedation, constipation, and urinary retention as well as cardiac toxicity.[4,26,29]

Topical therapies such as lidocaine and capsaicin can be used for individuals with localized pain or for those who cannot tolerate or do not desire systemic agents. Topical lidocaine (5%) patches can provide pain relief for patients with PHN; however, quality evidence supporting its clinical efficacy is limited.[40,41] Capsaicin is another topical agent that has been used in the treatment of PHN. Capsaicin 0.075% cream has been shown to have a moderate effect on pain relief, although it can cause burning upon application that limits its clinical use.[17,42] Capsaicin in the form of a high-concentration (8%) patch has demonstrated effective pain relief, however high-concentration topical capsaicin must be administered in a clinical setting often with the use of a local anesthetic.[43]

Opioids are considered to be second-line therapies and their use for the treatment of PHN remains controversial. Clinical data support that opioids (specifically oxycodone and morphine) can effectively treat the pain of PHN.[26,44,45] Tramadol has been shown to be less effective than strong opioids.[17] Both the side effects and safety concerns related to the use of opioids make them less desirable treatment options. Opioid use can lead to sedation, nausea, and constipation and carries the risks of abuse, physical dependence, and tolerance.[6,8]

Infusion therapies with medications such as lidocaine and ketamine have shown some benefit in the treatment of chronic neuropathic pain, although the current evidence does not support their use in PHN. Lidocaine infusion appears to be effective in relieving neuropathic pain and mechanical hyperalgesia in patients with complex regional pain syndrome (CRPS).[46] However, intravenous lidocaine has not demonstrated improved pain relief in the treatment of PHN.[47] Intravenous ketamine has been used successfully for the treatment of multiple neuropathic pain conditions including CRPS, spinal cord injury, fibromyalgia, and neuropathic cancer pain.[48] Limited research has shown a modest benefit in the use of intravenous ketamine for PHN.[49]

Injections

Interventional procedures including sympathetic nerve blocks, intrathecal glucocorticoid injections, and Botulinum toxin injections are alternative options for the

TABLE 20.1
A Summary of Pharmacologic Therapies for the Treatment of PHN.

Medication	Mechanism of Action	Initial and Titrating Dosage	Adverse Effects
ANTICONVULSANTS			
Gabapentin[4,8,19,26,73]	Inhibits voltage-gated calcium channels; prevents release of stimulatory neurotransmitters	100–300 mg at bedtime or in three divided doses; increase by 100–300 mg every 5 days to a total daily dose of 1800–3600 mg	Somnolence, dizziness, ataxia, peripheral edema, xerostomia, weight gain
Pregabalin[4,8,19,26,73]	Inhibits voltage-gated calcium channels; prevents release of stimulatory neurotransmitters	50 mg three times per day or 75 mg twice daily; increase to maximum total daily dose of 600 mg	Somnolence, dizziness, peripheral edema, xerostomia, weight gain
TRICYCLIC ANTIDEPRESSANTS			
Amitriptyline[4,8,19,69,73]	Inhibits reuptake of norepinephrine and serotonin	10–25 mg at bedtime; increase by 10–25 mg weekly to target dose of 75–150 mg per day	Sedation, xerostomia, constipation, urinary retention, cardiac toxicity
Nortriptyline[4,8,19,69,73]	Inhibits reuptake of norepinephrine and serotonin	10–25 mg at bedtime; increase by 10–25 mg weekly to target dose of 75–150 mg per day	Sedation, xerostomia, constipation, urinary retention, cardiac toxicity
OPIOIDS			
Morphine[4,8,19,73]	Mu opioid receptor agonist	15 mg every 6 h as needed; dose escalation per provider's discretion	Nausea/vomiting, constipation, dizziness, drowsiness, potential for dependence and abuse
Oxycodone[4,8,19,73]	Mu opioid receptor agonist	5 mg every 6 h as needed; dose escalation per provider's discretion	Nausea/vomiting, constipation, dizziness, drowsiness, potential for dependence and abuse
Tramadol[4,8,19,44,73]	Weak opioid agonist; serotonin and norepinephrine reuptake inhibitor	50 mg once or twice daily; dose escalation per provider's discretion	Nausea/vomiting, constipation, dizziness, drowsiness, increased risk of seizures
TOPICAL THERAPIES			
Capsaicin[4,8,17,19,26]	Vanilloid type I receptor agonist	0.075% cream (up to 3–4 applications per day); 8% patch (application time of 30–90 min)	Burning at the application site
Lidocaine[4,8,17,19,73]	Voltage-gated sodium channel blocker	5% patch; up to 3 patches per day for a maximum of 12 h	Local erythema, pruritus

treatment of PHN. The available evidence suggests that sympathetic nerve blocks are not beneficial for the pain of PHN.[3] Intrathecal glucocorticoid injections have demonstrated mixed results in the treatment of PHN. Although some clinical trials found improvement in pain, other studies identified no benefit.[3,50,51] Limited evidence suggests that subcutaneous injection with Botulinum toxin may be a promising treatment for PHN, however further studies are needed to evaluate its efficacy.[52,53]

Advanced Procedures

Advanced procedures utilized for the treatment of PHN include neuromodulatory approaches, intrathecal drug delivery, and low-level laser therapy. These treatments carry the risks of periprocedural complications and side effects.

Neuromodulation: Although there have been positive results with neuromodulatory strategies such as spinal cord stimulation (SCS), dorsal root ganglion (DRG) stimulation, and peripheral nerve stimulation, they are currently considered to be experimental treatments that have yet to be evaluated in controlled clinical trials.[54] Several small case series have demonstrated the efficacy of SCS in the short-term and long-term treatment of PHN in terms of reduction in both pain levels and requirement for opioid pain relievers.[54–56] SCS was most commonly performed at the thoracic levels, while a minority was performed at the cervical levels.[55] Reported complications include transient hypotension and urinary retention.[55] Unlike SCS, DRG stimulation directly targets the primary sensory neurons implicated in neuropathic pain conditions.[57] The evidence supporting the efficacy of DRG stimulation for patients with PHN has been limited to small studies and case reports that have demonstrated some positive results for pain, by often targeting the DRG above and below the affected dermatomal level.[58–60] Subcutaneous peripheral nerve stimulation for the relief of PHN involves the surgical implantation of a stimulating electrode in the trigeminal or thoracic region.[55,61] A few studies that have investigated peripheral nerve stimulation have demonstrated significant reductions in pain levels, again targeting affected trigeminal nerve or thoracic dermatome distribution.[54,55,61,62] No major complications have been reported with this technique.[55]

Intrathecal drug delivery: It can be used for intractable cases of PHN. Two FDA-approved medication options for intrathecal administration are morphine and ziconotide.[63] Intrathecal opioid therapy has been extensively studied and appears to be clinically effective in the management of chronic, severe noncancer pain.[63] However, there is currently insufficient evidence to support the use of intrathecal opioid therapy in PHN.[55,64] Additionally, patients have experienced opioid-related side effects and surgical complications from intrathecal opioid drug delivery.[64] Ziconotide is a novel, intrathecally administered N-type calcium channel blocker that has shown positive results in the treatment of chronic neuropathic pain.[65] As it does not interact with opioid receptors, ziconotide lacks opioid-induced systemic side effects.[65] No study has yet evaluated the efficacy of ziconotide intrathecal therapy explicitly in patients with PHN.

Low-level laser therapy (LLLT): LLLT, also known as photobiomodulation, may be considered as an alternative treatment option in the management of refractory PHN. LLLT involves the use of a laser that emits low-level red or near-infrared light and is thought to improve the function of injured nerves.[66] Limited research has shown that LLLT reduced pain levels in patients with PHN who had failed conventional treatments.[66,67]

Surgical Interventions

Invasive surgical procedures should be reserved for the most intractable cases of PHN. Surgical interventions have demonstrated limited benefit in the treatment of PHN and may impose significant complications. Dorsal root entry zone lesioning involves the selective destruction of neurons in the area where the dorsal root fibers enter the spinal cord, thus interrupting the sensory pathways. It appears to achieve initial pain reduction with subsequent pain relapse and has been associated with the development of motor deficits.[55,68] Other neurosurgical techniques such as electrical stimulation of the thalamus and anterolateral cordotomy may provide pain relief; however, these surgeries also carry substantial risks.[69] The surgical removal of painful skin in medically intractable PHN has been shown to be an ineffective treatment.[70]

Other

Nontraditional techniques for the treatment of PHN include acupuncture and psychological therapies. Although acupuncture is deemed to be safe, there is insufficient quality evidence to conclude whether it is effective in relieving pain for patients with PHN.[71] Mindfulness-based techniques have shown some success in alleviating pain intensity and psychological symptoms such as depression and anxiety in patients with PHN.[72]

REFERENCES

1. Campbell JN, Meyer RA. Mechanisms of neuropathic pain. *Neuron.* 2006;52(1):77–92.
2. Dworkin RH, et al. Pharmacologic management of neuropathic pain: evidence-based recommendations. *Pain.* 2007;132(3):237–251.
3. Dworkin RH, et al. Interventional management of neuropathic pain: NeuPSIG recommendations. *Pain.* 2013; 154(11):2249–2261.

4. Massengill JS, Kittredge JL. Practical considerations in the pharmacological treatment of postherpetic neuralgia for the primary care provider. *J Pain Res.* 2014;7:125–132.
5. Watson P. Postherpetic neuralgia. *Am Fam Physician.* 2011; 84(6):690–692.
6. Tontodonati M, et al. Post-herpetic neuralgia. *Int J Gen Med.* 2012;5:861–871.
7. Harpaz R, et al. Prevention of herpes zoster: recommendations of the Advisory Committee on Immunization Practices (ACIP). *MMWR Recomm Rep.* 2008;57(RR-5):1–30. quiz CE2-4.
8. Mallick-Searle T, Snodgrass B, Brant JM. Postherpetic neuralgia: epidemiology, pathophysiology, and pain management pharmacology. *J Multidiscip Healthc.* 2016;9: 447–454.
9. Yawn BP, et al. A population-based study of the incidence and complication rates of herpes zoster before zoster vaccine introduction. *Mayo Clin Proc.* 2007;82(11): 1341–1349.
10. Nagasako EM, et al. Rash severity in herpes zoster: correlates and relationship to postherpetic neuralgia. *J Am Acad Dermatol.* 2002;46(6):834–839.
11. Choo PW, et al. Risk factors for postherpetic neuralgia. *Arch Intern Med.* 1997;157(11):1217–1224.
12. Meier JL, Straus SE. Comparative biology of latent varicella-zoster virus and herpes simplex virus infections. *J Infect Dis.* 1992;166(Suppl 1):S13–S23.
13. Argoff CE, Katz N, Backonja M. Treatment of postherpetic neuralgia: a review of therapeutic options. *J Pain Symptom Manag.* 2004;28(4):396–411.
14. Gharibo C, Kim C. Neuropathic pain of postherpetic neuralgia. *Pain Med News.* 2011;9:84–92.
15. Wall PD. Neuropathic pain and injured nerve: central mechanisms. *Br Med Bull.* 1991;47(3):631–643.
16. Watson CP, et al. Post-herpetic neuralgia: 208 cases. *Pain.* 1988;35(3):289–297.
17. Argoff CE. Review of current guidelines on the care of postherpetic neuralgia. *Postgrad Med.* 2011;123(5):134–142.
18. Ragozzino MW, et al. Population-based study of herpes zoster and its sequelae. *Medicine.* 1982;61(5):310–316.
19. Johnson RW, Rice AS. Clinical practice. Postherpetic neuralgia. *N Engl J Med.* 2014;371(16):1526–1533.
20. Fields HL, Rowbotham M, Baron R. Postherpetic neuralgia: irritable nociceptors and deafferentation. *Neurobiol Dis.* 1998;5(4):209–227.
21. Bowsher D. Pathophysiology of postherpetic neuralgia: towards a rational treatment. *Neurology.* 1995;45(12 Suppl 8):S56–S57.
22. Nurmikko T, Bowsher D. Somatosensory findings in postherpetic neuralgia. *J Neurol Neurosurg Psychiatry.* 1990; 53(2):135–141.
23. Dworkin RH, Portenoy RK. Pain and its persistence in herpes zoster. *Pain.* 1996;67(2–3):241–251.
24. Drolet M, et al. The impact of herpes zoster and postherpetic neuralgia on health-related quality of life: a prospective study. *Can Med Assoc J.* 2010;182(16):1731–1736.
25. Coplan PM, et al. Development of a measure of the burden of pain due to herpes zoster and postherpetic neuralgia for prevention trials: adaptation of the brief pain inventory. *J Pain.* 2004;5(6):344–356.
26. Nalamachu S, Morley-Forster P. Diagnosing and managing postherpetic neuralgia. *Drugs Aging.* 2012;29(11):863–869.
27. Gilden D, et al. Neurological disease produced by varicella zoster virus reactivation without rash. *Curr Top Microbiol Immunol.* 2010;342:243–253.
28. Gilden DH, et al. Zoster sine herpete, a clinical variant. *Ann Neurol.* 1994;35(5):530–533.
29. Sampathkumar P, Drage LA, Martin DP. Herpes zoster (shingles) and postherpetic neuralgia. *Mayo Clin Proc.* 2009;84(3):274–280.
30. McElveen W.A. *Postherpetic Neuralgia Differential Diagnoses;* March 6, 2018 July 28, 2019. Available from: https:// emedicine.medscape.com/article/1143066-differential.
31. Haanpaa M, et al. NeuPSIG guidelines on neuropathic pain assessment. *Pain.* 2011;152(1):14–27.
32. Baron R, et al. A cross-sectional cohort survey in 2100 patients with painful diabetic neuropathy and postherpetic neuralgia: differences in demographic data and sensory symptoms. *Pain.* 2009;146(1–2):34–40.
33. Philip A, Thakur R. Post herpetic neuralgia. *J Palliat Med.* 2011;14(6):765–773.
34. Alper BS, Lewis PR. Treatment of postherpetic neuralgia: a systematic review of the literature. *J Fam Pract.* 2002;51(2): 121–128.
35. Wiffen PJ, et al. Gabapentin for chronic neuropathic pain in adults. *Cochrane Database Syst Rev.* 2017;6:CD007938.
36. Cappuzzo KA. Treatment of postherpetic neuralgia: focus on pregabalin. *Clin Interv Aging.* 2009;4:17–23.
37. Derry S, et al. Pregabalin for neuropathic pain in adults. *Cochrane Database Syst Rev.* 2019;1:CD007076.
38. Tzellos TG, et al. Gabapentin and pregabalin in the treatment of fibromyalgia: a systematic review and a meta-analysis. *J Clin Pharm Therapeut.* 2010;35(6):639–656.
39. Max MB, et al. Amitriptyline, but not lorazepam, relieves postherpetic neuralgia. *Neurology.* 1988;38(9): 1427–1432.
40. Wolff RF, et al. 5% lidocaine-medicated plaster vs other relevant interventions and placebo for post-herpetic neuralgia (PHN): a systematic review. *Acta Neurol Scand.* 2011;123(5):295–309.
41. Derry S, et al. Topical lidocaine for neuropathic pain in adults. *Cochrane Database Syst Rev.* 2014;(7):CD010958.
42. Watson CP, Evans RJ, Watt VR. Post-herpetic neuralgia and topical capsaicin. *Pain.* 1988;33(3):333–340.
43. Derry S, et al. Topical capsaicin (high concentration) for chronic neuropathic pain in adults. *Cochrane Database Syst Rev.* 2013;(2):CD007393.
44. Finnerup NB, et al. Pharmacotherapy for neuropathic pain in adults: a systematic review and meta-analysis. *Lancet Neurol.* 2015;14(2):162–173.
45. Raja SN, et al. Opioids versus antidepressants in postherpetic neuralgia: a randomized, placebo-controlled trial. *Neurology.* 2002;59(7):1015–1021.
46. Kandil E, Melikman E, Adinoff B. Lidocaine infusion: a promising therapeutic approach for chronic pain. *J Anesth Clin Res.* 2017;8(1).

47. Hempenstall K, et al. Analgesic therapy in postherpetic neuralgia: a quantitative systematic review. *PLoS Med.* 2005;2(7):e164.
48. Maher DP, Chen L, Mao J. Intravenous ketamine infusions for neuropathic pain management: a promising therapy in need of optimization. *Anesth Analg.* 2017;124(2):661−674.
49. Eide PK, et al. Relief of post-herpetic neuralgia with the N-methyl-D-aspartic acid receptor antagonist ketamine: a double-blind, cross-over comparison with morphine and placebo. *Pain.* 1994;58(3):347−354.
50. Kotani N, et al. Intrathecal methylprednisolone for intractable postherpetic neuralgia. *N Engl J Med.* 2000;343(21):1514−1519.
51. Rijsdijk M, et al. No beneficial effect of intrathecal methylprednisolone acetate in postherpetic neuralgia patients. *Eur J Pain.* 2013;17(5):714−723.
52. Ding XD, et al. Botulinum as a toxin for treating postherpetic neuralgia. *Iran J Public Health.* 2017;46(5):608−611.
53. Xiao L, et al. Subcutaneous injection of botulinum toxin a is beneficial in postherpetic neuralgia. *Pain Med.* 2010;11(12):1827−1833.
54. Kurklinsky S, et al. Neuromodulation in postherpetic neuralgia: case reports and review of the literature. *Pain Med.* 2018;19(6):1237−1244.
55. Texakalidis P, Tora MS, Boulis NM. Neurosurgeons' armamentarium for the management of refractory postherpetic neuralgia: a systematic literature review. *Stereotact Funct Neurosurg.* 2019;97(1):55−65.
56. Harke H, et al. Spinal cord stimulation in postherpetic neuralgia and in acute herpes zoster pain. *Anesth Analg.* 2002;94(3):694−700. table of contents.
57. Deer TR, et al. A prospective study of dorsal root ganglion stimulation for the relief of chronic pain. *Neuromodulation.* 2013;16(1):67−71. discussion 71-2.
58. Piedade GS, et al. *Cervical and High-Thoracic Dorsal Root Ganglion Stimulation in Chronic Neuropathic Pain. Neuromodulation.* 2019.
59. Lynch PJ, et al. Case report: successful epiradicular peripheral nerve stimulation of the C2 dorsal root ganglion for postherpetic neuralgia. *Neuromodulation.* 2011;14(1):58−61. discussion 61.
60. Kim ED, Lee YI, Park HJ. Comparison of efficacy of continuous epidural block and pulsed radiofrequency to the dorsal root ganglion for management of pain persisting beyond the acute phase of herpes zoster. *PLoS One.* 2017;12(8):e0183559.
61. Johnson MD, Burchiel KJ. Peripheral stimulation for treatment of trigeminal postherpetic neuralgia and trigeminal posttraumatic neuropathic pain: a pilot study. *Neurosurgery.* 2004;55(1):135−141. discussion 141-2.
62. Zibly Z, et al. Peripheral field stimulation for thoracic post herpetic neuropathic pain. *Clin Neurol Neurosurg.* 2014;127:101−105.
63. Sukul VV. Intrathecal pain therapy for the management of chronic noncancer pain. *Neurosurg Clin N Am.* 2019;30(2):195−201.
64. Zacest A, Anderson VC, Burchiel KJ. The glass half empty or half full-how effective are long-term intrathecal opioids in post-herpetic neuralgia? A case series and review of the literature. *Neuromodulation.* 2009;12(3):219−223.
65. Brookes ME, Eldabe S, Batterham A. Ziconotide monotherapy: a systematic review of randomised controlled trials. *Curr Neuropharmacol.* 2017;15(2):217−231.
66. Knapp DJ. Postherpetic neuralgia: case study of class 4 laser therapy intervention. *Clin J Pain.* 2013;29(10):e6−9.
67. Moore K,C, Hira N, Kramer PS, Jayakumar CS, Ohshiro T. Double blind crossover trial of low level laser therapy. *Prac Pain Manag.* 1988:1−7.
68. Awad AJ, et al. Experience with 25 years of dorsal root entry zone lesioning at a single institution. *Surg Neurol Int.* 2013;4:64.
69. Kost RG, Straus SE. Postherpetic neuralgia–pathogenesis, treatment, and prevention. *N Engl J Med.* 1996;335(1):32−42.
70. Petersen KL, Rowbotham MC. Relief of post-herpetic neuralgia by surgical removal of painful skin: 5 years later. *Pain.* 2007;131(1−2):214−218.
71. Wang Y, et al. Acupuncture for postherpetic neuralgia: systematic review and meta-analysis. *Medicine.* 2018;97(34):e11986.
72. Zhu X, et al. Effects of mindfulness-based stress reduction on depression, anxiety, and pain in patients with postherpetic neuralgia. *J Nerv Ment Dis.* 2019;207(6):482−486.
73. Dworkin RH, et al. Recommendations for the pharmacological management of neuropathic pain: an overview and literature update. *Mayo Clin Proc.* 2010;85(3 Suppl):S3−S14.

CHAPTER 21

Atypical Chest Wall Pain

HEENA S. AHMED, MD • KRISHNA B. SHAH, MD • DANIEL J. PAK, MD

INTRODUCTION

The initial evaluation for chest pain must rule out potentially life-threatening cardiac and pulmonary causes. However, the majority of chest pain cases are actually noncardiac in origin and typically involve the chest wall.[1,2]

A retrospective study of over 1300 emergency department visits for noncardiac chest pain found that 45% of the cases were musculoskeletal in origin.[3] Another prospective trial of 130 consecutive emergency department admissions found 30% had chest wall tenderness.[4] Chest wall pain is even more common in the outpatient setting, with up to 47% of cases categorized as noncardiac in nature.[5-7] In addition, 45% of patients who proceeded with a negative coronary angiography were found to have chest wall pain present.[8]

Chest wall pain is defined as pain along the xiphoid, costosternal junction, or sternum.[4] Chest wall pain may be an isolated musculoskeletal pain syndrome or can present as a result of rheumatic and nonrheumatic systemic causes, which makes early recognition essential for providing appropriate management.[4,9-12] The majority of chest wall pain syndromes are self-limiting in nature and amenable to conservative management.

ETIOLOGY AND PATHOGENESIS

The causes and pathophysiology of chest wall pain are poorly understood. It is commonly believed that chest wall pain is largely due to inflammation of the costal cartilages and sternal articulations, with costosternal and lower rib syndromes being the most common causes.[13] For patients with radicular symptoms along with a dermatomal distribution, it may be secondary to thoracic disc herniation or osteophyte compression, both of which can cause nerve root impingement or irritation, although these are relatively rare occurrences in the thoracic spine.[14,15]

Persistent chest wall pain is also seen following surgical procedures. The incidence of postmastectomy pain syndrome (PMPS) is 20%−72% following breast cancer-related procedures and is due to direct nerve injury during surgery or nerve entrapment from postoperative scar formation.[16,17] The anterior and lateral cutaneous branches of the intercostal nerves originating from the T3−6 nerve roots innervate the skin overlying the breast.[6] Moreover, the most commonly injured nerve during axillary dissection is the intercostobrachial nerve, which is the lateral branch of the second intercostal nerve that innervates the upper lateral breast quadrant.

Similarly, postthoracotomy pain syndrome (PTPS) occurs in approximately 30%−50% of patients who undergo thoracotomy procedures and presents as persistent pain along the thoracotomy scar.[18] PTPS is thought to be a result of injury to the intercostal nerves during surgical incision, rib retraction, and insertion of the surgical trocars.

Clinical Features

There are a variety of chest wall pain syndromes that present similarly with a few distinguishing characteristics (Table 21.1).

- *Costochondritis:*
  - Costochondritis is one of the most common causes of chest wall pain, with 30% of chest pain complaints in the emergency department being attributed to this diagnosis.[4] Patients complain of pain that worsens with upper body movement and deep breathing. Most commonly with an unknown cause, pain is typically diffuse and reproducible with palpation of the costosternal joints of the chest. The upper costochondral or costosternal junctions are most frequently involved.[13,14,16]
- *Lower Rib Pain Syndrome*
  - This condition occurs when the inferior ribs are displaced due to hypermobility of the false rib costal cartilages and is also known as "rib-tip" syndrome, "slipping rib," or "clicking rib" syndrome. Pain is localized to the lower chest or upper abdomen along the costal margin. Pain is

TABLE 21.1
Chest Wall Pain Syndromes.

Syndrome	Location of Pain
Costochondritis	Upper costochondral or costosternal junctions[4]
Lower rib pain syndrome	Lower chest or upper abdomen along the costal margin[18]
Sternalis syndrome	Directly over the sternum with pain radiating bilaterally[19]
Tietze's syndrome	Along the costosternal, costochondral, or sternoclavicular joints[20]
Xiphoidalgia	Localized tenderness over the xiphoid[21]
Posterior chest wall pain	Dermatomal distribution radiating from the thoracic spine[22]
Postmastectomy pain syndrome (PMPS)	May involve the surgical site, chest wall, axilla, or ipsilateral arm with neuropathic pain symptoms such as numbness, tingling, burning, allodynia, hyperalgesia[23]
Postthoracotomy pain syndrome (PTPS)	Pain along previous thoracotomy incision with associated neuropathic pain symptoms[23]

often reproducible on palpation. It may occur at any age, though it is more commonly seen in younger female athletes.[18]

- *Sternalis Syndrome*
  - Patients present with tenderness directly over the sternum with pain radiating bilaterally. This syndrome does not typically present with a diffuse distribution of pain and is thought to be due to myofascial pain.[19]
- *Tietze's Syndrome*
  - Patients present with pain along the costosternal, costochondral, or sternoclavicular joints that worsens with upper body movements. There is often nonsuppurative, localized swelling or edema present and most commonly occurs near the second and third ribs. Swelling or edema is a distinguishing feature of Tietze Syndrome and is

found to be self-limiting and benign.[20] This is often due to infectious, neoplastic, or rheumatologic processes.

- *Xiphoidalgia*
  - Often times a result of chest wall trauma, this rare condition presents with localized tenderness over the xiphoid. Typically, symptoms will present after a large meal, with chest movement, or lifting heavy objects.[21]
- *Posterior Chest Wall Pain*
  - Posterior chest pain typically arises from structures in the thoracic spine, including the intervertebral discs, facet joints, and costovertebral joints. Although pain is often localized either unilaterally or bilaterally to the posterior chest, patients may present with pain that radiates in a band-like, dermatomal distribution to the anterior chest with associated numbness and tingling.[22]
- *Postmastectomy Pain Syndrome*
  - Patients present with burning, electric shock-like, and stabbing pains with associated neuropathic symptoms (numbness, paresthesia) at the surgical site, chest wall, axilla, or ipsilateral arm.[23] Also a misnomer, symptoms often occur after breast cancer-related surgeries but can also be seen following radiation therapy or chemotherapy without signs of infection or recurrent disease.[17,24]
- *Post-Thoracotomy Pain Syndrome*
  - Much like PMPS, patients present with intense sharp pains with associated neuropathic symptoms along a previous thoracotomy incision.
- *Other rheumatologic causes*
  - Rheumatic and psoriatic arthritis as well as fibromyalgia are possible etiologies that should be considered, though isolated chest pain is rarely the presenting symptom.

DIAGNOSIS

It is important to note that cardiopulmonary (i.e., acute coronary syndrome, pulmonary embolism, pneumonia) and musculoskeletal chest pain syndromes can present similarly, so if patients complain of associated shortness of breath, nausea, dizziness, exertional chest pain, or sweating, then life-threatening etiologies need to be ruled out before diagnosing a chest wall pain syndrome.

Most chest wall pain syndromes are clinical diagnoses, and there are no gold standards for confirmatory diagnostic testing. As previously mentioned, reproducible pain on palpation and the location of pain provides important diagnostic information; distinguishing clinical features are described earlier. Chest or thoracic spine X-ray may be considered to rule out rib or spine fractures, respectively. Diagnosis of posterior chest pain is often supplemented with thoracic MRI to confirm the presence of intervertebral disc herniation, facet hypertrophy, or osteophytes that may potentially be a source of thoracic nerve root impingement.[25] PMPS and PTPS are also diagnosed clinically, with imaging studies generally considered unnecessary unless to rule out potential recurrent disease.[17,24]

PHYSICAL EXAM FINDINGS

As previously mentioned, chest wall pain syndromes are diagnosed after taking a comprehensive history and physical exam. Light and deep palpation along the sternum, xiphoid, costochondral/costosternal junctions, thoracic/lumbar spine, and paraspinal muscles may reproduce pain, and location/laterality of the symptoms should be noted.[13] Swelling or edema along the different joint lines may be present, which is a distinguishing feature for Tiezte's syndrome and also many rheumatologic disorders.[20] Furthermore, atypical features, such as weight loss and pain in the middle of the night, may indicate neoplastic or infectious sources. In addition to pain following surgery, patients with PMPS or PTPS may present with associated sensory changes in the distribution of the pain, including hyperesthesia, allodynia, burning, numbness, tingling.

TREATMENT
Conservative Therapy

As most chest wall pain syndromes are self-limiting in nature, reassurance and education of the syndrome should be provided to all patients. Activity restriction with temporary avoidance of aggravating activities should be encouraged, and the application of heat pads or cold compresses to pain sites has been shown to be helpful for many musculoskeletal pain disorders.[19,26] Physical therapy should focus on thoracic wall extensions, pectoralis stretches, scapular squeeze exercises, and chest wall stretches among other exercises.[17,18]

Pharmacologic

For all chest wall pain syndromes, the drug of choice is nonsteroidal antiinflammatory medications. Meloxicam, celebrex, and naproxen have been commonly used. These medications are not recommended for patients with acute or chronic kidney disease and a history of gastrointestinal ulcers or bleeds.[6,26] Paracetamol and topical agents, such as lidocaine, are also utilized when appropriate.

Posterior chest wall pain syndrome, PMPS, and PTPS can also be treated with neuropathic agents, including gabapentinoids (gabapentin, pregabalin), tricyclic antidepressants (amitriptyline, nortriptyline), and serotonin-norepinephrine reuptake inhibitors (duloxetine). Gabapentin is often considered first-line therapy given its relatively benign side-effect profile and can be initiated at 300 mg TID and titrated to patient response. Pregabalin is typically initiated at 50 mg BID and titrated to patient response.[26−28] Common side effects of neuropathic medications include altered mental status, weight gain, and sedation.[27,28]

Interventional Procedures
Subcutaneous local infiltration

For patients with pain refractory to the above conservative measures and costochondral pain limited to one or two joints, infiltration with local anesthetic and corticosteroid may be performed.[29,30] Ultrasound may be utilized for needle visualization to decrease the risk of lung puncture.

Interlaminar epidural steroid injection

For patients with posterior chest wall pain syndrome where nerve root impingement is suspected, an interlaminar epidural steroid injection can be performed under fluoroscopic guidance at the level of impingement.[31,32] Typically, 80 mg of particulate steroids, such as methylprednisolone or triamcinolone, with either normal saline or low concentration local anesthetic is administered.

Intercostal nerve block

Intercostal nerves innervate the skin and subcutaneous tissue of the lateral trunk and upper abdomen. For lower rib syndrome or PTPS where intercostal neuralgia is suspected, these nerves can be anesthetized by injection of local anesthetic and corticosteroid at the inferior border of the rib, typically at the midposterior axillary line.[33] Ultrasound or fluoroscopic guidance is recommended to avoid complications of vascular and lung injury. The level at which the block is performed depends on the location of the pain. If the pain occurs following breast surgery, the second to sixth intercostal spaces would be most effective. Reduction in pain occurs quickly and can last up to a few months. Patients may require repeat injections if the pain returns.[33−35]

Neuromodulation

Spinal cord stimulation can be used for refractory cases of PMPS and PTPS. Patients undergo a spinal cord stimulation trial with two leads with one lead at the midline and the other more laterally placed toward the ipsilateral side of the pain.[36] The leads are typically placed in the thoracic region between T1 and T4 vertebral bodies.[36] Either paresthesia, high-frequency, or burst stimulation should be utilized during the trial period to determine an optimal program for pain relief. Patients may undergo permanent implants after a successful trial with a greater than 50% reduction in pain.

REFERENCES

1. Chambers J, Bass C, Mayou R. Non-cardiac chest pain: assessment and management. *Heart Br Card Soc.* 1999; 82(6):656–657. https://doi.org/10.1136/hrt.82.6.656.
2. How J, Volz G, Doe S, Heycock C, Hamilton J, Kelly C. The causes of musculoskeletal chest pain in patients admitted to hospital with suspected myocardial infarction. *Eur J Intern Med.* 2005;16(6):432–436. https://doi.org/10.1016/j.ejim.2005.07.002.
3. Wertli MM, Dangma TD, Müller SE, et al. Non-cardiac chest pain patients in the emergency department: do physicians have a plan how to diagnose and treat them? A retrospective study. *PLoS One.* 2019;14(2):e0211615. https://doi.org/10.1371/journal.pone.0211615.
4. Disla E, Rhim HR, Reddy A, Karten I, Taranta A. Costochondritis. A prospective analysis in an emergency department setting. *Arch Intern Med.* 1994;154(21):2466–2469. https://doi.org/10.1001/archinte.154.21.2466.
5. Verdon F, Herzig L, Burnand B, et al. Chest pain in daily practice: occurrence, causes and management. *Swiss Med Wkly.* 2008;138(23–24):340–347.
6. Bosner S, Becker A, Hani MA, et al. Chest wall syndrome in primary care patients with chest pain: presentation, associated features and diagnosis. *Fam Pract.* 2010;27(4): 363–369. https://doi.org/10.1093/fampra/cmq024.
7. Hoorweg BB, Willemsen RT, Cleef LE, et al. Frequency of chest pain in primary care, diagnostic tests performed and final diagnoses. *Heart Br Card Soc.* 2017;103(21): 1727–1732. https://doi.org/10.1136/heartjnl-2016-310905.
8. Brunse MH, Stochkendahl MJ, Vach W, et al. Examination of musculoskeletal chest pain – an inter-observer reliability study. *Man Ther.* 2010;15(2):167–172. https://doi.org/10.1016/j.math.2009.10.003.
9. Almansa C, Wang B, Achem SR. Noncardiac chest pain and fibromyalgia. *Med Clin N Am.* 2010;94(2):275–289. https://doi.org/10.1016/j.mcna.2010.01.002.
10. Rodríguez-Henríquez P, Solano C, Peña A, et al. Sternoclavicular joint involvement in rheumatoid arthritis: clinical and ultrasound findings of a neglected joint. *Arthritis Care Res.* 2013;65(7):1177–1182. https://doi.org/10.1002/acr.21958.
11. Jurik AG. Seronegative anterior chest wall syndromes. A study of the findings and course at radiography. *Acta Radiol Suppl.* 1992;381:1–42.
12. Fortier M, Mayo JR, Swensen SJ, Munk PL, Vellet DA, Müller NL. MR imaging of chest wall lesions. *Radiographics.* 1994;14(3):597–606. https://doi.org/10.1148/radiographics.14.3.8066274.
13. Schumann JA, Parente JJ. *Costochondritis.* StatPearls Publishing; 2020. http://www.ncbi.nlm.nih.gov/books/NBK532931/. Accessed June 5, 2020.
14. Gregory PL, Biswas AC, Batt ME. Musculoskeletal problems of the chest wall in athletes. *Sports Med.* 2002; 32(4):235–250. https://doi.org/10.2165/00007256-200232040-00003.
15. Fam AG, Smythe HA. Musculoskeletal chest wall pain. *Can Med Assoc J.* 1985;133(5):379–389.
16. Wolf E. Costosternal syndrome: its frequency and importance in differential diagnosis of coronary heart disease. *Arch Intern Med.* 1976;136(2):189–191. https://doi.org/10.1001/archinte.136.2.189.
17. Caffo O, Amichetti M, Ferro A, Lucenti A, Valduga F, Galligioni E. Pain and quality of life after surgery for breast cancer. *Breast Cancer Res Treat.* 2003;80(1):39–48. https://doi.org/10.1023/A:1024435101619.
18. Foley CM, Sugimoto D, Mooney DP, Meehan WP, Stracciolini A. Diagnosis and treatment of slipping rib syndrome. *Clin J Sport Med.* 2019;29(1):18–23. https://doi.org/10.1097/JSM.0000000000000506.
19. Ayloo A, Cvengros T, Marella S. Evaluation and treatment of musculoskeletal chest pain. *Prim Care Clin Off Pract.* 2013; 40(4):863–887. https://doi.org/10.1016/j.pop.2013.08.007.
20. Aeschlimann A, Kahn MF. Tietze's syndrome: a critical review. *Clin Exp Rheumatol.* 1990;8(4):407–412.
21. Lipkin M, Fulton LA, Wolfson EA. The syndrome of the hypersensitive xiphoid. *N Engl J Med.* 1955;253(14):591–597. https://doi.org/10.1056/NEJM195510062531403.
22. Van Holsbeeck M, Van Melkebeke J, Dequeker J, Pennes DR. Radiographic findings of spontaneous subluxation of the sternoclavicular joint. *Clin Rheumatol.* 1992; 11(3):376–381. https://doi.org/10.1007/BF02207196.
23. Rietman JS, Dijkstra PU, Debreczeni R, Geertzen JH, Robinson DP, de Vries J. Impairments, disabilities and health related quality of life after treatment for breast cancer: a follow-up study 2.7 years after surgery. *Disabil Rehabil.* 2004;26(2): 78–84. https://doi.org/10.1080/09638280310001629642.
24. Miguel R, Kuhn AM, Shons AR, et al. The effect of sentinel node selective axillary lymphadenectomy on the incidence of postmastectomy pain syndrome. *Cancer Control.* 2001;8(5): 427–430. https://doi.org/10.1177/107327480100800506.
25. Kuhne M, Boniquit N, Ghodadra N, Romeo AA, Provencher MT. The snapping scapula: diagnosis and treatment. *Arthrosc J Arthrosc Relat Surg.* 2009;25(11): 1298–1311. https://doi.org/10.1016/j.arthro.2008.12.022.
26. Epstein SE. Chest wall syndrome. A common cause of unexplained cardiac pain. *J Am Med Assoc.* 1979;241(26): 2793–2797. https://doi.org/10.1001/jama.241.26.2793.

27. Wang W, Sun Y-H, Wang Y-Y, et al. Treatment of functional chest pain with antidepressants: a meta-analysis. *Pain Physician*. 2012;15(2):E131–E142.

28. Cannon RO, Quyyumi AA, Mincemoyer R, et al. Imipramine in patients with chest pain despite normal coronary angiograms. *N Engl J Med*. 1994;330(20):1411–1417. https://doi.org/10.1056/NEJM199405193302003.

29. Kamel M, Kotob H. Ultrasonographic assessment of local steroid injection in Tietze's syndrome. *Rheumatology*. 1997;36(5):547–550. https://doi.org/10.1093/rheumatology/36.5.547.

30. Howell JM. Xiphodynia: a report of three cases. *J Emerg Med*. 1992;10(4):435–438. https://doi.org/10.1016/0736-4679(92)90272-U.

31. Brown CW, Deffer PA, Akmakjian J, Donaldson DH, Brugman JL. The natural history of thoracic disc herniation. *Spine*. 1992;17(Supplement):S97–S102. https://doi.org/10.1097/00007632-199206001-00006.

32. Goodman BS, Posecion LWF, Mallempati S, Bayazitoglu M. Complications and pitfalls of lumbar interlaminar and transforaminal epidural injections. *Curr Rev Musculoskelet Med*. 2008;1(3–4):212–222. https://doi.org/10.1007/s12178-008-9035-2.

33. Baxter CS, Ajib FA, Fitzgerald BM. *Intercostal Nerve Block*. StatPearls Publishing; 2020. http://www.ncbi.nlm.nih.gov/books/NBK482273/. Accessed June 5, 2020.

34. Kang CM, Kim WJ, Yoon SH, Cho CB, Shim JS. Postoperative pain control by intercostal nerve block After augmentation mammoplasty. *Aesthetic Plast Surg*. 2017;41(5):1031–1036. https://doi.org/10.1007/s00266-017-0802-6.

35. Wurnig PN, Lackner H, Teiner C, et al. Is intercostal block for pain management in thoracic surgery more successful than epidural anaesthesia? *Eur J Cardio Thorac Surg*. 2002;21(6):1115–1119. https://doi.org/10.1016/s1010-7940(02)00117-3.

36. de Leon-Casasola OA. Spinal cord and peripheral nerve stimulation techniques for neuropathic pain. *J Pain Symptom Manag*. 2009;38(2):S28–S38. https://doi.org/10.1016/j.jpainsymman.2009.05.005.

CHAPTER 22

Esophagitis

JOEL EHRENFELD, MD • MATTHEW A. SPIEGEL, MD • NEEL D. MEHTA, MD

INTRODUCTION

Abdominal pain and chest pain represent the two most prevalent pain complaints to the US emergency departments each year at 8.6% and 5.2%, respectively.[1] Of those presenting with chest pain, the esophagus is a not uncommon etiology. Fruergaard et al., for example, demonstrated that 42% of patients admitted to a Coronary Care Unit were later found to have esophageal pain or discomfort, not acute coronary syndrome.[2] Accordingly, it is prudent for the modern pain clinician to be well versed in esophageal pain syndromes and their corresponding treatments. What follows is a generalized discussion of esophagitis, highlighting varied common pathophysiologies.

ETIOLOGIES AND PATHOGENESIS

Some of the more prevalent etiologies of esophagitis and esophageal injury include eosinophilia, infection, radiation, malignancy, motility disorders, alcohol, and traumatic/surgical. Gastroesophageal reflux disease (GERD) as a cause of esophagitis is a larger topic, and we will, therefore, do justice by discussing it elsewhere in this textbook.

Eosinophilic esophagitis (EoE) is an immune/antigen-mediated disorder characterized by esophageal dysfunction due to a pathologic eosinophilic infiltration.[3-5] Intramucosal eosinophils are hypothesized to be recruited via a chain reaction, which is initiated by antigenic proteins (most frequently food, less often inhaled particles) that trigger helper T-cells to release inflammatory cytokines (e.g., interleukin 5).[6,7]

Infectious esophagitis (IE) is more prevalent in immunocompromised hosts, for example, human immunodeficiency virus (HIV) and transplant patients (bone marrow > solid organ) but has also been described in patients on chronically inhaled fluticasone for COPD.[8-10] Although there are others, certainly the most frequented pathogens in IE are the herpes simplex virus (HSV), cytomegalovirus (CMV), and candida

species.[11] CMV specifically is most often seen in HIV patients with CD4 counts <50.[12]

Medication or "pill" induced esophagitis is thought to occur secondary to direct mucosal injury of the offending pill at a tight juncture within the esophagus. The most common site of esophageal anatomical narrowing is near the aortic arch. Frequent offenders include antibiotics, bisphosphonates, nonsteroidal antiinflammatory drugs (NSAIDS), aspirin, emepronium, alprenolol, pinaverium, potassium chloride, quinidine, and iron-containing compounds. The mechanism of injury is hypothesized to include caustic injury due to the acidity of the dissolving medications leading to hyperosmolar tissue destruction and vascular injury. Additionally, NSAIDs or aspirin may disturb the protective mucosal lining of the stomach and esophagus normally mediated by prostaglandins.[13] Risk factors for pill esophagitis include old age, large pill size, swallowing the pill with minimal or no fluid, patient positioning during pill swallowing, and abnormal esophageal anatomy.

Radiation therapy directed toward or near the esophagus may disrupt the normal process of cell turnover within the esophagus that can lead to mucosal thinning and denudation. Predictors of the likelihood that a patient might develop radiation esophagitis (RE) include the dose and technique used for radiation therapy, concurrent treatment with chemotherapy, and preexisting esophageal disease.[14]

Esophageal malignancy generally comes in the form of adenocarcinoma or squamous cell carcinoma (SCC). Obesity, GERD, smoking, and diets low in fruits and vegetables are all risk factors for esophageal adenocarcinoma. Barrett's esophagus, a form of metaplasia where chronic gastric acid exposure causes columnar to squamous metaplasia of the lower esophageal epithelium, is considered a complication of GERD. This metaplasia is then a risk factor for further damage, dysplasia, and thereby adenocarcinoma. Hereditary conditions such as Peutz–Jeghers syndrome along with others associated with mutations

Interventional Management of Chronic Visceral Pain Syndromes. https://doi.org/10.1016/B978-0-323-75775-1.00005-2

in the PTEN gene meanwhile pose an increased risk of esophageal SCC. Smoking and alcohol use, however, are the largest modifiable risk factors and account for nearly 90% of esophageal SCC in the United States.[15]

Esophageal motility disorders are classified by the Chicago classification based on relaxation at the esophago-gastric junction (EGJ) and pattern of peristalsis.[16] Dysfunction of peristalsis accompanied by impairment of relaxation at the EGJ is characteristic of achalasia. When relaxation at the EGJ is not impaired, diagnosis is based on the peristaltic pattern within the esophagus. The complete absence of peristalsis is usually a feature of scleroderma. Contrarily hyper-peristalsis suggests either a hypercontractile "jack-hammer" (formerly "nutcracker") esophagus (possibly due to a hyper-cholinergic state) or distal esophageal spasm.[17]

Alcohol consumption has been linked to GERD, although somewhat controversial. Conflicting data have been published over the years regarding the association between alcohol and reflux.[18-24] More recently, Pan et al. have published a meta-analysis demonstrating a clear link between the two; however, other large-scale studies have failed to demonstrate an association.[25-27] This has led some investigators to consider alcohol an intermittent trigger of reflux events in the short term, rather than a causative agent of longer-term persistent reflux or esophagitis.[28] Alcohol is hypothesized to cause reflux by decreasing lower esophageal sphincter (LES) tone or by reducing peristalsis within the lower esophagus.[29-33] Alternatively, animal studies have suggested that alcohol might have the ability to cause direct noxious injury to esophageal mucosa.[34]

Lastly, depending on size and location, penetrating esophageal injury has the potential to be catastrophic, and should be considered a surgical emergency until proven otherwise. Esophageal injury is most often (>50%) iatrogenic, being caused by proceduralists intervention. Most frequently this occurs during endoscopy, but can also be a complication of transesophageal echocardiogram or pneumatic dilation.[35-37] Other causes of esophageal perforation include (in decreasing frequency): Boerhaave's syndrome (full-thickness tear of the esophageal wall often caused by severe retching/emesis), foreign body ingestion, trauma (e.g., penetrating stab injuries), intraoperative injury, and malignancy.[35,38] This condition can have mortality rates upwards of 20%, largely in part due to the esophagus's real estate with adjacent proximity to other high acuity organs (trachea, heart, lungs).[38]

CLINICAL FEATURES

Clinical features of esophagitis generally present as some combination of heartburn, dysphagia, odynophagia, regurgitation, feelings of food impaction, and rarely hematemesis.[9,39-45] The pain is typically described as retrosternal, chest or upper abdominal, and may or may not radiate to the back.[9,39,45-48] Herpes labialis and oral vesicles are specifically more suspicious of HSV IE. In HSV, the vesicles eventually coalesce to form well-circumscribed ulcers but usually smaller than those identified in CMV.[9]

Harmful clinical features of radiation on esophageal tissue may be seen as early as 2–3 weeks from commencing therapy and as late as 3 months after completion of therapy. Early/acute effects will be similar to those seen in other causes of esophagitis while later effects of RE usually relate to strictures, motility alterations, perforation, and/or fistula. A small percentage of esophageal cancer is detected early via routine surveillance. For a majority of patients, however, oncologic symptoms prompt clinician visits and evaluation. As malignancy progresses, it may present with signs of esophageal lumen obstruction (dysphagia to solids) due to frank mass plus the red flag of unwarranted weight loss. Contrarily, insidious dysphagia of both solids and liquids is more suggestive of an esophageal motility disorder (e.g., achalasia). Sudden acute chest pain that radiates to the back or left shoulder is often the cardinal symptom of the dreaded esophageal rupture.[38] A triad of chest pain emesis and subcutaneous emphysema is known as Mackler's triad and should be very suspicious for an esophageal perforation.[38,49] Along the lines of emphysema, any penetrating esophageal injury may also demonstrate Hamman's sign on mediastinal auscultation that is a crunching sound felt to result from the heart beating against air-filled tissues.[50] Finally, other ominous indications of esophageal penetration may involve rapid development of a systemic inflammatory response (tachycardia, fever) or bacterial-related sepsis.[38]

DIAGNOSIS

Diagnostic evaluation of esophagitis begins with a thorough history and physical examination primarily of the oral/labial region. Further assessment may consist of lab work, endoscopy, biopsy, and occasionally barium esophagram or other imaging (CT, MRI).

Eosinophilic esophagitis is histologically defined by an eosinophilic predominance and is primarily a diagnosis of exclusion.[3,45,51,52] Characteristic EoE endoscopic findings include linear furrows (longitudinal creases), esophageal trachealization (mucosal stacked rings), changes to vascular patterns in the subepithelium, small caliber esophagus, white papules/exudates (eosinophil microabscesses), and strictures.[45,53,54] Barium studies for assessment of anatomical changes and esophageal dysfunction may be helpful as well.[55,56] In 2018, the international consensus for EoE diagnostic criteria was updated to include the following: symptoms of esophageal dysfunction, biopsy demonstrating ≥15 eosinophils per high power field (~60 eosinophils/mm^2), and rule out of alternative causes of esophageal eosinophilia.[45,57]

Biopsies in HSV IE should reveal multinucleated giant cells with ground glass nuclei and eosinophilic inclusions.[9] CMV lesions meanwhile appear as shallow lower esophageal erosions/ulcerations on endoscopic exam. Histological analysis of CMV uncovers cytomegalic cells and intracytoplasmic or intranuclear inclusions. White oral thrush is suspicious of candida esophagitis and similarly Candida appears as white plaques on endoscopy. Biopsies show yeasts with pseudohyphae while cultures should grow out the Candida species (usually albicans, but glabrata, krusei, and tropicalis are occasionally seen).

Regarding pill esophagitis, diagnosis is frequently made by history and clinical suspicion alone. Invasive diagnostic studies are rarely warranted except in patients with severe or rare findings (e.g., hematemesis). Upper endoscopy and biopsy may help rule out other causes. If esophageal compression is suspected based on exam, a barium esophagram may be clinically useful to further delineate patients' anatomy.

In radiation esophagitis, endoscopic exam may reveal ulcers, mucositis, and/or strictures while biopsy should show evidence of fibrotic tissue with chronic inflammation and epithelial thickening.

Early endoscopic findings of esophageal malignancies often appear as plaque or ulcers while later stages may show circumferential masses causing strictures and increased luminal obstruction. Diagnosis is typically confirmed via direct endoscopic biopsy or histological examination of metastases.

Diagnostic workup of suspected motility disorders begins with upper endoscopy that may demonstrate retained food products and increased resistance to passing the endoscope at the EGJ. Endoscopy is often followed by manometry which, in achalasia, may show absent peristalsis in the lower two-thirds of the esophagus and above average integrated relaxation pressure at the LES. Manometry in the jackhammer esophagus would show sequential abnormally elevated esophageal contraction pressure in the setting of normal LES relaxation. When the manometric findings are equivocal, barium swallow is suggested, which on patients with achalasia would demonstrate delayed emptying, aperistalsis, narrowing at the EGJ, and abnormal esophageal dilation.

Radiographic evidence is instrumental to the diagnosis of esophageal traumatic perforation.[38] Plain chest radiographs, for example, may demonstrate pneumomediastinum, subcutaneous emphysema, pneumothorax, lung collapse, and pleural effusion.[38] Meanwhile, a water-soluble contrast swallow study (plain films or computed tomography) should reveal obvious leak often in need of urgent or emergent repair.[38,58,59]

PHYSICAL EXAM

There are no pathognomonic findings for esophagitis and most patients will have unremarkable findings. As previously mentioned, the examination of the oral cavity may reveal thrush, suggesting the presence of candidiasis, which is commonly associated with esophageal candidiasis. The presence of oral herpetic lesions may also indicate herpetic esophagitis. Patients with EoE may present with signs of atopy, such as wheezing on lung auscultation and atopic dermatitis. Abdominal exam is typically benign without positive findings.

TREATMENT

Esophagitis treatment is often divided into curing the underlying etiology (e.g., antivirals in HSV) and treating the symptomatology (e.g., esophageal dilation, stents, Heller myotomy/fundoplication).[60,61] As the supportive options apply to most etiologies, what follows will touch on the more directed curative therapies.

The prevalence of food allergies is higher in patients diagnosed with eosinophilic esophagitis. Accordingly, prevention via avoiding the known triggering allergen is the first line, as it is effective and inexpensive.[45] Next line therapy, is generally suggested as an 8-week course with a proton pump inhibitor (PPI).[57] For EoE suffering patients still refractory, topical steroids are the therapy standard as they have been found to improve 95% of cases and systemic corticosteroids are reserved for the most extreme cases given their undesirable adverse effects.[45,62] Specifically, fluticasone and nebulized budesonide are the topical agents of choice, where patients are instructed to swallow as opposed to inhale the medication.[3,63,64] It is often suggested to continue corticosteroid therapy as maintenance in the hope of avoiding relapse. There are experimental agents being studied for the treatment of EoE, such as mono-clonal antibodies targeting various interleukins, prosta-glandin antagonists, and montelukast.[65–69]

Oral acyclovir (7–10 days) is the mainstay in HSV treatment with immunocompromised patients often-times necessitating longer treatments (14–21 days). Intravenous (IV) acyclovir is traditionally reserved for HSV in-patients with severe odynophagia. In patients with high clinical suspicion of CMV esophagitis, empiric treatment with ganciclovir > foscarnet should commence immediately, rather than wait for patho-logic confirmation. IV induction is often recommen-ded given patients' moderate-to-severe odynophagia but with symptomatic improvement may be transi-tioned to oral. The induction phase generally lasts 3–6 weeks. Furthermore, as perhaps alluded to, the pa-tient population that tends to develop CMV esophagi-tis is frequently not on or not compliant with HIV antiretroviral therapy (ART). Therefore, it is a first-rate recommendation to commence treatment (the exception being if there is concomitant CMV retinitis in which case ART risks immune reconstitution inflam-matory syndrome). Maintenance therapy with oral val-ganciclovir is typically reserved for patients with recurrences or those with concurrent CMV retinitis. Candida esophagitis is treated with typical antifungals such as fluconazole (alternatively voriconazole, posa-conazole, or itraconazole) for a 14–21-day course. Due to their increased cost and IV preparation, Echino-candins (capsofungin, micafungin, anidulafungin) are generally considered the second line. Amphotericin is a known toxic drug and such is reserved for drug-resistant cases and during pregnancy (azoles are known teratogens and echinocandins have not been studied in pregnancy).[70,71]

Prevention is the best treatment for "stuck pill" esophagitis. In patients with known difficulty swallow-ing, liquid formulations may be preferred to tablets or capsules. Patients should be guided to take their medication with at least 8oz of water and remain upright for at least 30 min after ingestion.

Although cessation of radiation is likely to improve symptoms in radiation caused esophagitis, this approach is likely to interfere with malignancy outcomes.

Surgical resection is the recommended treatment when patients present with early esophageal malig-nancy as it can be curative. However, once there exist metastases to other organs or lymph nodes, resection may be less advised. Radiation and chemotherapeutics may be used as neoadjuvants (to decrease tumor size preoperatively) or as adjuvant treatment in patients who are poorer surgical candidates.

In suspected achalasia, patients are often treated with 4 weeks of a PPI before any diagnostic workup. For confirmed achalasia, nitroglycerin or isosorbide dinitrate (not available in the US) may be prescribed before meals. Unfortunately, pharmacotherapy is often insufficient for achalasia but may be an attractive option for those that are not surgical candidates. Injected botulinum toxin and pneumatic dilation at the LES may be offered as interventional options in achalasia, where laparoscopic Heller myotomy with fundoplication offer the most invasive options. Recently, peroral endoscopic myotomy has been gain-ing popularity as an ostensibly less invasive option for patients with achalasia. During this endoscopic proced-ure, an incision is made through the mucosa of the esophagus and the endoscope is tunneled from the submucosa of the esophagus into the gastric cardia. Once there, the muscularis propria can be severed with endoscopic tools and decreased LES pressures achieved. As this endoscopic myotomy is not accompa-nied by antireflux measures such as fundoplication, there is potential for resultant GERD postoperatively. In jackhammer esophagus, it is recommended to first control heartburn symptoms with 3 months of PPI ± H2-antagonists. Peppermint oil serves to relax the esophageal smooth muscle that may provide symptom-atic relief. The second line for esophageal smooth mus-cle relaxation is calcium channel blockers such as diltiazem. For scleroderma related disease, a promotil-ity agent (e.g., metoclopramide) may be of more utility. Patients with scleroderma who exhibit esophageal stric-tures or webs are offered pneumatic dilation treatment. In scleroderma patients exhibiting bad reflux, surgical correction via Nissen fundoplication is the procedure of choice after more conservative options like PPIs, promotility agents, and dilations have been exhausted.

Akin to pill esophagitis, as mentioned earlier for pill esophagitis, alcohol-related reflux is best treated with prevention through abstinence. Alcohol is considered a trigger of symptoms in these cases, and patients are counseled to avoid it.[28]

Esophageal perforation should be regarded with some trepidation as patients may be critically ill.[38,72] First recommendation is that all patients be immediately nil per os and transferred to a higher acuity setting with near continuous oxygen monitoring.[73] In instances of contained perforation or limited injury, conservative nonoperative treatment modalities may suffice with broad-spectrum antibiotics, IV hydration, PPIs, and possibly nutritional support.[44] Conversely, in patients that are critically ill or with larger/mal-positioned esophageal perforations, immediate surgical

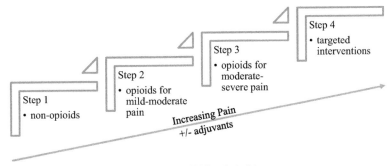

FIG. 22.1 WHO pain ladder.

repair may be warranted. When the perforation is due to a more distal stricture, a myotomy ± fundoplication might be indicated. T-tubes (shaped like the letter "T") is a surgical option that creates an esophagocutaneous fistula that permits drainage, allowing time for the local tissue to heal and is typically removed after 4—6 weeks.[38,74] Occasionally, prompt partial or complete esophageal resection may be obligatory, but in this urgent/emergent setting, mortality remains high (15%—40%).[38,75]

PAIN TREATMENT

Esophageal nociception is carried by two varieties of pain fibers. The general somatic afferent myelinated small diameter A∂ fibers transmit fast somatosensory sharp and abrupt pain.[76—78] The general visceral afferent unmyelinated smaller diameter C-fibers transmit slow visceral dull or burning discomfort that is less well localized and often attributed to heat (gastric acidity) or chemicals.[77—79] These afferent neurons are carried with the vagal and spinal (C1—L2) nerves.[77,80,81]

Coffee, caffeine, alcohol, spicy foods, and foods at extremes of temperature may all exacerbate esophageal pain and should be avoided. Bland pureed soft foods are the ideal. Proton-pump inhibitors and competitive H2 receptor antagonists may be of benefit in decreasing heartburn-type discomfort.

Further pain therapeutics are advised for in-line with the World Health Organization' (WHO) pain relief ladder, which was originally designed for cancer-related pain, but now is widely applied to all types of pain.[82] In the ladder model, nonopioids are described as first line (e.g., NSAIDs, acetaminophen), mild opioids (e.g., codeine, tramadol) are second line, and stronger opioids (e.g., morphine, hydromorphone) are reserved for severe refractory pain.[83] Along any step of the ladder, adjuvants may be added as appropriate (e.g., gabapentinoids, steroids, antidepressants). This three-step approach has been described as effective in 80% —90% of patients.[83] In patients where this pain ladder proves insufficient, a fourth step (Fig. 22.1) has been proposed that concerns itself with interventional pain approaches, which in our esophageal-related pain discussion may include high thoracic epidurals and intrathecal drug-delivery systems.[82]

REFERENCES

1. Rui P, Kang K, Ashmann J. *National Hospital Ambulatory Medical Care Survey: 2016 Emergency Department Summary Tables*; 2016. Available from: https://www.cdc.gov/nchs/data/nhamcs/web_tables/2016_ed_web_tables.pdf.
2. Fruergaard P, Launbjerg J, Hesse B, et al. The diagnoses of patients admitted with acute chest pain but without myocardial infarction. *Eur Heart J*. 1996;17:1028—1034.
3. Liacouras CA, Furuta GT, Hirano I, et al. Eosinophilic esophagitis: updated consensus recommendations for children and adults. *J Allergy Clin Immunol*. 2011;128: 3—20.e6.   https://doi.org/10.1016/j.jaci.2011.02.040. Available from:.
4. Furuta GT. Eosinophils in the esophagus: acid is not the only cause. *J Pediatr Gastroenterol Nutr*. 1998;26: 468—471. Available from: http://www.ncbi.nlm.nih.gov/pubmed/9552148.
5. Ahmad M, Soetikno RM, Ahmed A. The differential diagnosis of eosinophilic esophagitis. *J Clin Gastroenterol*. 2000;30:242—244. Available from: http://www.ncbi.nlm.nih.gov/pubmed/10777180.
6. Hogan SP, Mishra A, Brandt EB, Foster PS, Rothenberg ME. A critical role for eotaxin in experimental oral antigen-induced eosinophilic gastrointestinal allergy. *Proc Natl Acad Sci USA*. 2000;97:6681—6686.
7. Watts MM, Saltoun C, Greenberger PA. Eosinophilic esophagitis. *Allergy asthma Proc*. 2019;40:462—464. Available from: http://www.ncbi.nlm.nih.gov/pubmed/31690395.
8. Kanda N, Yasuba H, Takahashi T, et al. Prevalence of esophageal candidiasis among patients treated with inhaled fluticasone propionate. *Am J Gastroenterol*. 2003; 98:2146—2148. Available from: http://www.ncbi.nlm.nih.gov/pubmed/14572559.

9. Canalejo E, García Durán F, Cabello N, García Martínez J. Herpes esophagitis in healthy adults and adolescents: report of 3 cases and review of the literature. *Medicine).* 2010;89:204−210.

10. Généreau T, Rozenberg F, Bouchaud O, Marche C, Lortholary O. Herpes esophagitis: a comprehensive review. *Clin Microbiol Infect.* 1997;3:397−407.

11. Sutton FM, Graham DY, Goodgame RW. Infectious esophagitis. *Gastrointest Endosc Clin N Am.* 1994;4: 713−729. Available from: http://www.ncbi.nlm.nih.gov/pubmed/7812643.

12. Raffi F. Cytomegalovirus infections in AIDS. *Rev Prat.* 1995;45:733−738. Available from: http://www.ncbi.nlm.nih.gov/pubmed/7754312.

13. Wallace JL. Prostaglandins, NSAIDs, and gastric mucosal protection: why doesn't the stomach digest itself? *Physiol Rev.* 2008;88:1547−1565.

14. Maguire PD, Sibley GS, Zhou SM, et al. Clinical and dosimetric predictors of radiation-induced esophageal toxicity. *Int J Radiat Oncol Biol Phys.* 1999;45:97−103.

15. Engel LS, Chow WH, Vaughan TL, et al. Population attributable risks of esophageal and gastric cancers. *J Natl Cancer Inst.* 2003;95:1404−1413.

16. Kahrilas PJ, Bredenoord AJ, Fox M, et al. The Chicago classification of esophageal motility disorders, v3.0. *Neurogastroenterol Motil.* 2015;27:160−174. Available from: http://www.ncbi.nlm.nih.gov/pubmed/25469569.

17. Korsapati H, Bhargava V, Mittal RK. Reversal of asynchrony between circular and longitudinal muscle contraction in nutcracker esophagus by atropine. *Gastroenterology.* 2008; 135:796−802. Available from: http://www.ncbi.nlm.nih.gov/pubmed/18675815.

18. Anderson LA, Cantwell MM, Watson RGP, et al. The association between alcohol and reflux esophagitis, barrett's esophagus, and esophageal adenocarcinoma. *Gastroenterology.* 2009;136:799−805. https://doi.org/10.1053/j.gastro.2008.12.005. Available from:.

19. Mohammed I, Nightingale P, Trudgill NJ. Risk factors for gastro-oesophageal reflux disease symptoms: a community study. *Aliment Pharmacol Ther.* 2005;21:821−827. Available from: http://www.ncbi.nlm.nih.gov/pubmed/15801917.

20. Nocon M, Labenz J, Willich SN. Lifestyle factors and symptoms of gastro-oesophageal reflux − a population-based study. *Aliment Pharmacol Ther.* 2006;23:169−174. Available from: http://www.ncbi.nlm.nih.gov/pubmed/16393294.

21. Locke GR, Talley NJ, Fett SL, Zinsmeister AR, Melton LJ. Risk factors associated with symptoms of gastroesophageal reflux. *Am J Med.* 1999;106:642−649. Available from: http://www.ncbi.nlm.nih.gov/pubmed/10378622.

22. Veugelers PJ, Porter GA, Guernsey DL, Casson AG. Obesity and lifestyle risk factors for gastroesophageal reflux disease, Barrett esophagus and esophageal adenocarcinoma. *Dis esophagus Off J Int Soc Dis Esophagus.* 2006;19: 321−328. Available from: http://www.ncbi.nlm.nih.gov/pubmed/16984526.

23. Ryan P, Hetzel DJ, Shearman DJ, McMichael AJ. Risk factors for ulcerative reflux oesophagitis: a case-control study. *J Gastroenterol Hepatol.* 1995;10:306−312. Available from: http://www.ncbi.nlm.nih.gov/pubmed/7548808.

24. Avidan B, Sonnenberg A, Schnell TG, Sontag SJ. Risk factors for erosive reflux esophagitis: a case-control study. *Am J Gastroenterol.* 2001;96:41−46. Available from: http://www.ncbi.nlm.nih.gov/pubmed/11197285.

25. Pan J, Cen L, Chen W, Yu C, Li Y, Shen Z. Alcohol consumption and the risk of gastroesophageal reflux disease: a systematic review and meta-analysis. *Alcohol Alcohol.* 2019;54:62−69.

26. Hallan A, Bomme M, Hveem K, Møller-Hansen J, Ness-Jensen E. Risk factors on the development of new-onset gastroesophageal reflux symptoms. A population-based prospective cohort study: the HUNT study. *Am J Gastroenterol.* 2015;110:393−400. quiz 401.

27. Nilsson M, Johnsen R, Ye W, Hveem K, Lagergren J. Lifestyle related risk factors in the aetiology of gastro-oesophageal reflux. *Gut.* 2004;53:1730−1735.

28. Ness-Jensen E, Lagergren J. Tobacco smoking, alcohol consumption and gastro-oesophageal reflux disease. *Best Pract Res Clin Gastroenterol.* 2017;31:501−508. Available from: http://www.ncbi.nlm.nih.gov/pubmed/29195669.

29. Pehl C, Wendl B, Pfeiffer A, Schmidt T, Kaess H. Low-proof alcoholic beverages and gastroesophageal reflux. *Dig Dis Sci.* 1993;38:93−96.

30. Pehl C, Pfeiffer A, Wendl B, Kaess H. Different effects of white and red wine on lower esophageal sphincter pressure and gastroesophageal reflux. *Scand J Gastroenterol.* 1998;33:118−122.

31. Kaufman SE, Kaye MD. Induction of gastro-oesophageal reflux by alcohol. *Gut.* 1978;19:336−338.

32. Vitale GC, Cheadle WG, Patel B, Sadek SA, Michel ME, Cuschieri A. The effect of alcohol on nocturnal gastroesophageal reflux. *J Am Med Assoc.* 1987;258:2077−2079.

33. Hogan WJ, Viegas de Andrade SR, Winship DH. Ethanol-induced acute esophageal motor dysfunction. *J Appl Physiol.* 1972;32:755−760.

34. Bor S, Bor-Caymaz C, Tobey NA, Abdulnour-Nakhoul S, Orlando RC. Esophageal exposure to ethanol increases risk of acid damage in rabbit esophagus. *Dig Dis Sci.* 1999;44:290−300.

35. Brinster CJ, Singhal S, Lee L, Marshall MB, Kaiser LR, Kucharczuk JC. Evolving options in the management of esophageal perforation. *Ann Thorac Surg.* 2004;77: 1475−1483. Available from: http://www.ncbi.nlm.nih.gov/pubmed/15063302.

36. Kavic SM, Basson MD. Complications of endoscopy. *Am J Surg.* 2001;181:319−332. Available from: http://www.ncbi.nlm.nih.gov/pubmed/11438266.

37. Bufkin BL, Miller JI, Mansour KA. Esophageal perforation: emphasis on management. *Ann Thorac Surg.* 1996;61: 1447−1451. discussion 1451-2 Available from: http://www.ncbi.nlm.nih.gov/pubmed/8633957.

38. Søreide JA, Viste A. Esophageal perforation: diagnostic work-up and clinical decision-making in the first 24 hours. *Scand J Trauma Resusc Emerg Med.* 2011;19:66. Available from: http://www.ncbi.nlm.nih.gov/pubmed/22035338.

39. Straumann A, Bussmann C, Zuber M, Vannini S, Simon H-U, Schoepfer A. Eosinophilic esophagitis: analysis of food impaction and perforation in 251 adolescent and adult patients. *Clin Gastroenterol Hepatol.* 2008;6:598−600. Available from: http://www.ncbi.nlm.nih.gov/pubmed/18407800.

40. Achem SR, Almansa C, Krishna M, et al. Oesophageal eosinophilic infiltration in patients with noncardiac chest pain. *Aliment Pharmacol Ther.* 2011;33:1194−1201. Available from: http://www.ncbi.nlm.nih.gov/pubmed/21466568.

41. Kapel RC, Miller JK, Torres C, Aksoy S, Lash R, Katzka DA. Eosinophilic esophagitis: a prevalent disease in the United States that affects all age groups. *Gastroenterology.* 2008; 134:1316−1321. Available from: http://www.ncbi.nlm.nih.gov/pubmed/18471509.

42. Généreau T, Lortholary O, Bouchaud O, et al. Herpes simplex esophagitis in patients with AIDS: report of 34 cases. The cooperative study group on herpetic esophagitis in HIV infection. *Clin Infect Dis.* 1996;22:926−931. Available from: http://www.ncbi.nlm.nih.gov/pubmed/8783688.

43. Sgouros SN, Bergele C, Mantides A. Eosinophilic esophagitis in adults: a systematic review. *Eur J Gastroenterol Hepatol.* 2006;18:211−217. Available from: http://www.ncbi.nlm.nih.gov/pubmed/16394804.

44. Pasha SF, DiBaise JK, Kim HJ, et al. Patient characteristics, clinical, endoscopic, and histologic findings in adult eosinophilic esophagitis: a case series and systematic review of the medical literature. *Dis esophagus Off J Int Soc Dis Esophagus.* 2007;20:311−319. Available from: http://www.ncbi.nlm.nih.gov/pubmed/17617880.

45. Watts MM, Saltoun C, Greenberger PA. Eosinophilic esophagitis. *Allergy Asthma Proc.* 2019;40:462−464.

46. Achem SR, Almansa C, Krishna M, et al. Oesophageal eosinophilic infiltration in patients with noncardiac chest pain. *Aliment Pharmacol Ther.* 2011;33:1194−1201.

47. Kapel RC, Miller JK, Torres C, Aksoy S, Lash R, Katzka DA. Eosinophilic esophagitis: a prevalent disease in the United States that affects all age groups. *Gastroenterology.* 2008; 134:1316−1321.

48. Généreau T, Lortholary O, Bouchaud O, et al. Herpes simplex esophagitis in patients with AIDS: report of 34 cases. The cooperative study group on herpetic esophagitis in HIV infection. *Clin Infect Dis.* 1996;22:926−931.

49. Mackler SA. Spontaneous rupture of the esophagus; an experimental and clinical study. *Surg Gynecol Obstet.* 1952;95:345−356. Available from: http://www.ncbi.nlm.nih.gov/pubmed/14950670.

50. Hadjis T, Palisaitis D, Dontigny L, Allard M. Benign pneumopericardium and tamponade. *Can J Cardiol.* 1995;11: 232−234. Available from: http://www.ncbi.nlm.nih.gov/pubmed/7889442.

51. Furuta GT. Eosinophils in the esophagus: acid is not the only cause. *J Pediatr Gastroenterol Nutr.* 1998;26:468−471.

52. Ahmad M, Soetikno RM, Ahmed A. The differential diagnosis of eosinophilic esophagitis. *J Clin Gastroenterol.* 2000;30:242−244.

53. Kim HP, Vance RB, Shaheen NJ, Dellon ES. The prevalence and diagnostic utility of endoscopic features of eosinophilic esophagitis: a meta-analysis. *Clin Gastroenterol Hepatol.* 2012;10:988−996.e5. https://doi.org/10.1016/j.cgh.2012.04.019. Available from:.

54. Hawari R, Pasricha PJ. Images in clinical medicine. *Eosinophilic esophagitis. N Engl J Med.* 2007;356:e20. Available from: http://www.ncbi.nlm.nih.gov/pubmed/17507698.

55. Gentile N, Katzka D, Ravi K, et al. Oesophageal narrowing is common and frequently under-appreciated at endoscopy in patients with oesophageal eosinophilia. *Aliment Pharmacol Ther.* 2014;40:1333−1340. Available from: http://www.ncbi.nlm.nih.gov/pubmed/25287184.

56. Menard-Katcher C, Swerdlow MP, Mehta P, Furuta GT, Fenton LZ. Contribution of esophagram to the evaluation of complicated pediatric eosinophilic esophagitis. *J Pediatr Gastroenterol Nutr.* 2015;61:541−546. Available from: http://www.ncbi.nlm.nih.gov/pubmed/25988559.

57. Dellon ES, Liacouras CA, Molina-Infante J, et al. Updated international consensus diagnostic criteria for eosinophilic esophagitis: proceedings of the AGREE conference. *Gastroenterology.* 2018;155:1022−1033.e10. https://doi.org/10.1053/j.gastro.2018.07.009. Available from:.

58. Vial CM, Whyte RI. Boerhaave's syndrome: diagnosis and treatment. *Surg Clin North Am.* 2005;85:515−524. ix Available from: http://www.ncbi.nlm.nih.gov/pubmed/15927648.

59. Sajith A, O'Donohue B, Roth RM, Khan RA. CT scan findings in oesophagogastric perforation after out of hospital cardiopulmonary resuscitation. *Emerg Med J.* 2008;25: 115−116. Available from: http://www.ncbi.nlm.nih.gov/pubmed/18212156.

60. Robles-Medranda C, Villard F, le Gall C, et al. Severe dysphagia in children with eosinophilic esophagitis and esophageal stricture: an indication for balloon dilation? *J Pediatr Gastroenterol Nutr.* 2010;50:516−520. Available from: http://www.ncbi.nlm.nih.gov/pubmed/19934772.

61. Schoepfer AM, Gonsalves N, Bussmann C, et al. Esophageal dilation in eosinophilic esophagitis: effectiveness, safety, and impact on the underlying inflammation. *Am J Gastroenterol.* 2010;105:1062−1070. Available from: http://www.ncbi.nlm.nih.gov/pubmed/19935783.

62. Sgouros SN, Bergele C, Mantides A. Eosinophilic esophagitis in adults: a systematic review. *Eur J Gastroenterol Hepatol.* 2006;18:211−217.

63. Remedios M, Campbell C, Jones DM, Kerlin P. Eosinophilic esophagitis in adults: clinical, endoscopic, histologic findings, and response to treatment with fluticasone propionate. *Gastrointest Endosc.* 2006;63:3−12. Available from: http://www.ncbi.nlm.nih.gov/pubmed/16377308.

64. Aceves SS, Furuta GT, Spechler SJ. Integrated approach to treatment of children and adults with eosinophilic esophagitis. *Gastrointest Endosc Clin N Am.* 2008;18: 195−217. xi Available from: http://www.ncbi.nlm.nih.gov/pubmed/18061112.

65. Straumann A, Hoesli S, Bussmann C, et al. Anti-eosinophil activity and clinical efficacy of the CRTH2 antagonist OC000459 in eosinophilic esophagitis. *Allergy.* 2013;68: 375−385. Available from: http://www.ncbi.nlm.nih.gov/pubmed/23379537.

66. Hirano I, Dellon ES, Hamilton JD, et al. Efficacy of dupilumab in a phase 2 randomized trial of adults with active eosinophilic esophagitis. *Gastroenterology*; 2019. Available from: http://www.ncbi.nlm.nih.gov/pubmed/31593702.

67. Hirano I, Collins MH, Assouline-Dayan Y, et al. RPC4046, a monoclonal antibody against IL13, reduces histologic and endoscopic activity in patients with eosinophilic esophagitis. *Gastroenterology*. 2019;156:592−603.e10. Available from: http://www.ncbi.nlm.nih.gov/pubmed/30395812.

68. Spergel JM, Rothenberg ME, Collins MH, et al. Reslizumab in children and adolescents with eosinophilic esophagitis: results of a double-blind, randomized, placebo-controlled trial. *J Allergy Clin Immunol*. 2012;129:456−463, 463.e1-3 Available from: http://www.ncbi.nlm.nih.gov/pubmed/22206777.

69. Attwood SEA, Lewis CJ, Bronder CS, Morris CD, Armstrong GR, Whittam J. Eosinophilic oesophagitis: a novel treatment using Montelukast. *Gut*. 2003;52:181−185. Available from: http://www.ncbi.nlm.nih.gov/pubmed/12524397.

70. Pursley TJ, Blomquist IK, Abraham J, Andersen HF, Bartley JA. Fluconazole-induced congenital anomalies in three infants. *Clin Infect Dis*. 1996;22:336−340. Available from: http://www.ncbi.nlm.nih.gov/pubmed/8838193.

71. Benson CA, Kaplan JE, Masur H, et al. Treating opportunistic infections among HIV-infected adults and adolescents: recommendations from CDC, the National Institutes of Health, and the HIV Medicine Association/Infectious Diseases Society of America. *MMWR Recomm Reports*. 2004;53:1−112. Available from: http://www.ncbi.nlm.nih.gov/pubmed/15841069.

72. Wolfson D, Barkin JS. Treatment of Boerhaave's syndrome. *Curr Treat Options Gastroenterol*. 2007;10:71−77. Available from: http://www.ncbi.nlm.nih.gov/pubmed/17298767.

73. Sepesi B, Raymond DP, Peters JH. Esophageal perforation: surgical, endoscopic and medical management strategies. *Curr Opin Gastroenterol*. 2010;26:379−383. Available from: http://www.ncbi.nlm.nih.gov/pubmed/20473156.

74. Qadir I, Zafar H, Khan MZ, Sharif HM. T-tube management of late esophageal perforation. *J Pak Med Assoc*. 2011;61:418−420. Available from: http://www.ncbi.nlm.nih.gov/pubmed/21465993.

75. Schenfine J, Griffin SM. *Oesophageal Emergencies*. Oesophagogastric Surgery—A Companion to Spec Surg Pract. 2006:365−393.

76. Burgess PR, Perl ER. Myelinated afferent fibres responding specifically to noxious stimulation of the skin. *J Physiol*. 1967;190:541−562. Available from: http://www.ncbi.nlm.nih.gov/pubmed/6051786.

77. Lynn RB. Mechanisms of esophageal pain. *Am J Med*. 1992;92:11S−19S. Available from: http://www.ncbi.nlm.nih.gov/pubmed/1595755.

78. Miwa H, Kondo T, Oshima T, Fukui H, Tomita T, Watari J. Esophageal sensation and esophageal hypersensitivity — overview from bench to bedside. *J Neurogastroenterol Motil*. 2010;16:353−362.

79. Bessou P, Perl ER. Response of cutaneous sensory units with unmyelinated fibers to noxious stimuli. *J Neurophysiol*. 1969;32:1025−1043. Available from: http://www.ncbi.nlm.nih.gov/pubmed/5347705.

80. Clerc N. Afferent innervation of the lower esophageal sphincter of the cat. Pathways and functional characteristics. *J Auton Nerv Syst*. 1984;10:213−216. Available from: http://www.ncbi.nlm.nih.gov/pubmed/6481088.

81. Sengupta JN. Esophageal sensory physiology. *GI Motil*. 2006.

82. Pergolizzi JV, Raffa RB. The WHO pain ladder: do we need another step? *Pract Pain Manag*. 2015;14.

83. WHO's cancer pain ladder for adults. *World Heal Organ*; 2019. Available from: https://www.who.int/cancer/palliative/painladder/en/.

CHAPTER 23

Gastroesophageal Reflux Disease

JAVIER SANCHEZ, MD • NEEL D. MEHTA, MD

INTRODUCTION

Gastroesophageal reflux disease (GERD) is defined as a "condition which develops when the reflux of gastric contents causes troublesome symptoms or complications."[1] The estimated prevalence of GERD in North America is 20% (specifically defined as heartburn and/or regurgitation occurring at least once a week),[2] and it has been increasing due to the obesity epidemic.[3] The true prevalence is likely higher as many patients take over the counter acid reducing medications without seeking formal medical care.

The economic impact of GERD is very high, totaling $15–$20 billion a year in direct and indirect costs.[4] The direct costs of GERD are an estimated $9–$10 billion per year. These costs include inpatient and outpatient visits, diagnostic procedures, and medications (with proton pump inhibitors accounting for the highest share of the cost). Indirect costs are a result of decreased quality of life, workplace absenteeism, and decrease in productivity.

A subset of patients with GERD present with noncardiac chest pain (NCCP).[5] NCCP is a recurring angina-like retrosternal chest pain that is not due to cardiac causes and is a chronic disorder that reduces the quality of life of the patient but has no impact on mortality. NCCP contributes significantly to poor quality of life and increased economic burden, as patients often continue to have symptoms for years and frequently undergo multiple and repeated workups to rule out cardiac origins of chest pain.[6] The estimated prevalence of NCCP is 25%. It affects both males and females equally. Prevalence generally decreases with increasing age. Patients with NCCP are younger, consume more alcohol, smoke, and are more likely to suffer from anxiety compared to patients with ischemic heart disease.

ETIOLOGY AND PATHOGENESIS

The etiology and pathogenesis of GERD are multifactorial. In approximately 60% of patients, the lower esophageal sphincter (LES) is mechanically incompetent. In the remaining 40%, reflux occurs secondary to transient relaxations in the LES that are not triggered by swallowing, but rather likely secondary to gastric distention.[7] About 30% of patients with GERD have a defect in esophageal peristalsis resulting in ineffective esophageal motility and delayed gastric emptying.[8] Hiatal hernias can contribute to the development of GERD as well, as there can be loss of external compression around the LES paired with external compression of a distended stomach.[9] Conditions that produce increased intraabdominal pressure (e.g., obesity), as well as a decrease in intrathoracic pressure (e.g., obstructive sleep apnea, which frequently coexists with obesity), can create an unfavorable pressure gradient that the LES may not be able to counterbalance, thus resulting in reflux. In addition to these mechanical factors, the acidity of gastric reflux can contribute to the severity of symptoms, as well as the volume and frequency of reflux episodes. GERD also commonly occurs in pregnancy, likely secondary to a combination of mechanical factors (weight gain, increase in intraabdominal pressure) and physiologic factors (increased progesterone).[7]

GERD is the most common esophageal cause of NCCP in patients with and without coronary artery disease. The mechanism by which GERD causes NCCP, however, is poorly understood.[6] One proposed mechanism involves peripheral sensitization of esophageal afferents leading to increased sensation of physiologic and pathologic stimuli. In one study, healthy subjects exposed to acid in the distal esophagus experienced a decrease in the pain threshold in the proximal esophagus. In response to the same stimulus, subjects with NCCP experienced a more profound sensitization of the upper esophagus that lasted longer than in healthy subjects, and additionally had a decrease in the pain threshold in the anterior chest wall, or development of secondary somatic allodynia, suggesting central sensitization as a likely mechanism.[10,11]

Interventional Management of Chronic Visceral Pain Syndromes. https://doi.org/10.1016/B978-0-323-75775-1.00013-1

CLINICAL FEATURES

Patients with GERD frequently present with heartburn and regurgitation, and less commonly dysphagia, which is usually secondary to ineffective peristalsis. Patients may also present with atypical symptoms of GERD such as NCCP, chronic cough, aspiration pneumonia, pulmonary fibrosis, hoarseness, globus, and dental erosions.[2,7] NCCP is characterized by recurrent angina-like retrosternal chest pain in the absence of cardiac causes of chest pain.[12]

DIAGNOSIS

The diagnosis of GERD in patients who present with typical symptoms such as heartburn or regurgitation is often done clinically. In these patients, a trial of empiric proton-pump inhibitor (PPI) therapy is recommended.[5] A good response to a PPI trial confirms the presumptive diagnosis in this setting. However, this strategy is not without limitations, as a PPI trial has a sensitivity of 78% and specificity of 54%.[13] Additional diagnostic testing, including esophagogastroduodenoscopy, esophageal manometry, and esophageal pH monitoring may be required in patients who do not respond to a trial of PPI therapy or who present with atypical or worrisome symptoms. Upper GI endoscopy is performed to assess for evidence of mucosal damage and is indicated in patients presenting with GERD with alarm symptoms, as only 50%–60% of patients with GERD have evidence of mucosal damage (positive predictive value 53%).[5] Upper GI endoscopy can be useful to exclude other pathologies such as eosinophilic esophagitis, gastritis, peptic ulcer disease, Barrett's esophagus, esophageal strictures, and malignancy.

Esophageal manometry is of limited use in the diagnosis of GERD, but can be used to confirm proper placement of a pH probe, to rule out primary motility disorders such as achalasia, and for surgical planning.[5]

Esophageal pH monitoring is considered the gold standard for the diagnosis of GERD. An esophageal pH probe is placed while the patient is not taking acid reducing medications. Measurements are taken 5 cm above the LES, and the patient keeps a symptom diary that is correlated to pH measurements. The test is less useful in correlating episodes of reflux to NCCP because of the low likelihood of patients having an episode of chest pain during the test. The test may be more useful for those patients that are being considered for antireflux surgery.[5] A barium swallow has very little use in the diagnosis of GERD. It has a low sensitivity (20%), and the presence of barium reflux is of questionable significance as a proportion of subjects with normal pH esophageal pH will have spontaneous barium reflux.[5]

In patients who present with NCCP secondary to GERD, it is prudent to rule out cardiac causes of chest pain such as coronary artery disease and pericarditis. Patients should be referred to a cardiologist for testing that may include electrocardiography, echocardiography, stress testing, and other diagnostic modalities to rule out a cardiac etiology.[14]

DIFFERENTIAL DIAGNOSIS

The differential diagnosis of GERD includes esophageal motility disorders such as achalasia, esophageal strictures, malignancy, gastritis, peptic ulcer disease, esophagitis (eosinophilic, viral, or fungal), coronary artery disease (i.e., angina pectoris), and pericarditis. Table 23.1 illustrates the multiple causes of noncardiac chest pain.

TABLE 23.1
Causes of Noncardiac Chest Pain.

Organ System	Cause
Gastrointestinal	GERD Barrett's esophagus Esophageal motility disorders (e.g., diffuse esophageal spasms, achalasia) Hypersensitive esophagus Schatski rings Eosinophilic esophagitis Infectious esophagitis Pill (drug-induced) esophagitis Mallory–Weiss syndrome, Boerhaave syndrome Gastroduodenal ulcers Pancreatitis, biliary colic, cholangitis
Respiratory	Lung embolism Pneumonia Pneumothorax
Neurological	Nerve compression Zoster neuralgia, postherpetic neuralgia
Orthopedic/ Rheumatologic	Degenerative disc disease, spinal stenosis, nerve root compression Inflammatory arthritis Costochondritis
Psychiatric	Depression Chronic pain disorders

PHYSICAL EXAM

Most patients with mild to moderate GERD will present with an unremarkable physical exam. Those with severe disease may have voice hoarseness, chronic cough, evidence of dental erosions, and wheezing on lung auscultation. Cardiac exam should otherwise be normal. Most patients should also present with a benign abdominal exam.

TREATMENT

The primary treatment of GERD-related NCCP is the treatment of the underlying GERD. Approaches range from conservative measures, such as lifestyle modifications, to surgery. Table 23.2 summarizes the various treatment modalities available for noncardiac chest pain.

LIFESTYLE MODIFICATIONS

Primary treatment modalities of GERD consist in reducing the number of episodes of reflux and reducing the acidity of the refluxate. Lifestyle modifications are often

TABLE 23.2
Summary of Management Strategies for GERD-Related Noncardiac Chest Pain.

Therapeutic Category	Therapeutic Modality
Lifestyle modifications	Elevation of the head of the bed Avoidance of late meals Avoidance of alcohol and tobacco Avoidance of chocolate, coffee, carbonated beverages, and other known triggers Weight loss
Medical management	Antacids H2-receptor antagonists Proton pump inhibitors Neuromodulators
Endoscopic procedures	Endoscopic botulinum toxin injection RFA of LES Transoral incisionless fundoplication
Surgical management	Laparoscopic fundoplication Roux-en-Y gastric bypass Linx magnetic ring
Alternative therapies	Cognitive behavioral therapy Hypnotherapy

recommended and include elevation of the head of the bed at night, avoiding late-night meals, and avoiding alcohol, tobacco, and certain foods such as chocolate, coffee, and carbonated beverages that are known triggers of acid reflux. In patients who are obese, weight loss is recommended, and should it be successful often leads to complete resolution of symptoms.[2,5,7,15,16]

PHARMACOLOGIC TREATMENT

The mainstay of treatment for GERD is acid-reducing medications, such as H2 receptor antagonists and PPIs. The efficacy of H2 receptor antagonists in controlling GERD-related NCCP is 42%−52%. PPIs have been more efficacious in treating GERD and are considered the first line of treatment.[2,5,7,17] In a systematic review of eight randomized controlled trials (RCT) evaluating the efficacy of PPIs in NCCP, the efficacy of treatment was more effective than the placebo. Furthermore, the efficacy improved significantly for the subset of patients that were GERD-positive.[18] PPIs reduce symptoms by decreasing the acidity of refluxed contents but do not actually decrease the number of reflux episodes, so regurgitation symptoms may not be well controlled. Side effects of treatment with PPIs include increased risk of C diff infection, community-acquired pneumonia, hip fractures, vitamin B12 deficiency, and hypomagnesemia. PPI use has also been associated with severe cardiac events such as MI due to potential effects on vascular function, and in patients taking clopidogrel because of decreased inhibition of platelet aggregation.[7]

Few other drug categories are recommended in the treatment of GERD, or GERD-related NCCP.[19] Prokinetic agents such as metoclopramide are not frequently used due to side effects such as tardive dyskinesias and are usually limited to patients with severe gastroparesis. In one RCT, although the use of baclofen significantly decreased reflux episodes and esophageal pH, it was associated with worsening of chest pain at the 2-week follow-up.[14]

Pain modulators have classically been used for non-GERD-related NCCP.[16,18] Tricyclic antidepressants exhibit central neuromodulatory and visceral analgesic effects. These effects have been demonstrated in both healthy subjects and patients with NCCP. In one study, imipramine administered at a dose of 75 mg daily was shown to significantly increase the pain threshold in healthy men during esophageal balloon distention. In another study, patients with NCCP receiving imipramine had a significant (52%) reduction in chest pain. However, another study failed to show any benefits for amitriptyline. In general, tricyclic antidepressants have been shown to provide continued symptomatic relief during long-term use. Trazodone, a tetracyclic antidepressant, has also been shown to provide symptomatic relief in some studies. Selective serotonin reuptake inhibitors such as sertraline and paroxetine have been studied as well. In one single-blinded placebo-controlled trial, sertraline produced significant reductions in pain. In a similar double-blinded placebo-controlled trial paroxetine showed improvement in a physician-rated scale but not in patient self-reported pain scores. The effects of both drugs are likely secondary to visceral analgesic effects.

Adenosine analogues such as theophylline have been studied and shown to increase pain thresholds in 75% of patients with functional chest pain.[20] However, the evidence is limited, and its use may be limited by side effects and toxicity. Anxiolytics such as alprazolam and clonazepam have been shown to reduce episodes of chest pain in patients with NCCP and panic disorder. Serotonin receptor inhibitors such as ondansetron have been shown to increase esophageal perception thresholds for pain in patients with NCCP. Tegaserod, a 5-HT4 receptor agonist has shown similar properties. Octreotide, a synthetic analog of somatostatin, has been shown to increase pain perception thresholds in the rectum and sigmoid colon in healthy subjects and patients with IBS.[19]

Gabapentin has been recently studied for the treatment of cough associated with GERD but does not seem to have a role in the treatment of GERD-related NCCP.[21] Pregabalin, a centrally acting modulator of voltage-sensitive calcium channels, has been shown to reduce pain and esophageal hypersensitivity in healthy subjects after acid infusion to the distal esophagus but has otherwise not been studied in patients with NCCP.[19]

GERD in pregnancy can be treated with lifestyle modifications and H2 receptor antagonists. PPIs are not routinely used as they are Category C.[7]

ADVANCED PROCEDURES

Botulinum toxin injections into the lower esophageal sphincter have been described for the treatment of NCCP.[18,19] Botulinum toxin interacts selectively with cholinergic neurons to inhibit the release of acetylcholine at the presynaptic terminal. Some studies have shown variable efficacy for this treatment in patients with NCCP and an esophageal motility disorder, but these studies are limited by small numbers and are primarily not placebo controlled. In the only available double-blind placebo-controlled trial, botulinum toxin

significantly improved dysphagia but had no effect on chest pain or GERD-related symptoms.[22] In summary, there may be some benefit for patients with NCCP and esophageal motility disorders, but it's use in GERD-related NCCP is limited.

Radiofrequency ablation (RFA) of the LES and endoscopic suturing of the LES (otherwise known as transoral incisionless fundoplication) have also been described. These therapies are limited to a patient population that excludes patients with hiatal hernias of more than 2 cm, esophageal dysmotility disorders Barret's esophagus, Grade C or D esophagitis, esophageal strictures, and BMI>35[7]. Evidence for these techniques is limited. In a randomized control trial, RFA of the LES was not shown to be better than treatment with PPIs.[23] A meta-analysis of four trials similarly found no benefit compared to therapy with PPIs.[24] Transoral incisionless fundoplication is useful in reducing regurgitation based on one RCT, but results deteriorate over time.[25,26] RFA of the LES and endoscopic suturing of the LES are not widely accepted—while the Society of American Gastrointestinal and Endoscopic Surgeons recommends these therapies, the American College of Gastroenterologists guidelines state that these should not be considered as alternatives to medical therapy or surgical intervention.[7]

SURGICAL INTERVENTIONS

Surgery is generally reserved for patients with severe symptoms that are refractory to medical management. This includes patients who are unable to tolerate PPIs or who do not wish to take them for the rest of their lives as well as patients with large hiatal hernias or patients who are morbidly obese and unable to lose weight with lifestyle modifications. The primary method of intervention is laparoscopic fundoplication. In patients who are obese, fundoplication has a high failure rate, and Roux-en-Y gastric bypass is favored. Surgery can be very effective, but a significant portion of patients continue to take PPIs after surgery.[2,7,17] A recent Cochrane review of RCTs comparing medical therapy versus surgery showed considerable uncertainty in the balance of risks versus benefits.[27] Recently, a magnetic ring has been introduced into the market.[17] This device is placed laparoscopically around the distal end of the esophagus and augments the lower esophageal sphincter tone. Initial studies have shown an overall reduction in acid exposure and reduction in usage of PPIs, but a significant rate of side effects such as dysphagia in up to 68% of patients. The long-term efficacy of this device remains to be determined.

ALTERNATIVE THERAPIES

Patients with NCCP may also be referred for cognitive behavioral therapy (CBT) or hypnotherapy. CBT has shown mixed results, with some studies showing a reduction in pain intensity compared to usual care at a cardiology department and other studies showing a reduction in the frequency of episodes of pain despite no reduction in the intensity of pain. One small study showed significant benefits using Johrei, a process of transmission of healing energy, but the findings have yet to be validated. Another study showed a potential benefit for hypnotherapy in patients with NCCP. Overall, studies on alternative therapies are small and evidence is limited, but there may be a role for these therapies in selected patients with refractory symptoms or coexisting anxiety or depression.[18]

REFERENCES

1. Clarrett DM, Hachem C. Gastroesophageal Reflux Disease (GERD). *Mo Med.* 2018 May–Jun;115(3):214–218. PMID: 30228725; PMCID: PMC6140167.
2. Kellerman R, Kintanar T. Gastroesophageal reflux disease. *Prim Care Clin Off Pract.* 2017;44(4):561–573. https://doi.org/10.1016/j.pop.2017.07.001.
3. El-Serag HB, Sweet S, Winchester CC, Dent J. Update on the epidemiology of gastro-oesophageal reflux disease: a systematic review. *Gut.* 2014;63(6):871–880. https://doi.org/10.1136/gutjnl-2012-304269.
4. Gawron AJ, French DD, Pandolfino JE, Howden CW. Economic evaluations of gastroesophageal reflux disease medical management. *Pharmacoeconomics.* 2014;32(8):745–758. https://doi.org/10.1007/s40273-014-0164-8.
5. Katz PO, Gerson LB, Vela MF. Guidelines for the diagnosis and management of gastroesophageal reflux disease. *Am J Gastroenterol.* 2013;108(3):308–328. https://doi.org/10.1038/ajg.2012.444.
6. Fass R, Achem SR. Noncardiac chest pain: epidemiology, natural course and pathogenesis. *J Neurogastroenterol Motil.* 2011;17(2):110–123. https://doi.org/10.5056/jnm.2011.17.2.110.
7. Patti MG. An evidence-based approach to the treatment of gastroesophageal reflux disease. *JAMA Surg.* 2016;151(1):73–78. https://doi.org/10.1001/jamasurg.2015.4233.
8. Diener U, Patti MG, Molena D, Fisichella PM, Way LW. Esophageal dysmotility and gastroesophageal reflux disease. *J Gastrointest Surg.* 2001;5(3):260–265. http://www.ncbi.nlm.nih.gov/pubmed/11360049.
9. Gordon C, Kang JY, Neild PJ, Maxwell JD. The role of the hiatus hernia in gastro-oesophageal reflux disease. *Aliment Pharmacol Ther.* 2004;20(7):719–732. https://doi.org/10.1111/j.1365-2036.2004.02149.x.
10. Sarkar S, Thompson DG, Woolf CJ, Hobson AR, Millane T, Aziz Q. Patients with chest pain and occult gastroesophageal reflux demonstrate visceral pain hypersensitivity which may be partially responsive to acid suppression. *Am J Gastroenterol.* 2004;99(10):1998–2006. https://doi.org/10.1111/j.1572-0241.2004.40174.x.
11. Sarkar S, Aziz Q, Woolf CJ, Hobson AR, Thompson DG. Contribution of central sensitisation to the development of non-cardiac chest pain. *Lancet.* 2000;356(9236):1154–1159. https://doi.org/10.1016/S0140-6736(00)02758-6.
12. Fass R. Chest pain of esophageal origin. *Curr Opin Gastroenterol.* 2002;18(4):464–470. https://doi.org/10.1097/00001574-200207000-00011.
13. Numans ME, Lau J, de Wit NJ, Bonis PA. Short-term treatment with proton-pump inhibitors as a test for gastroesophageal reflux disease: a meta-analysis of diagnostic test characteristics. *Ann Intern Med.* 2004;140(7):518–527. https://doi.org/10.7326/0003-4819-140-7-200404060-00011.
14. Cossentino MJ, Mann K, Armbruster SP, Lake JM, Maydonovitch C, Wong RKH. Randomised clinical trial: the effect of baclofen in patients with gastro-oesophageal reflux—a randomised prospective study. *Aliment Pharmacol Ther.* 2012;35(9):1036–1044. https://doi.org/10.1111/j.1365-2036.2012.05068.x.
15. Frieling T. Non-cardiac chest pain. *Visc Med.* 2018. https://doi.org/10.1159/000486440.
16. Nguyen TMT, Eslick GD. Systematic review: the treatment of noncardiac chest pain with antidepressants. *Aliment Pharmacol Ther.* 2012;35(5):493–500. https://doi.org/10.1111/j.1365-2036.2011.04978.x.
17. Sandhu DS, Fass R. Current trends in the management of gastroesophageal reflux disease. *Gut Liver.* 2018;12(1):7–16. https://doi.org/10.5009/gnl16615.
18. Burgstaller JM, Jenni BF, Steurer J, Held U, Wertli MM. Treatment efficacy for non-cardiovascular chest pain: a systematic review and meta-analysis. *PLoS One.* 2014;9(8). https://doi.org/10.1371/journal.pone.0104722.
19. Maradey-Romero C, Fass R. New therapies for non-cardiac chest pain. *Curr Gastroenterol Rep.* 2014;16(6). https://doi.org/10.1007/s11894-014-0390-4.
20. Rao SSC, Mudipalli RS, Remes-Troche JM, Utech CL, Zimmerman B. Theophylline improves esophageal chest pain — a randomized, placebo-controlled study. *Am J Gastroenterol.* 2007;102(5):930–938. https://doi.org/10.1111/j.1572-0241.2007.01112.x.
21. Dong R, Xu X, Yu L, et al. Randomised clinical trial: gabapentin vs baclofen in the treatment of suspected refractory gastro-oesophageal reflux-induced chronic cough. *Aliment Pharmacol Ther.* 2019;49(6):714–722. https://doi.org/10.1111/apt.15169.
22. Vanuytsel T, Bisschops R, Farré R, et al. Botulinum toxin reduces dysphagia in patients with nonachalasia primary esophageal motility disorders. *Clin Gastroenterol Hepatol.* 2013. https://doi.org/10.1016/j.cgh.2013.03.021.
23. Corley DA, Katz P, Wo JM, et al. Improvement of gastroesophageal reflux symptoms after radiofrequency energy: a randomized, sham-controlled trial. *Gastroenterology.* 2003. https://doi.org/10.1016/S0016-5085(03)01052-7.

24. Lipka S, Kumar A, Richter JE. No evidence for efficacy of radiofrequency ablation for treatment of gastroesophageal reflux disease: a systematic review and meta-analysis. *Clin Gastroenterol Hepatol.* 2015. https://doi.org/10.1016/j.cgh.2014.10.013.

25. Hunter JG, Kahrilas PJ, Bell RCW, et al. Efficacy of transoral fundoplication vs omeprazole for treatment of regurgitation in a randomized controlled trial. *Gastroenterology.* 2015. https://doi.org/10.1053/j.gastro.2014.10.009.

26. Witteman BPL, Conchillo JM, Rinsma NF, et al. Randomized controlled trial of transoral incisionless fundoplication vs. proton pump inhibitors for treatment of gastroesophageal reflux disease. *Am J Gastroenterol.* 2015. https://doi.org/10.1038/ajg.2015.28.

27. Wileman SM, McLeer S, Campbell MK, et al. Laparoscopic fundoplication versus medical management for gastro-oesphageal reflux disease (GORD) in adults. In: *Cochrane Database of Systematic Reviews.* John Wiley & Sons, Ltd.; 2001. https://doi.org/10.1002/14651858.cd003243.

Index

Note: Page numbers followed by "f" indicate figures and "t" indicate tables.

Printed and bound by CPI Group (UK) Ltd, Croydon, CR0 4YY

03/10/2024

01040300-0019